Ultrasound Diagnostics of Thyroid Diseases

Vladimir P. Kharchenko • Peter M. Kotlyarov
Mikhail S. Mogutov • Yury K. Alexandrov
Alexander N. Sencha • Yury N. Patrunov
Denis V. Belyaev

Ultrasound Diagnostics of Thyroid Diseases

Springer

Vladimir P. Kharchenko, MD
Russian Radiology Research Center
86, Profsoyuznaya st.
117997 Moscow
Russia
Kharchenko_vp@mail.ru

Peter M. Kotlyarov, MD
Russian Center of Roentgenradiology
86, Profsoyuznaya st.
117997 Moscow
Russia
Kotlyarov_pm@mail.ru

Mikhail S. Mogutov, MD
Yaroslavl Railway Clinic
Suzdalskoye Shosse 21
150030 Yaroslavl
Russia
mogmikhail@mail.ru

Yury K. Alexandrov, MD
State Medical Academy
Revolucionnaya ulitsa 5
150000 Yaroslavl
Russia
yka2000@mail.ru

Alexander N. Sencha, MD
Yaroslavl Railway Clinic
Suzdalskoye Shosse 21
150030 Yaroslavl
Russia
senchavyatka@mail.ru

Yury N. Patrunov, MD
Yaroslavl Railway Clinic
Suzdalskoye Shosse 21
150030 Yaroslavl
Russia
unipatr@mail.ru

Denis V. Belyaev, MD
Yaroslavl Railway Clinic
Suzdalskoye Shosse 21
150030 Yaroslavl
Russia
belyaevdv@mail.ru

ISBN: 978-3-642-12386-3 e-ISBN: 978-3-642-12387-0

DOI: 10.1007/978-3-642-12387-0

Springer Heidelberg Dordrecht London New York

Library of Congress Control Number: 2010932938

Cover design: eStudio Calamar, Figueres/Berlin

Printed on acid-free paper

Springer is part of Springer Science+Business Media (www.springer.com)

Preface

Thyroid disease is the second most common type of endocrine pathology, only surpassed in prevalence by diabetes mellitus. Thyroid abnormalities are found in 8–20% of adults worldwide. In the endemic regions, the prevalence of such abnormalities is thought to be higher and exceeds 50%. Thyroid malignancies constitute 1–3% of all cancers with an average incidence in the world of 1.1 in 100,000 men and 3.8 in 100,000 women in 2008. Among the population of radionuclide polluted regions, this figure reaches 14 in 100,000. Recent research reveals a trend toward an increased incidence of thyroid pathology, including thyroid cancer, practically in all regions of the globe.

The diagnosis of thyroid diseases has been constantly improving due to the scientific development and technological advances in diagnostic equipment. The diagnostic value of visualization of the thyroid gland is method-dependent. In this regard, proper selection of a diagnostic procedure permits precise diagnosis while minimizing the cost and reducing the time to diagnosis. Minimally invasive surgical intervention is a promising tool in the treatment of thyroid diseases. Its feature is selective manipulation of the thyroid lesions and concomitant avoidance of damage to the surrounding tissue. The use of US guidance during such procedure allows to assess the operation course, predict the efficacy, and provide patient follow-up.

In this book we presented and analyzed certain debatable and unresolved problems and prospects of early, specific, and differential diagnosis of thyroid disease with the use of complex US. Our findings are based on the literature data and our extensive experience. We conducted analysis of more than 100,000 US examinations with the pathology of the thyroid and parathyroid glands, performed during 1995–2008, as well as the results of over 5,000 diagnostic and 2,000 therapeutic US guided minimally invasive manipulations with correlation to surgical findings and morphological structure. This analysis allowed us to generate a weighted opinion regarding the current role and limitations of a sonographic study of the thyroid, which we present here.

Moscow

Yaroslavl

V.P. Kharchenko
P.M. Kotlyarov
M.S. Mogutov
Y.K. Alexandrov
A.N. Sencha
Y.N. Patrunov
D.V. Belyaev

Acknowledgements

We wish to acknowledge

Vladimir V. Mitkov, MD, PhD
Moscow, Russia

Alexey V. Pavlov, MD, PhD
Yaroslavl, Russia

Leonid A. Zharikov
Moscow, Russia

Alexey V. Danilov, MD, PhD
Dartmouth, Hanover, NH, USA

Olga I. Jdanovskaya
Yaroslavl, Russia

for the help in working on the book.

Contents

Abbreviations

AIT	Autoimmune thyroiditis
AITD	Autoimmune thyroid disease
AT	Acute thyroiditis
ATC	Anaplastic thyroid carcinoma
BSA	Body surface area
CCA	Common carotid artery
CDI	Color Doppler imaging (Color flow imaging, CFI; Color flow mapping, CFM)
CEUS	Contrast-enhanced ultrasound
CPD	Color pixel density
CT	Computed tomography
EDV	End-diastolic velocity
FNAB	Fine needle aspiration biopsy
FTC	Follicular thyroid carcinoma
HPT	Hyperparathyroidism
HU	Hounsfield unit
ICD	International Classification of Diseases
IJV	Internal jugular vein
ITA	The inferior thyroid artery
MIM	Minimally invasive modality
MRI	Magnetic resonance imaging
MTC	Medullary thyroid carcinoma
PDI	Power Doppler imaging (mapping)
PEI	Percutaneous ethanol injection
PET	Positron emission tomography
PGA	Percutaneous glucocorticoid administration
PI	Pulsatility index
PI	Pulsatory index
PLA	Percutaneous laser ablation
PSV	Peak systolic velocity
PTC	Papillary thyroid carcinoma
PTH	Parathyroid hormone
PW	Pulse wave Doppler
RI	Resistance index
4D	Real time three-dimensional image reconstruction
RSI	Relative signal intensity

SAT Subacute thyroiditis
SI Solbiati index
SPECT Single photon emission computed tomography
3D Three-dimensional reconstruction of the image
3DPD Three-dimensional reconstruction of the image in vascular regimen (3D power Doppler imaging)
THI Tissue harmonic imaging
TSH Thyroid stimulating hormone
US Ultrasound
UTA The upper thyroid artery

1 Diagnosing Thyroid Pathology with Radiological Methods

Thyroid diseases are clinically diagnosed based on both individual features and sets of symptoms. According to evidence-based medicine, a disease should be diagnosed using objective diagnostic modalities. However, the diagnostic methods used should be cost-effective. The rational sequence of examinations employed is thus important. Normally, simple, cheap, and noninvasive methods are performed before complex, expensive, and invasive modalities.

Thyroid pathology is traditionally evaluated by *visual inspection* and *palpation* (Figs. 1.1 and 1.2). The World Health Organization recommends palpation as the basic method of epidemiological research in endemic regions. This method is undoubtedly needed by endocrinologists and surgeons. Nevertheless, its sensitivity to the enlargement and to structural abnormalities of the thyroid gland does not meet the needs of modern diagnostics.

Clinical surveys have shown that 5–10% of the general population have thyroid pathologies, including nodular lesions in 2.5–3% of cases. Palpation yields false-positive results in 8.7–10.9% of cases, and false-negative results in 18.5%. It is least informative for small lesions. Thyroid nodules smaller than 1 cm in size are barely defined, except for isthmus nodules. Palpation reveals only 4% of nodules that are smaller than 11 mm in size, 65% of nodules 11–30 mm in size, and 95% of nodules larger than 30 mm in size. According to Kasatkina et al. (1999), the sensitivity of palpation is 63%, its specificity is 67%, and its diagnostic accuracy is 65%. Differences in palpation techniques and patient gender do not affect its accuracy. According to Tan and Gharib (1997), the general sensitivity of palpation for defining thyroid nodules is 38%. Up to 55% of lymph nodes with a tumor or inflammatory involvement that are sonographically visualized cannot be palpated. In general, the sensitivity of palpation for diagnosing the pathology of the lymph nodes of the neck is about 73%. According to Zabolotskaya (1999), the sensitivity of palpation in the diagnosis of metastatic lymph nodes of the neck is 69%, its specificity is 87%, and its accuracy is 80%.

Patients with palpated lesions, vegetative, or somatic disorders that are characteristic of thyroid diseases should undergo detailed instrumental examination.

The following methods are utilized in the diagnosis of thyroid diseases (Dedov et al. 1999):

1. Preoperative

   Primary:

   - Palpation of the thyroid gland and the lymph nodes of the neck
   - Thyroid US
   - US-guided fine needle aspiration biopsy with cytology
   - Determination of thyroid hormones and TSH in blood

   Additional:

   - Determination of antithyroid antibodies
   - Thyroid radionuclide scan
   - X-ray of the mediastinum with contrasted esophagus
   - Computed tomography (CT)
   - Magnetic resonance imaging (MRI)
   - Thyroid lymphography
   - X-ray fluorescence analysis of intrathyroidal iodine concentration

2. Intraoperative

   - Intraoperative thyroid US
   - Urgent histological investigation in cases of suspected thyroid malignancy

V.P. Kharchenko et al., *Ultrasound Diagnostics of Thyroid Diseases*,
DOI: 10.1007/978-3-642-12387-0_1, © Springer-Verlag Berlin Heidelberg 2010

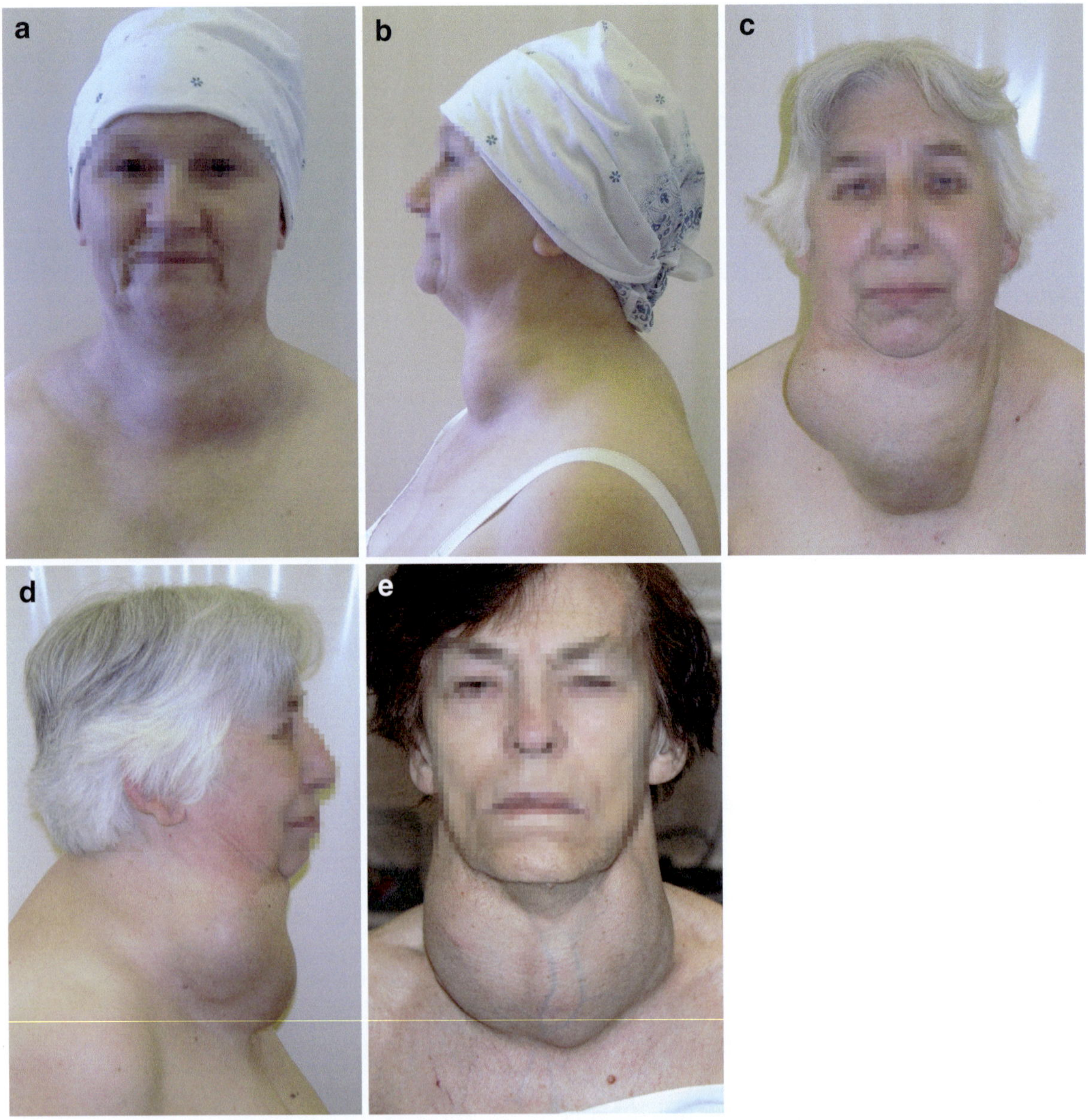

Fig. 1.1 (**a–e**) Visual inspection. Thyroid gland enlargement (**a**) visual enlargement of thyroid isthmus and left lobe, front view (**b**) the same patient, side view (**c**) visual enlargement of thyroid isthmus and right lobe, front view (**d**) the same patient, side view (**e**) visual enlargement of both thyroid lobes, front view

3. Postoperative
   Mainly:
   - Histological investigation of the resected thyroid tissue

   Additionally:
   - Immunohistochemical investigation of the tumor (definition of tumor markers)

Radiological methods, such as US, thyroid radionuclide scan, CT, MRI, and X-ray, are especially valuable for diagnosing thyroid diseases. Modern examination of the thyroid gland involves applying various methods in an optimal combination and sequence to reveal morphological and functional changes. From a practical point of view, the correct diagnostic scheme allows unnecessary procedures to be avoided, making the examination informative, prompt, and cost-effective.

Sonographic examination is readily available, noninvasive, and highly informative. Thus, US is the leading modality after physical examination (Fig. 1.3). Its

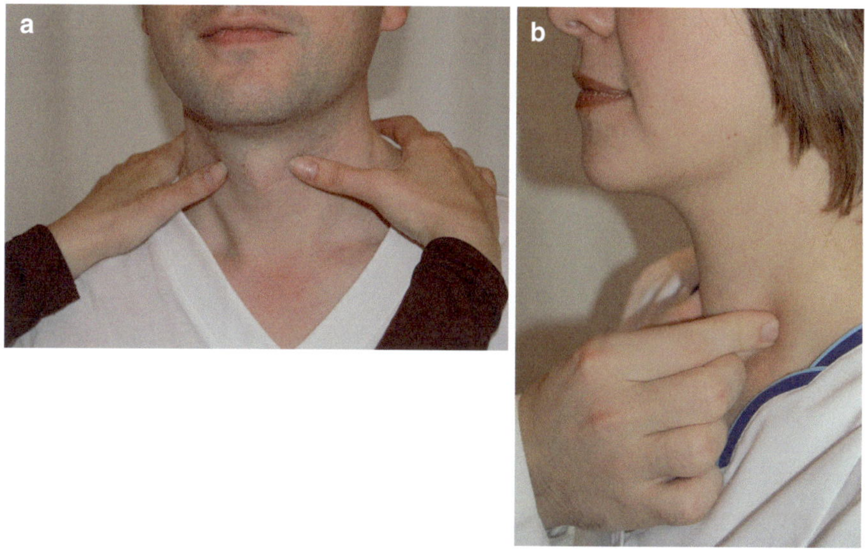

Fig. 1.2 (**a**, **b**) Thyroid palpation (**a**) thyroid palpation with thumbs (**b**) thyroid palpation with index finger

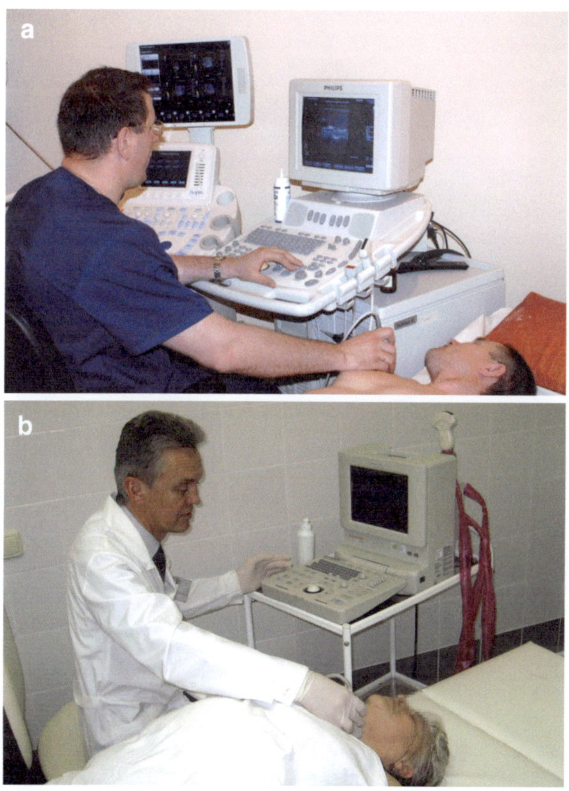

Fig. 1.3 (**a**, **b**) Thyroid US with (**a**) stationary equipment and (**b**) portable scanners

safety and comparatively low cost are additional factors in favor of the wide use of sonography for diagnosing thyroid diseases (Table 1.1). Since the first report of the application of US for diagnostic purposes was published, no scientifically proven adverse effect resulting from the medical use of US has been reported. It is possible that harmful effects may be identified in the future. However, the evidence available indicates that the benefits of US to patients are much greater than the risks, if any exist. Diagnostic doses of ultrasound do not accumulate, and the US examinations are short enough not to cause any significant biological effect. Hence, US can be performed several times without any limitations on the time interval between sessions. This enables the pathology to be assessed dynamically.

Modern US scanners can detect fluid lesions 1 mm or more and solid lesions 2 mm or more in size in the thyroid gland. Sonography can be effective in the detection of retrosternal goiter when it is in the upper mediastinum. However, localization of the goiter below the bifurcation of the trachea limits the possibilities of US. One disadvantage of thyroid sonography is its high dependence on operator skill. The variability in the results obtained when different US specialists examine the same patient is 10–30%. The information value and reproducibility of the method depend significantly on the quality of the equipment and the experience of the operator.

The use of color Doppler imaging (CDI), power Doppler imaging (PDI), and 3D reconstruction technology significantly improves the efficacy of US. This is very important for thyroid cancer and the early definition of metastases in regional lymph nodes (Tables 1.1 and 1.2).

Table 1.1 Information value of US in thyroid cancer

References	Sensitivity (%)	Specificity (%)	Diagnostic accuracy (%)
Kasatkin et al. (1989)	82.5	79.2	80.6
Anguissola et al. (1991)	96	81%	–
Urso et al. (1996)	100	88.2	–
Messina et al. (1996)	90	–	–
Agapitov et al. (1996)	69	91	84
Erdem (1997)	80	80	
Tsyb et al. (1997)	87.6	61.7	82.6
Pripachkina (1997)	89.2	92.1	89.8
Vetshev et al. (1998)	46.2	98.4	–
Harchenko et al. (1999)	90–95	55–65	80–89
Chumakov et al. (1999)	98	90	99
Markova (2001)	85.4	78.8	78.6
Semenov et al. (2006)	–	–	16.7
Miheeva (2007)	73.5	97.9	–
Maksimova and Kozel (2007)	63.9	38.1	54.4
Abalmasov and Ionova (2007)	80	91.1	89.1
Markova and Bashilov (2007)	88.8	74.5	81.0
Sencha et al. (2008)	94.2	77.8	92.7
Moon et al. (2008)	Up to 56.6	Up to 96.1	

Table 1.2 Efficacy of ultrasonography for thyroid cancer metastases in the lymph nodes of the neck

References	Sensitivity (%)	Specificity (%)	Diagnostic accuracy (%)
Bruneton et al. (1984)	93	91	92
Gritzmann et al. (1987)	92	84	89
Choi et al. (1995)	84	80	–
Tsyb et al. (1997)	96	72	89
Allahverdieva et al. (2005)	96.4	91	94
Abbasova et al. (2005)	100	90	93
Sencha et al. (2008)	80.6	84.2	81.5

Vetshev et al. (1997) and Karwowski et al. (2002) suggest *intraoperative US* as a reference method (Fig. 1.4). The authors report that intraoperative sonography detects additional lesions in 25% of cases. The nodules that had not been identified preoperatively were located mainly at the depth of the parenchyma and were 0.4 ± 0.07 cm in size. Histological investigations revealed thyroid cancer in 14.3% of such cases. Additional lesions 2–3 mm in size were found in 50% of patients with multinodular goiter. According to Harchenko et al.

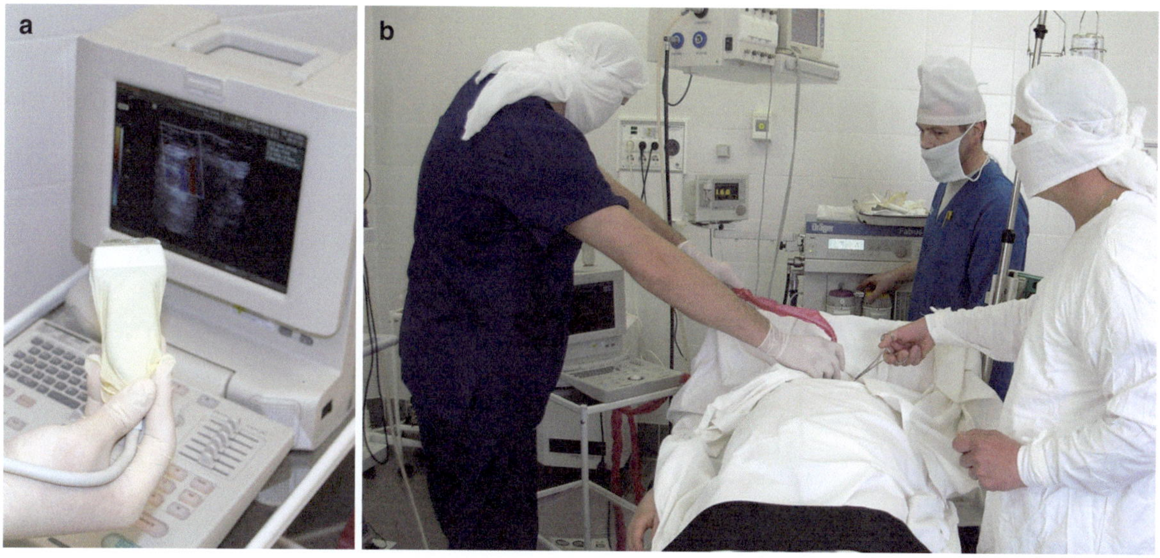

Fig. 1.4 (**a**, **b**) Intraoperative US (**a**) the simplest sterile cover for the US probe made of sterile surgical glove (**b**) thyroid US during the surgery

(2008), intraoperative US led to a change in the planned volume of thyroid surgery in 17.65% of cases.

Trofimova et al. (1999) utilize intraoperative US for precise neck examination after thyroid excision and lymph node dissection. This improves the radicality of the surgery. Alexandrov et al. (2001–2005) also point out the difference between the results of preoperative US and intraoperative findings. The authors suggest that sonography performed by a qualified sonographer on a high-quality scanner prior to the surgery may be of benefit for correcting surgical tactics.

Radionuclide scan (scintigraphy) is a method that involves acquiring a two-dimensional image which reflects the distribution of a radionuclide in organs. Thyroid scintigraphy is based on selective isotope absorption by the thyroid gland. Radionuclide scans permit the size of the thyroid to be defined, as well as its form, functional activity, localization of the lesions, and the detection of the thyroid ectopy. The method has a smaller resolution and produces less sharp images than US, CT, or MRI. However, scintigraphy provides information on the functional activity of the thyroid gland that cannot be obtained with any other visualizing modality (Figs. 1.5–1.7).

Radioiodine (^{123}I, ^{131}I), technetium (^{99m}Tc), cesium (^{137}Cs), gallium citrate (^{67}Ga), selenium (^{75}Se), thallium (^{201}Tl), and some other isotopes can be used for thyroid scans.

Thyroid scintigraphy may be indicated in the following cases of nodular goiter (Dedov et al. 2003):

1. Low TSH (for differential diagnosis of the diseases accompanied by thyrotoxicosis)
2. Suspicion of compensated functional autonomy (with normal TSH), especially in elderly and middle-aged patients

Besides, scintigraphy supplies valuable information in cases of thyroid ectopia (in the tongue root, pharynx, anterior mediastinum, and so on). It is the main modality used to verify the origin of the lesion in such circumstances.

Scintigraphy (or single photon emission computed tomography, or positron emission tomography, PET) is necessary for patients undergoing radioiodine therapy. It is indicated for patients with operated thyroid cancer and with suspected metastasis to various localizations.

The lesions are traditionally divided into "hot," "warm," and "cold," depending on the accumulation of radionuclide in the nodule and its functional activity. The minimum size of a nodule that can be detected is thought to be 1 cm. According to Nelson et al. (1978), nodules smaller than 2 cm in size are spotted in 41%, and nodules larger than 2 cm in 85% of cases.

Functionally inactive (cold) nodules are characterized by the absence or the significantly depressed accumulation of radionuclide. This can be seen in

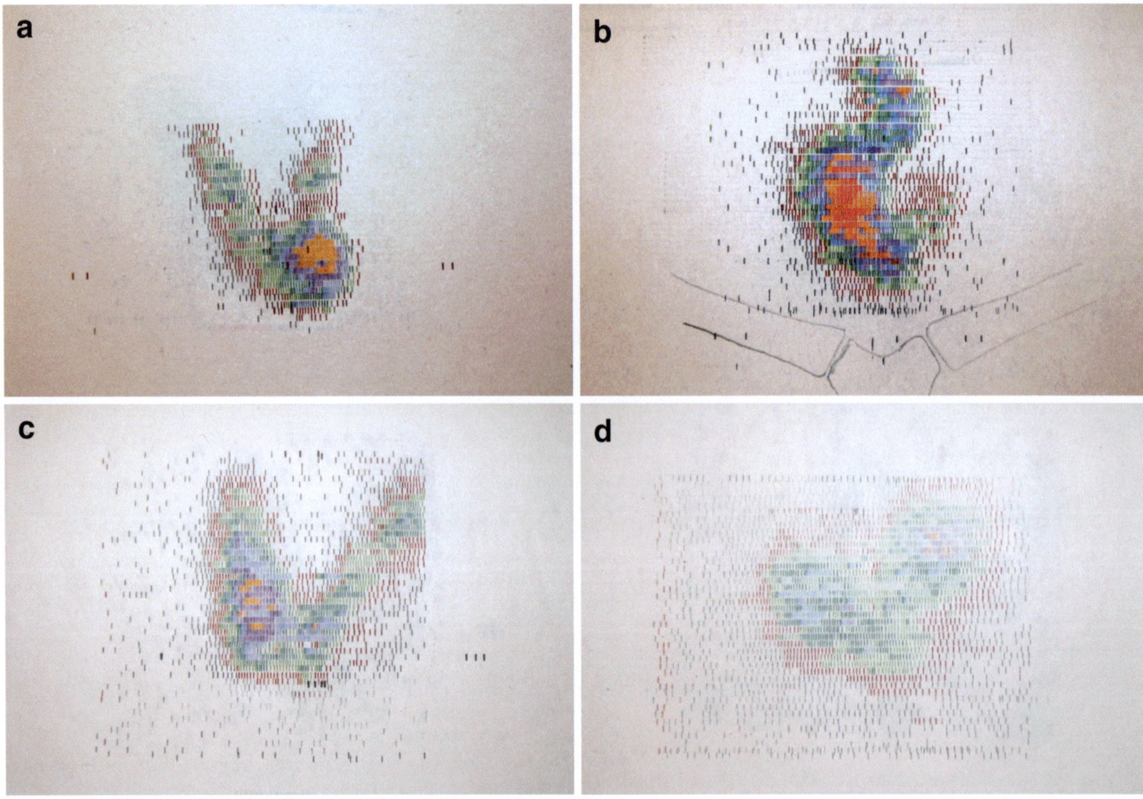

Fig. 1.5 (a–d) Scintiscans with ^{131}I showing nodular goiter (a) "hot" nodule in the lower segment of the left lobe (b) high iodine uptake predominantly by the right and pyramid lobes (c) "hot" nodule in the right lobe and "cold" nodule in the left lobe (d) diffusely enlarged thyroid

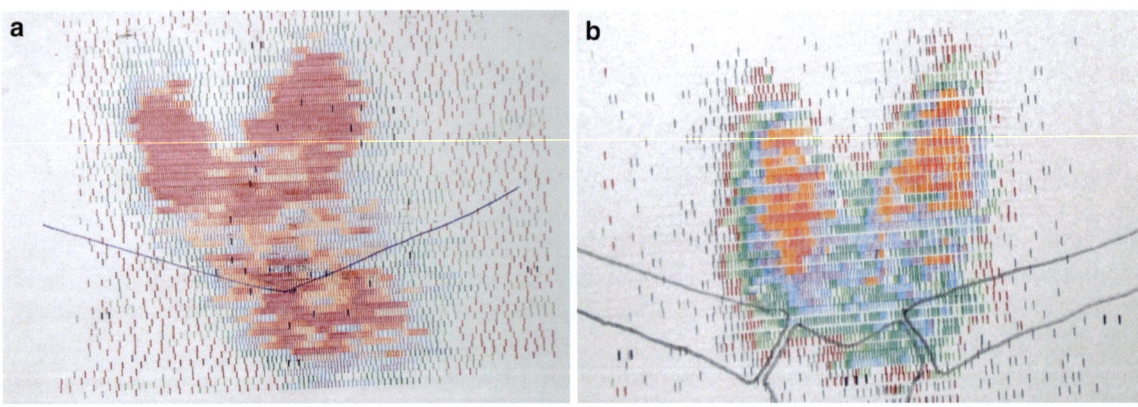

Fig. 1.6 (a, b) Scintiscans with ^{131}I showing substernal goiter (a) iodine uptake showing substernal part of the thyroid gland below the left lobe (b) partly substernal position of the thyroid

cases of nodular goiter, thyroiditis, cysts of the thyroid or parathyroid glands, nonspecific strumitis, and thyroid cancer (up to 20–25% of cases: McDougall 2006). Hot nodules almost exclusively trap isotopes, so the surrounding tissue appears isotope-free. Hot nodules often correspond to a colloidal proliferative goiter with increased functional activity, toxic adenoma, fetal or papillary A-cell adenoma, and sometimes autoimmune thyroid disease.

Identification of warm nodules is more difficult. These nodules can be considered a type of hot nodule, but, in contrast to hot nodules, the surrounding normal

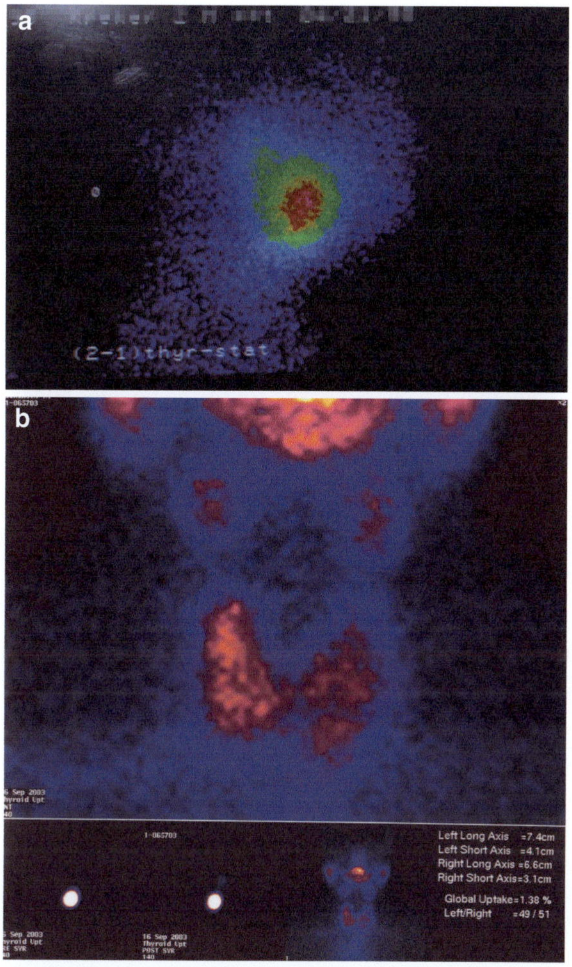

Fig. 1.7 Scans with ^{99m}Tc pertechnetate in nodular goiter

thyroid tissue remains unchanged or shows negligible functional depression. Isotope accumulation in such nodules may be similar to that seen in the surrounding parenchyma. This may result in false-negative data.

Data on the diagnostic value of scintigraphy are controversial (Table 1.3). Hot nodules were originally thought to exclude thyroid malignancy. Thyroid cancer was characterized by cold nodules (Mironov 1993). It was later proved that thyroid cancer can be associated with both functioning and nonfunctioning nodules (Goch 1997; Rubello et al. 2000). According to Harchenko et al. (1998), radionuclide scan data in cases of autoimmune thyroid disease are not specific either.

Scintigraphy involves the use of radioactive materials and exposes a patient to internal radiation. Thus, it should not be used in pregnant or nursing women, in children, and in people that have undergone previous irradiation.

Scintigraphy is now considered to be of no significant value for differentiating between benign and malignant thyroid lesions.

Scintigraphy is most valuable when combined with other diagnostic modalities, US in particular (Harchenko 1998). Raber et al. (1997) recommend that it should be combined with FNAB. They report that 38% of cold nodules are malignant, and consider FNAB to be indicated for all cold lesions.

Scintigraphy may be useful for monitoring the thyroid lesions after minimally invasive procedures (MIP). Paracchi et al. (1998) report that data on iodine uptake is important when following up thyroid adenomas after percutaneous ethanol injections. Radionuclide scans reveal the extinction of hot nodules in cases with good PEI results. Persistent accumulation of ^{131}I in the nodule corresponds to PEI insufficiency, and an additional PEI is then required to achieve the necessary effect.

MRI gives precise information on neck anatomy. It is capable of revealing lesions of 1–2 mm or larger (Kolokasidis 1999; Kabala 2007). It allows the dislocation of neck organs by the enlarged thyroid gland to be gauged, the margins and the capsule of the lesion to be assessed, the merging of lesions into surrounding

Table 1.3 Efficacy of scintigraphy in thyroid cancer

References	Sensitivity (%)	Specificity (%)	Diagnostic accuracy (%)
Mironov and Kasatkin (1993)	80	40	–
Severskaja (2002) (^{131}I, ^{99m}Tc)	96	14.3	44.9
Severskaja (2002) (MIBI)	71.4	43.3	59.7
Ahmedova et al. (2003) (^{99m}Tc)	33.3	77.7	68.1
Miheeva (2007) (^{99m}Tc pertechnetril)	73.5	97.9	–
Miheeva (2007) (^{99m}Tc pertechnetril)	55	76.9	–
Harchenko et al. (2008) (^{99m}Tc pertechnetril)	85.4	38.9	72.7

structures to be clarified, and lymph nodes to be detected and categorized.

MRI confers many advantages, such as the following:

1. High resolution, accuracy, 3D reconstruction, and the possibility of viewing planes that are usually inaccessible
2. The possibility of detecting and assessing the inner structure of the lesion (hemorrhage, cysts, etc.)
3. No ionizing radiation is involved, which is especially important in children and in cases of multiple repeated examinations

Thyroid MRI is indicated in the following cases (Harchenko et al. 2008):

1. All thyroid pathologies with a suspected substernal component
2. Big goiter
3. Discordant or disputable results from US or other visualization modalities

Thyroid MRI enables T1- and T2-weighted imaging with complete acquisition sequences in all projections (axial, sagittal, coronary) (Figs. 1.8–1.11). The normal thyroid gland appears isointense in comparison with neck muscles on T1-weighted images, and shows an enhanced signal on T2-weighted images. It may appear homogeneous or slightly heterogeneous (Pinskij 2005).

Abalmasov et al. (2002) suggest the following types of thyroid lesions in T1-weighted images:

1. Purely homogeneous nodules that are hypointense or isointense in relation to normal thyroid tissue. The relative signal intensity (RSI) is 0.91 ± 0.03. These can correspond morphologically to thyroid cancer, microfollicular adenoma, and microfollicular nodular goiter.
2. Relatively homogeneous nodules. The nodule periphery is often moderately hyperintensive in comparison with the center. Its RSI is 1.19 ± 0.03. These nodules are characteristic for mixed nodular goiter, follicular and microfollicular adenomas, and thyroid cancer (Table 1.4).
3. Nodules that have hyperintense foci with relative intensity values of 1.90 ± 0.07 against an iso- or moderately hyperintense background. The foci have rather accurate margins. Sometimes the whole nodule may appear hyperintense. Such nodules may be observed in cases of microfollicular or mixed nodular goiter and follicular adenoma.
4. Significantly hyperintense homogeneous nodules with RSI 2.54 ± 0.08. These have well-defined regular borders and correspond exclusively to colloid cysts.
5. Homogeneous hypointense nodules with RSI 0.82 ± 0.01 represent noncolloid cysts in a mixed nodular goiter, follicular cancer, or microfollicular adenoma.

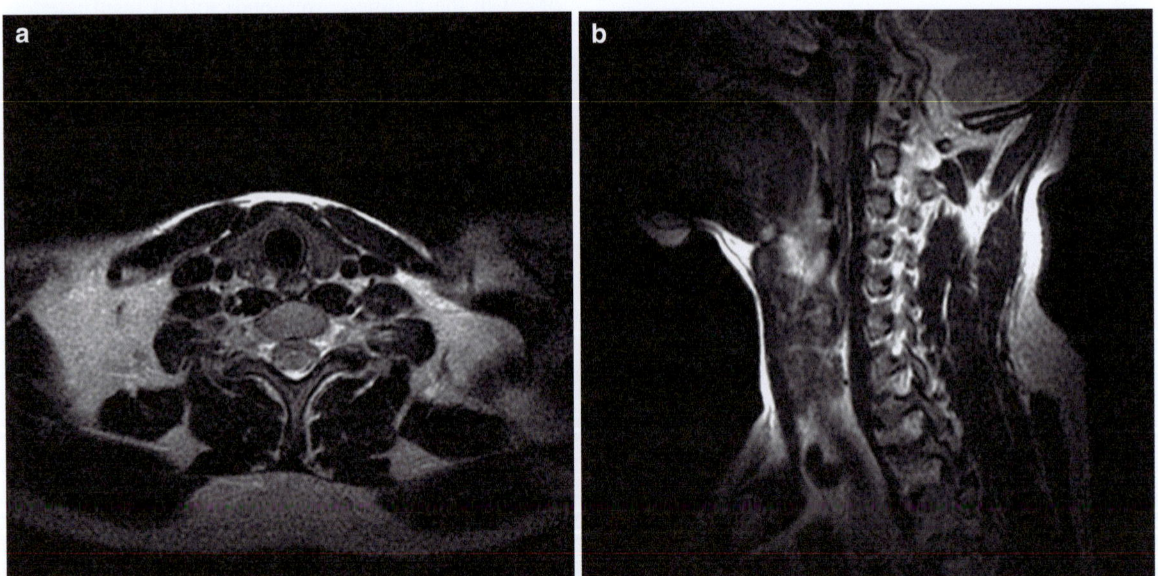

Fig. 1.8 **(a–d)** MRI. Normal thyroid (T1) **(a, c)** transverse scan **(b, d)** sagittal scan

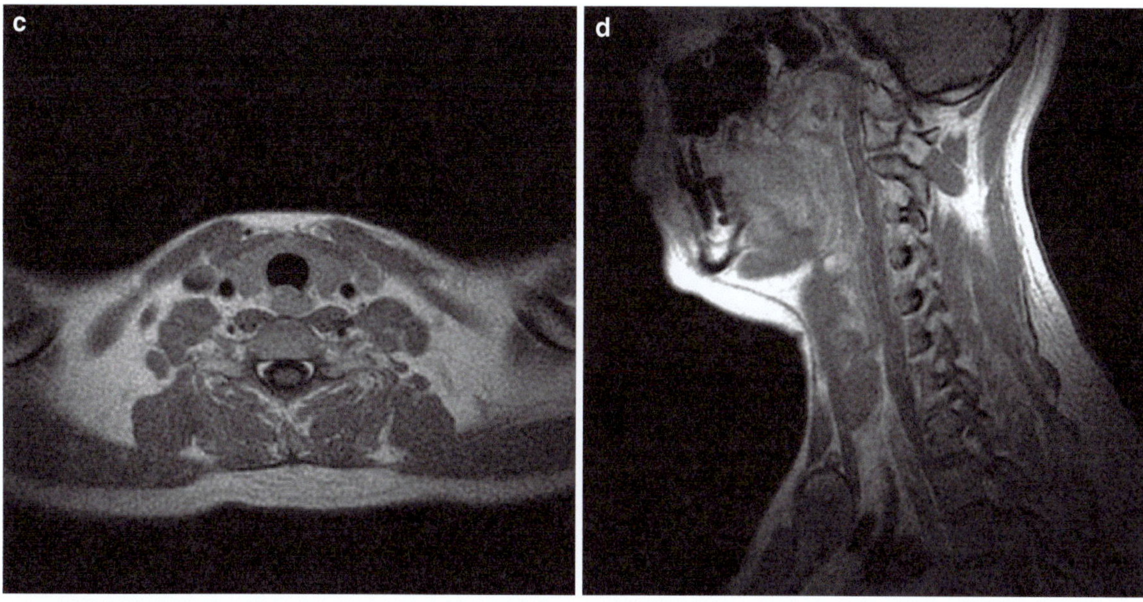

Fig. 1.8 (**c–d**) (continued)

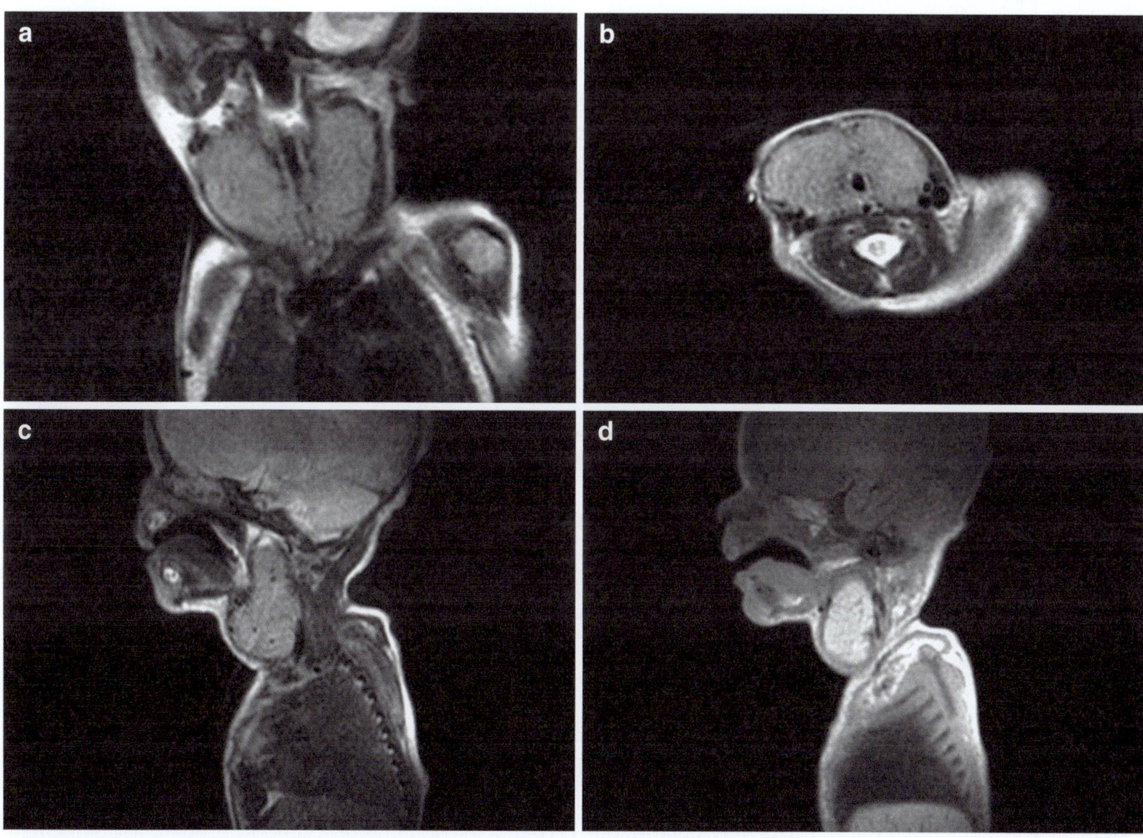

Fig. 1.9 (**a–d**) MRI. Diffuse (congenital) hyperplasia of the thyroid gland (T1) (**a**) front plane, (**b**) transverse plane, (**c**) sagittal plane

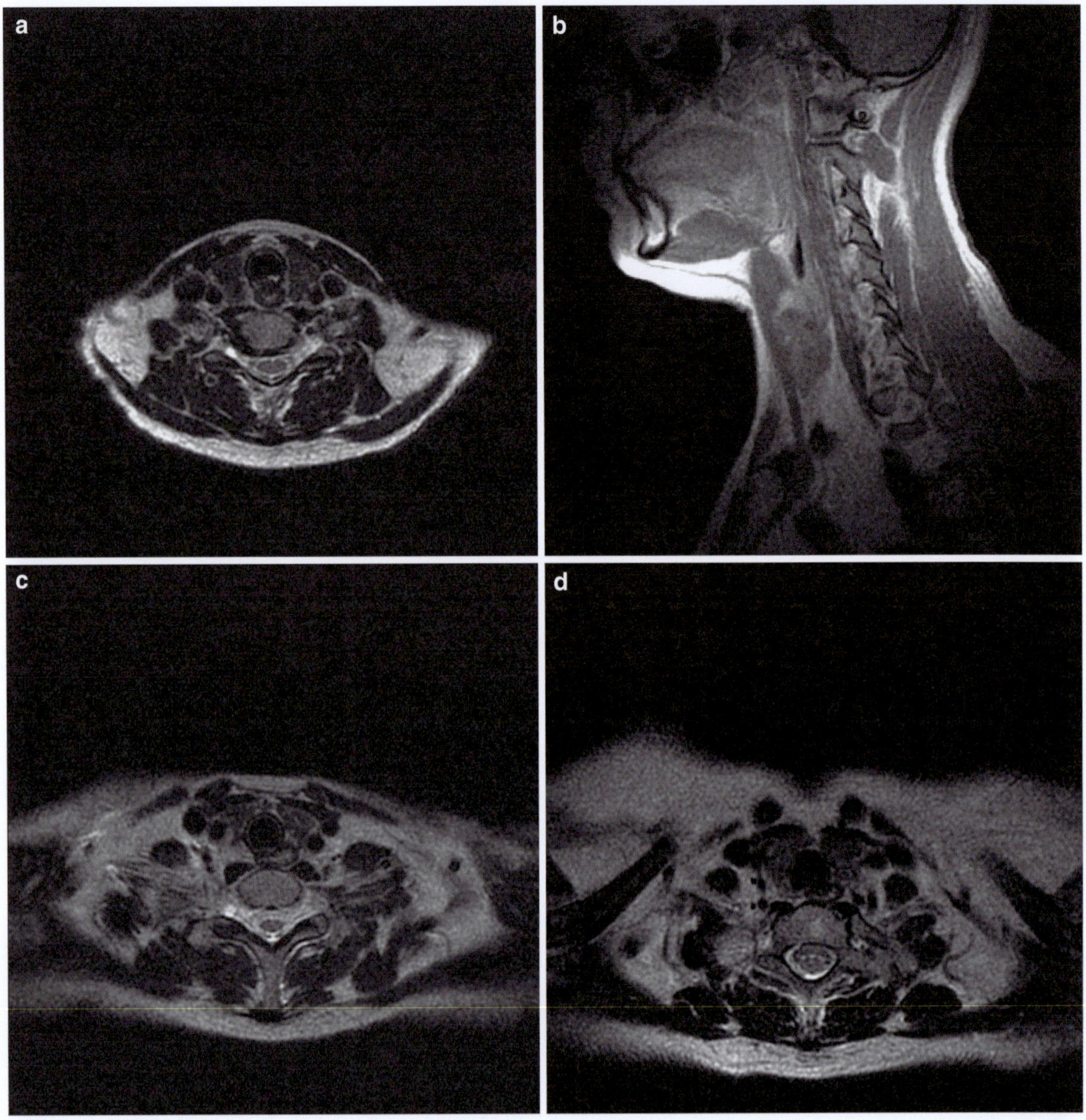

Fig. 1.10 (**a–d**) MRI. Autoimmune thyroid disease (T1) heterogeneous thyroid structure (**a, c, d**) transverse scan (**b**) sagittal scan

A high diagnostic value of MRI in defining the neoplastic expansion of thyroid cancer is reported by Noma et al. (1988). Pinsky et al. (2005) remark that MRI allows neck lymph nodes 1–2 mm or larger to be spotted. According to the authors, a hyperintense signal within the lymph nodes on T1–T2-weighted images increases the probability of metastases, even in cases with an unknown primary tumor. MRI may be utilized for the guidance of fine needle aspiration biopsy. Nevertheless, the question of whether the characteristics of the pathological process can be determined using MRI is still open. Despite all of its advantages, the high cost of MRI tests means that strict indications for thyroid MRI need to be implemented (Kolokasidis 1999; Harchenko et al. 2008).

Contrast-enhanced MRI significantly improves the sharpness and contrast of the image. It increases MRI efficacy in 72.73% of cases of thyroid pathology (Harchenko et al. 2008). It permits better assessment of the contours, the size, the structure of parenchyma of the thyroid gland, and changes in surrounding structures.

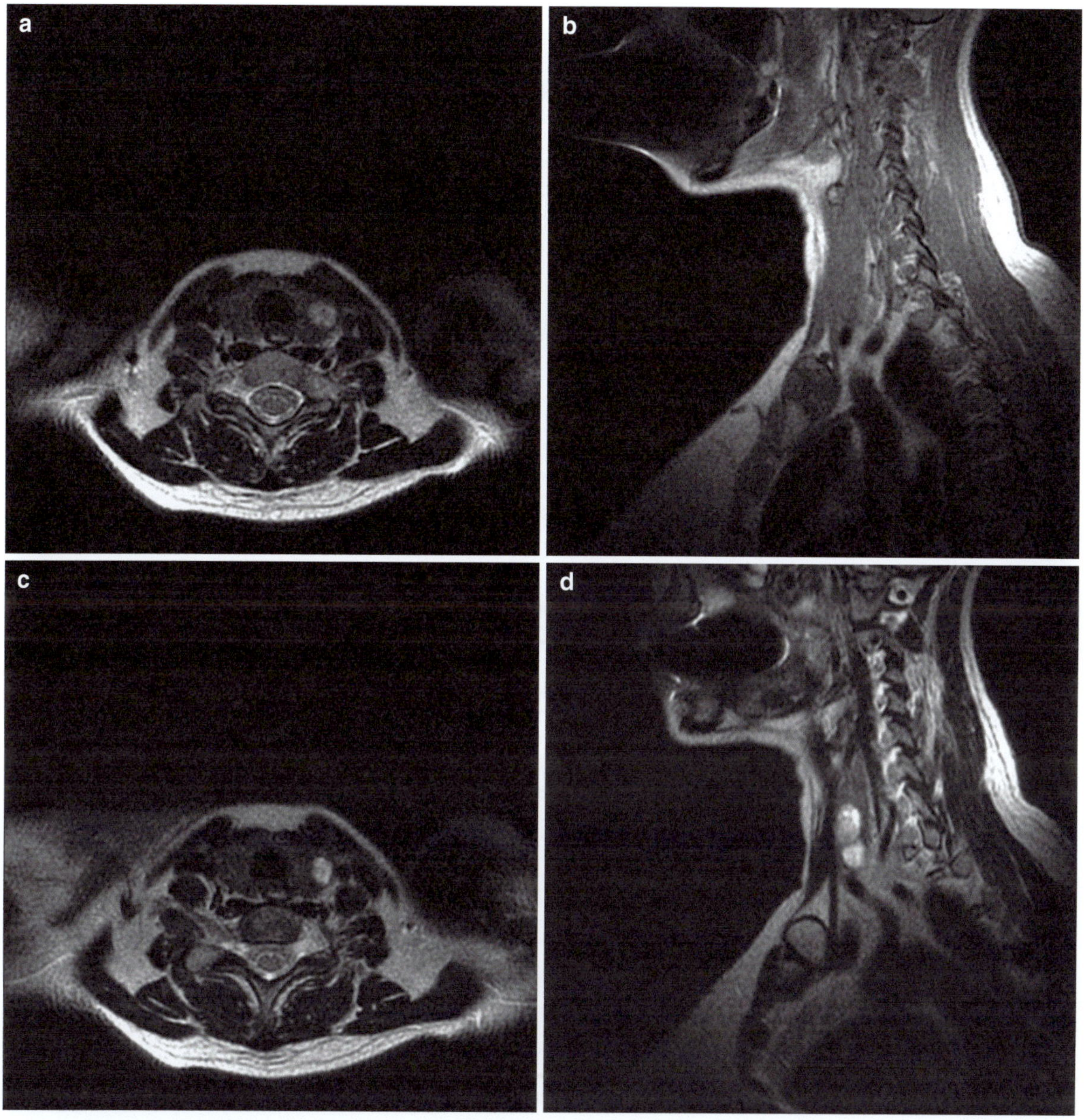

Fig. 1.11 (**a–d**) MRI. Thyroid cancer (T1) hyperintence focus within the thyroid lobe (**a, c**) transverse scan (**b, d**) sagittal scan

Table 1.4 MRI efficacy in thyroid cancer

References	Sensitivity (%)	Specificity (%)	Diagnostic accuracy (%)
Ahmedova et al. (2003)	93.8	98.5	97.6
Bahtin et al. (2006)	95.6	91.2	94.6
Harchenko et al. (2008)	76.5	42.9	66.7

Generally, the typical location of the thyroid gland does not require the use of X-ray CT. Friedman et al. (1988) and Dedov et al. (1994) underline that CT appears necessary for a retrosternal location of the thyroid in order to assess the range of the neoplastic process, the tumor invasion, the relation of the thyroid to surrounding organs, and to reveal metastases to lymph nodes (Figs. 1.12–1.14).

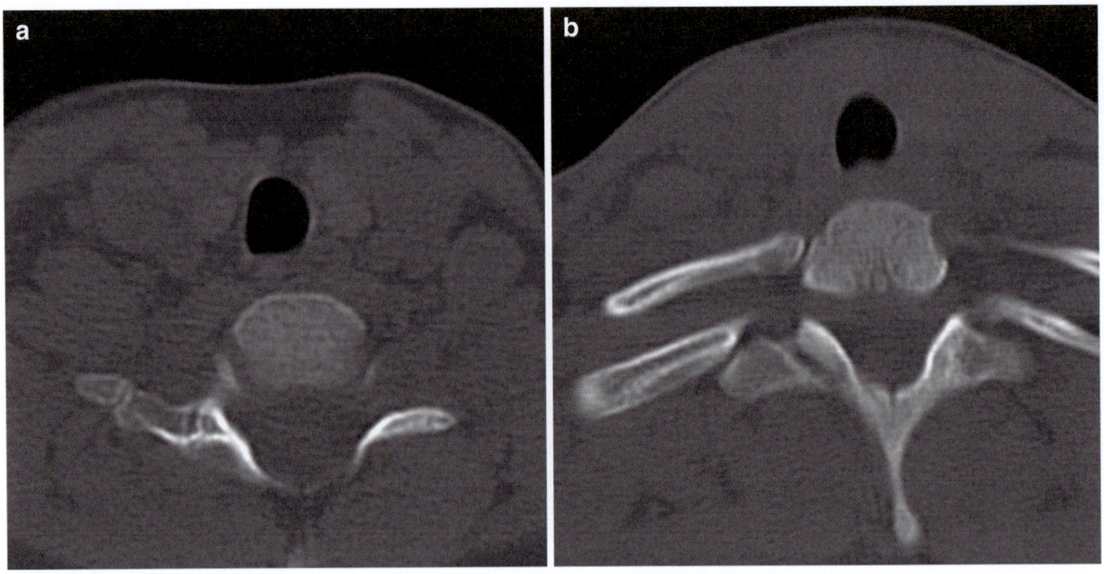

Fig. 1.12 CT. Substernal goiter. Diffuse thyroid enlargement

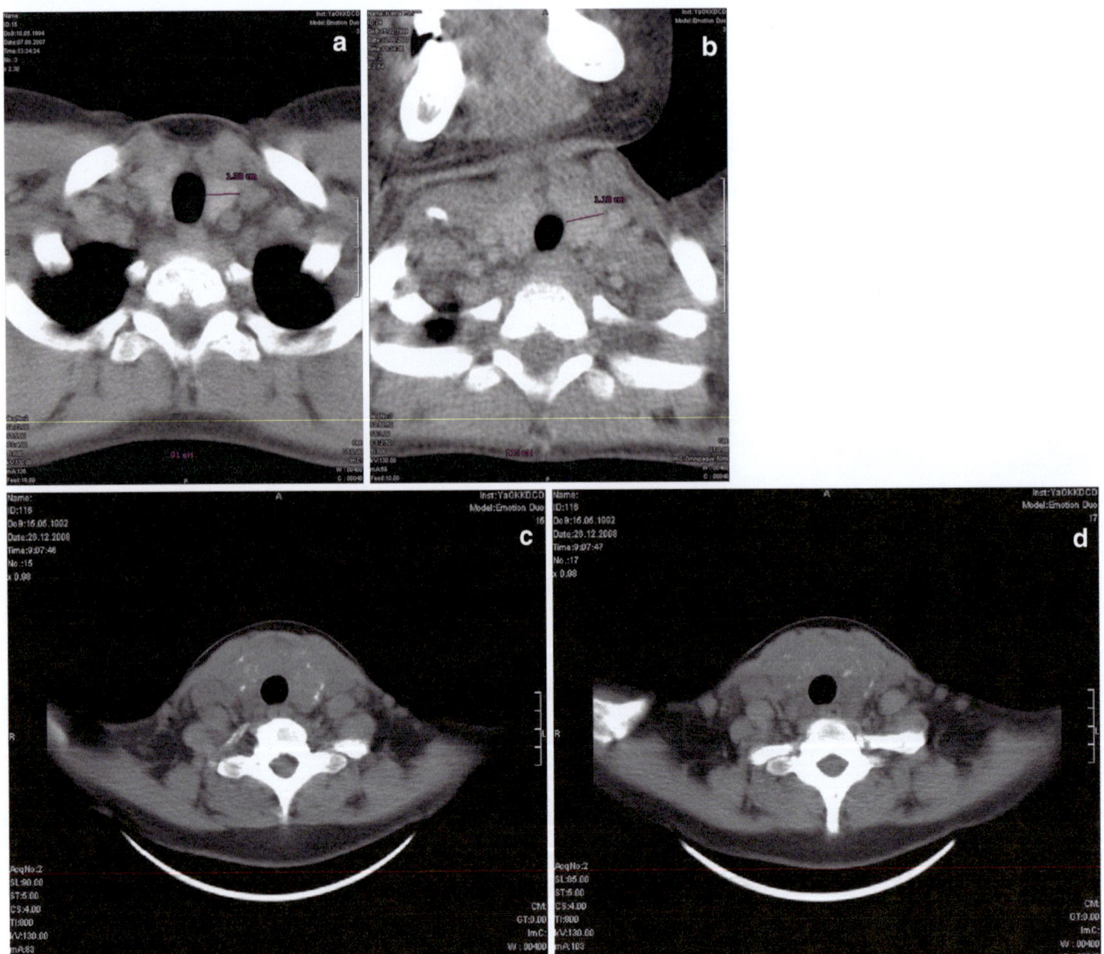

Fig. 1.13 (**a–d**) CT. Thyroid cancer (**a, b**) the suspicious region is measured (**c, d**) - microcalcifications can be detected as small hyperdense foci

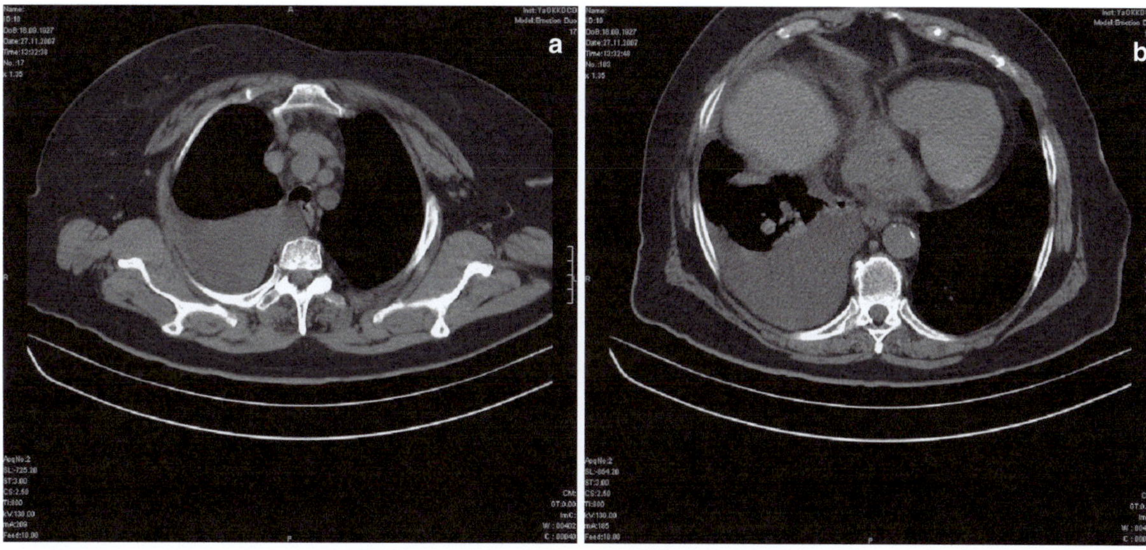

Fig. 1.14 CT. Thyroid cancer metastases in paratracheal (**a**) and mediastinal (**b**) lymph nodes

The basic indications for thyroid CT are as follows (Harchenko et al. 2008):

- Suspected cancer of the retrosternally located thyroid
- Big goiter
- The enlargement of paratracheal lymph nodes and the presence of any radiologically proved lesion in the mediastinum

The CT is of great value for tumors of ectopic or aberrant thyroid glands. It is also performed to diagnose metastatic lesions in cervical vertebrae (Kolokasidis 1999).

Glazer et al. (1982) suggest that the following CT criteria indicate a lesion of the mediastinum belonging to thyroid tissue:

1. Continuous anatomical connection with the cervical thyroid
2. Focal calcifications
3. Comparatively high CT density (HU)
4. Increase in CT density after intravenous contrast administration
5. Long persistence of tissue contrast after contrast administration

Contrast improves the quality of the CT scan in 65% of cases (Kharchenko et al. 2008).

The sensitivity of CT scan to thyroid cancer is 66.7%, its specificity is 50.0%, and its diagnostic accuracy is 66.7% (Kharchenko et al. 2008). According to Ahmedova and Filatova (2003), the sensitivity of contrast CT for thyroid cancer compounds is 88%, its specificity is 100%, and its diagnostic accuracy is 96.4%.

Nevertheless, CT is not a method of choice for thyroid pathology due to the high radiation dose imparted to the patient, and the presence of several efficient alternative methods. Additionally, the complexity of correlation between morphological structure and density limits the application of CT to the detection and categorization of thyroid tumors.

Biopsy with cytologic investigation (Fig. 1.15) is a unique preoperative method for assessing morphological structures of thyroid lesions. Cytology traditionally aims to confirm or to deny malignancy. Morphological examination permits early detection and differentiation of the thyroid pathology prior to clinical manifestation. Visualization methods significantly facilitate percutaneous diagnostic interventions and allow small, deeply located lesions 3–4 mm or larger in size to be punctured. Real-time biopsy guidance makes the US advantageous. US-guided thyroid puncture can be performed in outpatients, and in most cases does not demand anesthesia.

The biopsy permits differentiation of thyroid lesions with high accuracy. Special attention is paid to thyroid malignancy (Table 1.5). The FNAB is especially valuable in cases with combinations of nodules with diffuse thyroid changes.

The diagnostic value of thyroid cytology is 55–70%. Errors oc cur in 10–60% of cases, and suspicious or uncertain changes in 10–30% of patients (Romanchishen 1992; Holm et al. 1996).

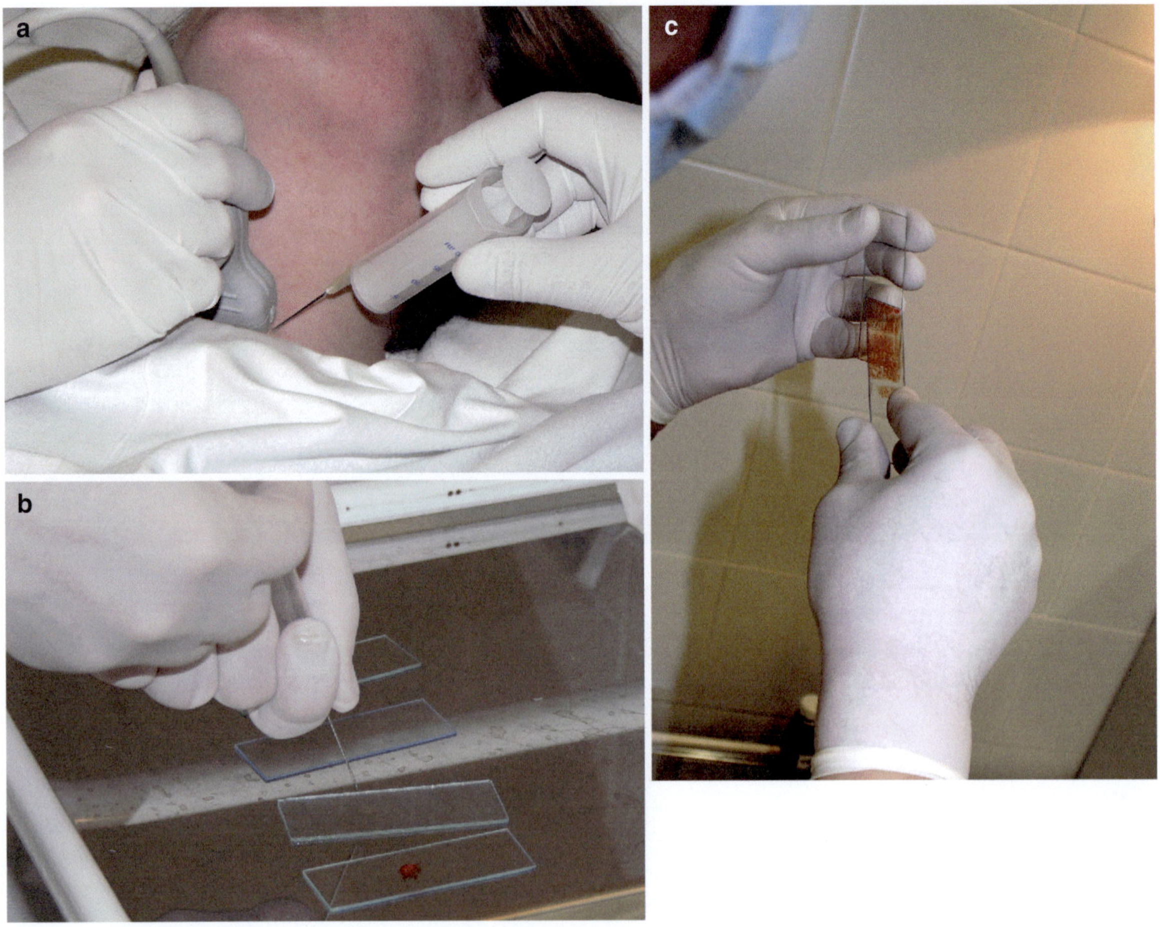

Fig. 1.15 (**a–c**) FNAB of the thyroid gland (**a**) position of the needle and US probe (**b**) flowing out the aspirate on the slides (**c**) making smears

According to Severskaya (2002), false-negative results of cytologic examinations are registered in 5.7% of cases, false positive in 6.7%, uninformative in 15%, and uncertain in 24%. According to Olshansky et al. (1996), cytological investigation allows the diagnosis of malignant tumor to be verified in 91.1% of cases (Figs. 1.16 and 1.17; Table 1.6). Gharib et al. (1984) found that an ambiguous cytologic report after FNAB was received for 20% of patients. That led to a differential diagnosis between various thyroid pathologies, although 20% of these patients received a final diagnosis of malignancy during surgery.

Baskin et al. (1987) underline the special difficulties of cytological examinations in cases of well-differentiated follicular cancer and follicular adenoma. According to Severskaya (2002), the probability of thyroid cancer with a cytological picture of a follicular tumor is 23%. Hence, some authors integrate all follicular thyroid tumors into the family of follicular neoplasias (Vetshev et al. 1997).

The indications for *X-ray* in thyroid pathology are very limited now, as there are several better methods. X-ray is not specific for thyroid diseases, but chest radiography is mandatory for the detection of metastases in lungs, mediastinum, bones, and in cases of rare thyroid tumor localizations.

Routine chest examination is of small benefit due to the low density of thyroid lesions. Thyroid pathology can be assessed based on indirect attributes (Fig. 1.18), such as the following (Vlasov 2006):

- Dilation of the mediastinum or changes in its shape (smoothing of the arches or extra protrusions)
- Displacement, narrowing, compression, or invasion of trachea or esophagus
- Changes in the retrotracheal space
- Calcification

Table 1.5 Efficacy of FNAB in thyroid cancer

References	Sensitivity (%)	Specificity (%)	Diagnostic accuracy (%)
Altivilla et al. (1990)	71	100	–
Kumar et al. (1992)	98.5	–	–
Horvath et al. (1993)	80	93	92
Brom-Ferral et al. (1993)	95	100	–
Sanchez et al. (1994)	78	–	–
Cochand-Priollet et al. (1997)	95	87.7	89
Vetshev et al. (1997)	23.1	96.4	–
Alexandrov et al. (1997)	90.7	97.3	96.3
Carmeci et al. (1998)	100	100	–
Ravetto et al. (2000)	92	76	–
Ogawa et al. (2001)	84	99	–
Karstrup et al. (2001)	83	77	80
Semikov (2004)	69.7	–	–
Grineva et al. (2005)	95.89	52.46	63.18
Abalmasov and Ionova (2007)	81.5	–	–
Nabieva (2008)	92.7	75	91.5
Kiyaev (2008)	97.2	80	–

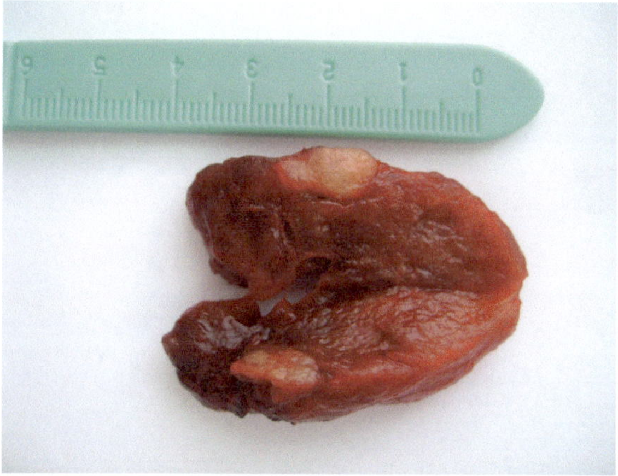

Fig. 1.16 Macroscopic view of papillary thyroid cancer

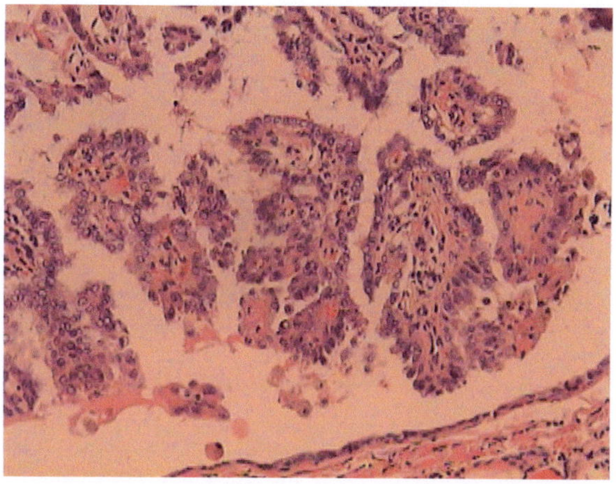

Fig. 1.17 FNAB. Papillary thyroid cancer (Romanowsky-stained smears; original magnification ×1000)

Table 1.6 Efficacy of cytologic examination for thyroid cancer

References	Sensitivity (%)	Specificity (%)	Diagnostic accuracy (%)
Edith de los Santos et al. (1990)	100	–	55
Severskaya (2002)	81.4	91.1	86.2

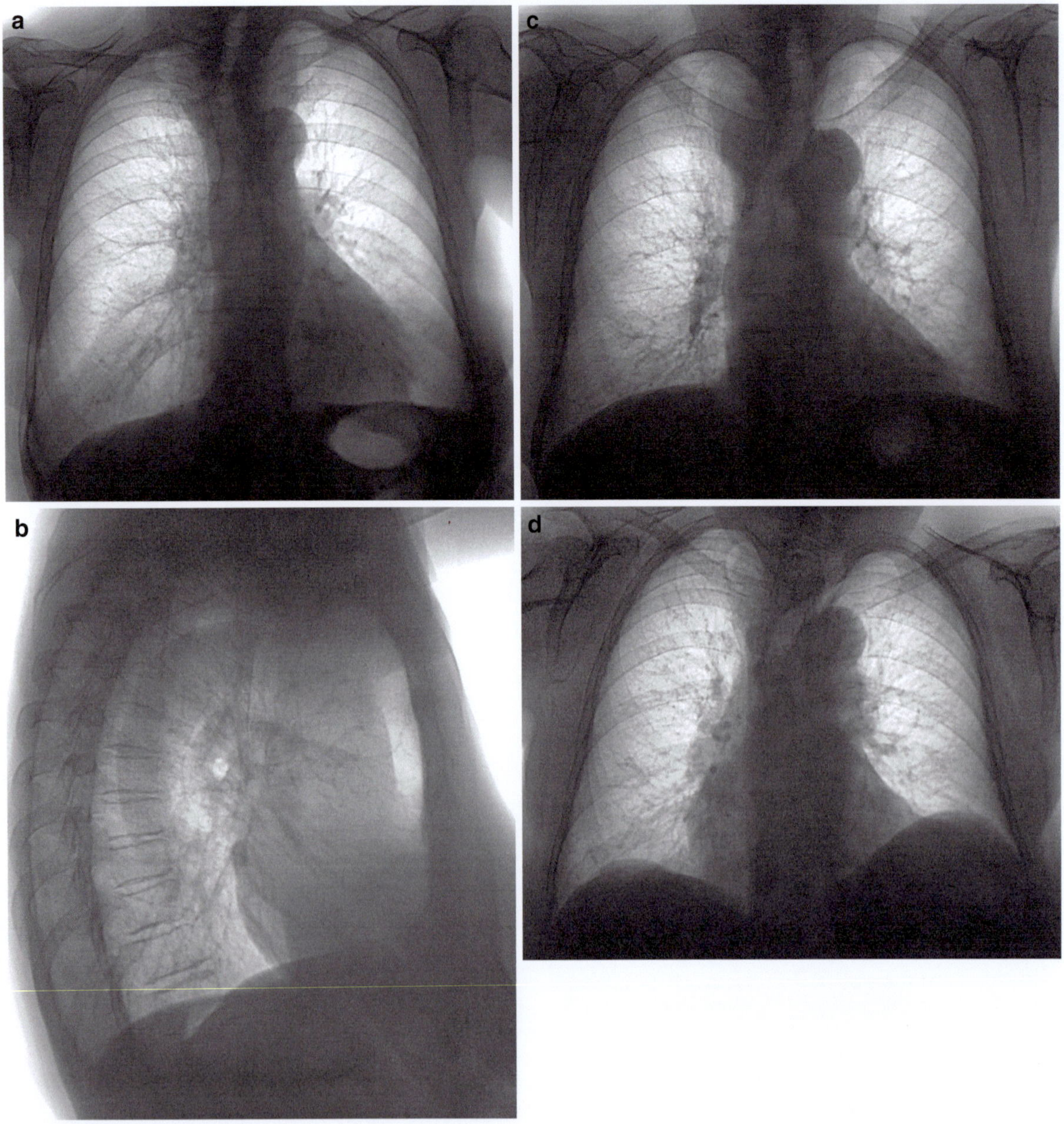

Fig. 1.18 (**a–d**) Anterior (**a, c, d**) and sagittal (**b**) projections of the chest. Dilation of the mediastinal shadow

Soft-tissue radiography of the neck and cervical trachea tomography permit estimation of thyroid size, the level of the inferior poles, the presence of calcifications in the gland or its lesions, tracheal displacement, the width of the tracheal lumen, and the status of the tracheal walls (Pinsky et al. 1999).

Contrast radiography of the esophagus is valuable in big thyroid masses, especially those located in lateral compartments, in substernal goiter, and in cancer recurrence (Fig. 1.19).

Indications for chest X-ray with barium-contrasted esophagus in cases of thyroid pathology are as follows:

- Big nodular goiter
- Substernal nodular goiter with compression of the trachea or the esophagus
- Thyroid cancer
- Riedel's thyroiditis
- Lymphosarcoma of the thyroid

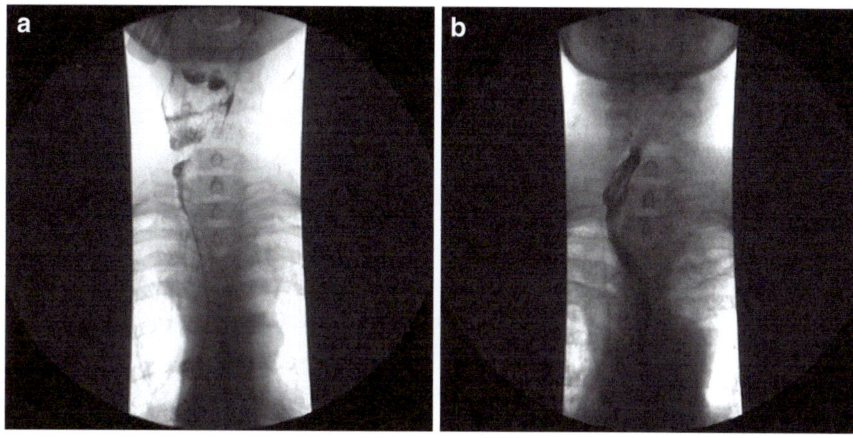

Fig. 1.19 Chest X-ray with contrasted esophagus. Displacement and compression of the esophagus

Esophagus radiography can reveal esophageal displacement and compression, or the invasion of its walls.

One contrast X-ray examination for thyroid diseases is percutaneous thyrolymphography (Scierski 1980).

Thermography was widely utilized to diagnose thyroid diseases in the 1990s. This was based on recording the temperature over the nodule or the tumor of the thyroid gland.

Paches et al. (1995) and Kalinin et al. (2004) found that thermography is of low diagnostic value for cancer and the differential diagnosis of thyroid masses. They suggest that thermographic representation is linked not to histological structure, but to the blood supply of the examined region. Combination with scintigraphy or sonography significantly increases the diagnostic possibilities of thermography (Vnotchenko et al. 1993). According to Kamardin et al. (1983), the sensitivity of thermography for diagnosing metastases and cancer recurrence is 92%, its specificity is 89%, its general efficacy is 89.3%, its positive predictive value is 70%, and its negative predictive value is 97%. Romanchishen (2003) confirms the high diagnostic efficacy of thermography for revealing of thyroid cancer recurrence and metastases if combined with radionuclide scan. According to Pinsky et al. (1999), thermography can be beneficial in combination with other methods, but has no diagnostic value if used independently.

Electroimpedance tomography was introduced several years ago. It is based on measuring the electrical resistance of certain body areas by applying electrodes to the skin. This method is now used in breast studies. It enables the anatomical uniformity of the mammary gland and the presence of solid lesions to be assessed. The data obtained are related to the physiological status of the tissues. The method allows planes of body parts to be created through mathematical reconstruction. Prototypes of probes for diagnosing thyroid diseases have been developed. The advantages of this method include complete harmlessness, low cost of equipment, and simplicity of the examination. The disadvantages are low resolution, which significantly deteriorates with depth from body surface, and poor dynamic visualization.

Vetshev et al. (2001) developed the method of intraoperative laser autofluorescent spectroscopy, aimed at improving instant thyroid pathology diagnostics during surgery. The authors suggest criteria for the differential diagnosis of benign and malignant lesions. The sensitivity of the method for malignant thyroid tumors can reach 95.4%, and its specificity 97.6%. The method allows morphological changes in the thyroid gland during an operation to be characterized. Thus, it aids the assessment of the optimum volume of surgical intervention. The authors report that this method resulted in an expansion beyond the planned operating volume in 18.2% of patients. This helped to avoid reoperation after the results of the scheduled histological examination were received.

PET utilizes biologically active molecules which contain short-lived isotopes. As a radioisotope decays it emits a positron. Further annihilation of the positron with an electron results in the simultaneous generation of two gamma quanta moving in opposite directions. Thus, it enables the exact coordinates of the source of the quanta to be determined, allowing an image to be created via mathematical reconstruction methods. The procedure is usually used in combination with other modalities: US, CT, MRI, thyroid hormone test, or ^{131}I scintigraphy of the whole body (Blinov 2005).

Other methods of diagnosing thyroid diseases include dynamic thyrolymphoscintigraphy, pneumothyroidography, arteriography, rheothyrography, polarography, and some other procedures.

None of the diagnostic methods can claim absolute reliability and accuracy. When choosing the diagnostic modality for thyroid diseases, it is important to consider all of its advantages and disadvantages. The methods exhibit different efficacies for different thyroid diseases, and their efficacies also depend on concomitant diseases, previous treatment, patient age, and other factors.

Incorrect assessments and exam results of low value depend on a number of parameters, most frequently on the human factor. Paches and Propp (1995) report that despite modern diagnostics, approximately 50% of patients with thyroid cancer receive a wrong diagnosis, and 60% are only diagnosed at a late stage. Initial stages are misdiagnosed in 50–100% of cases. The preoperative diagnosis is correct in 14–88.5%, and more often in 25–40% of cases. The greatest difficulties arise with early or small cancers. According to Bakanidze (2002), basic diagnostic and tactical errors (which, in patients with thyroid cancer, can correspond to 41.6% of cases) by general practitioners include unreasonably long observations (10.8%), conservative therapy (8.1%), the incorrect use of diagnostic methods (24.9%), and nonconventional surgery on the thyroid or the regional lymph nodes.

Employing several diagnostic modalities is the most effective approach, and one that permits the character and the severity of the pathology to be assessed. Modern complex diagnostics do not assume the use of all possible methods. It is necessary to find a rational range and sequence of diagnostic techniques to obtain the maximum information in each case.

Complex Ultrasound Diagnosis of Thyroid Diseases

2

2.1 Ultrasound Modalities

The first US examination of small parts was reported by Howry in 1955. Thyroid sonography (A- and B-scan) was first introduced in 1966–1967 (Fujimoto et al. 1967). It has been widely practiced since the 1970s and is now one of the most popular radiological methods for diagnosing thyroid diseases.

The method is based on differences between the abilities of different tissues to reflect US waves (cyclic sound pressure of an elastic medium with a frequency greater than 20,000 Hz). Modern US scanners permit real-time imaging of organs with constant monitoring of their motion.

Thyroid US has the following advantages:

- It is relatively simple, rapid to perform, and inexpensive.
- It is painless and noninvasive.
- This is no need for any special preparation of the patient before the examination.
- There are no contraindications.
- It is harmless and safe for the patient and staff. US can be used repeatedly in children, pregnant and nursing women, as well as seriously ill patients with severe concomitant pathology.
- Patients can be examined regardless of their medications, including thyroid blocking agents.
- It is a high-resolution technique.
- The differential diagnosis is based on sonographic options, such as Doppler modalities, 3D image reconstruction, and others.
- It supports documentation of video data and static images, as well as easy transmission via modern communication channels with virtual consultations.
- It provides easy guidance for minimally invasive modalities, such as FNAB, PEI, PLA, PGA, and others.

A patient is indicated for thyroid ultrasound in the following cases:

- Complaints that are often a consequence of thyroid pathology: dyspnea, cough, irritability, palpitation, precordial discomfort
- Palpated masses in the anterior neck
- Thyroid pathology detected by other methods
- Cardiovascular pathology, predominantly heart rhythm abnormalities
- Persistent diseases of ENT organs (such as larynx, pharynx, trachea), dysphonia, or aphonia
- Dysphagia
- Monitoring of the efficacy of treatment of thyroid diseases
- Postoperative follow-up

Sonography can be utilized as a screening method for thyroid diseases. It permits early detection of patients who are at an increased risk of developing a thyroid disease. Screening is an effective initial stage of evaluation within a target population (Parshin et al. 1999). It helps to pinpoint a possible thyroid abnormality at an early stage, and includes the elements of differential diagnosis that result in subsequent thorough examination and timely treatment in appropriate cases. The advantages of US as a screening method are patient safety, reproducibility, reduced dependence on the quality of the equipment and operator skill, speed, availability, and low cost. The disadvantage of US screening is its comparatively low diagnostic accuracy. A negative screening study does not guarantee the absence of the disease, and sometimes a positive study does not necessarily prove that a thyroid pathology is present. In practice, one example of screening is thyroid US performed by a general practitioner with a simple (e.g., only grayscale) scanner. The exam aims to divide patients into two generalized categories:

V.P. Kharchenko et al., *Ultrasound Diagnostics of Thyroid Diseases*,
DOI: 10.1007/978-3-642-12387-0_2, © Springer-Verlag Berlin Heidelberg 2010

those whose thyroids are grossly normal, and those with suspicious abnormalities in their thyroids.

Patients with thyroid abnormalities are subject to further complex qualified US. Complex US assumes the detection and certain differential diagnosis of diffuse changes and focal lesions, which is necessary to determine subsequent tactics.

US options utilized for the diagnosis of thyroid diseases include the following:

1. Grayscale
2. Tissue harmonics
3. Adaptive coloring
4. CDI
5. PDI
6. Grayscale 3D
7. Vascular 3D
8. 4D
9. Panoramic scan
10. Spectral pulsed wave Doppler
11. Others (multislice view, volume CT view, contrast US, US elastography, etc.)

Grayscale (B-mode, 2D mode) is a well-known basic type of scanning that provides an image of the thyroid in typically 256 shades of gray (Fig. 2.1).

The *harmonic (the second harmonic, tissue harmonic imaging or THI, tissue harmonic echo)* is an algorithm that allocates the harmonic component of fluctuations after the base US impulse has passed though the tissues (Fig. 2.2). It is often available as an option on grayscale scanners with standard probes.

THI enables the diagnosis of 70.8% of patients with thyroid pathologies (Miheeva 2007). THI emphasizes the US signs of thyroid cancer (visualization improves

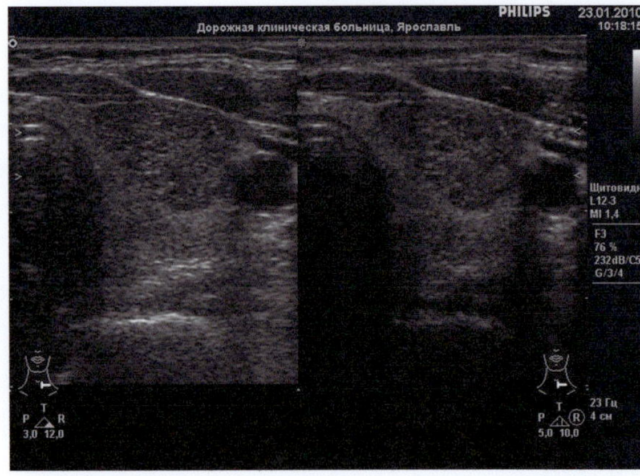

Fig. 2.2 Thyroid sonograms. THI

in about 28–30% of cases). It permits a more accurate definition of lesion margins, calcifications, and nodule structure. According to Belashkin et al. (2003), THI improves the visualization quality and defines features of colloid nodules in 80% of cases.

Adaptive coloring utilizes a color map in order to stain a grayscale image. The density of staining depends on the strength of the reflected echo (Fig. 2.3). Color inversion of the image is possible. The option is often added to grayscale scanners with standard probes.

This option improves the subjective perception of an US image. Thus, it helps in the detection of isoechoic thyroid lesions, and in the definition of nodule contours and posterior acoustic changes, especially in small lesions (up to 0.5–0.7 cm in size).

The vascularity of an abnormal thyroid can be characterized by Doppler modalities. The following aspects require special attention:

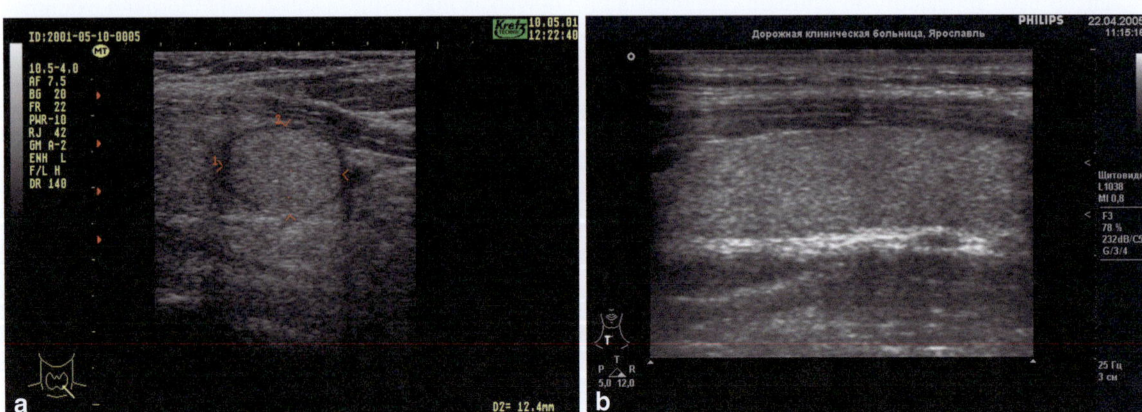

Fig. 2.1 (a, b) Thyroid sonograms. Grayscale mode (a) thyroid nodule (b) longitudinal scan of normal thyroid lobe

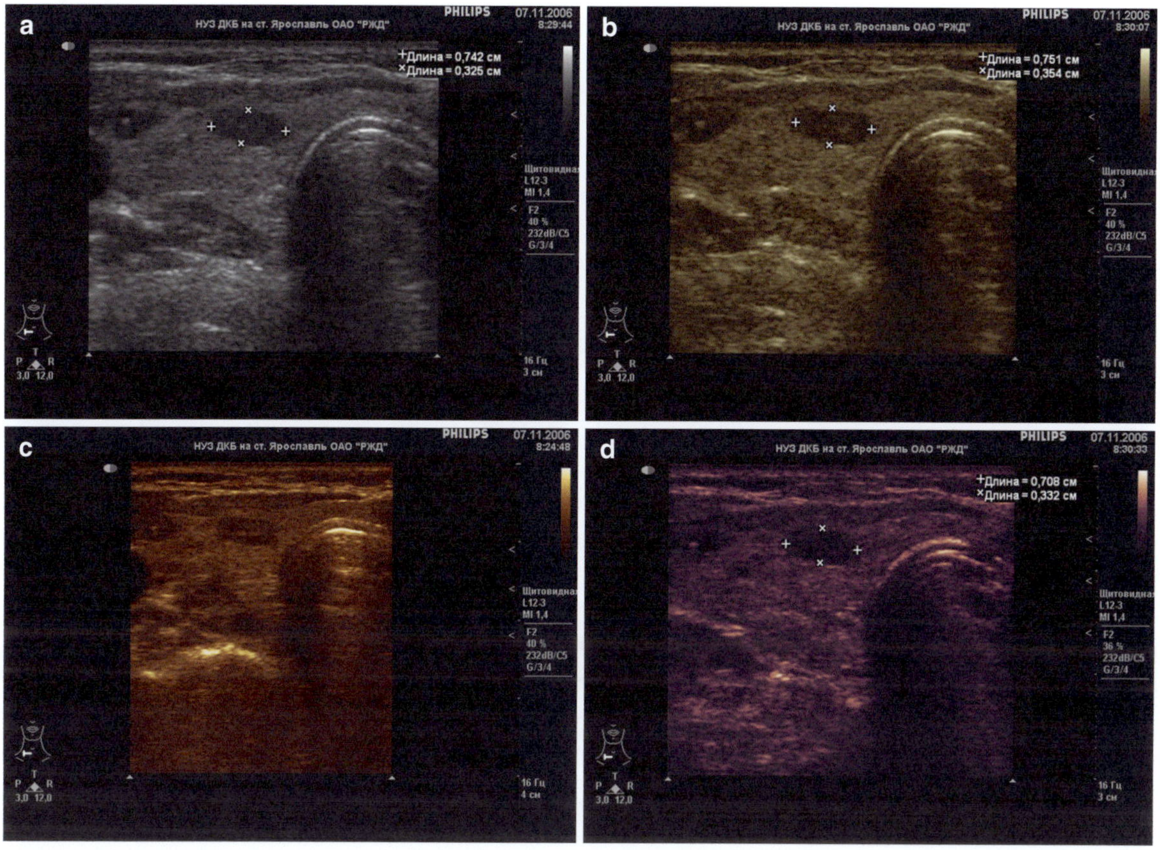

Fig. 2.3 (**a–d**) Thyroid sonograms. Adaptive coloring (**a**) conventional gray scale mode (**b**) different varieties of image color

- Blood flow in superior and inferior thyroid arteries
- Vascularity of the parenchyma of the thyroid
- Vascularity of the lesions

Color Doppler imaging (CDI; color flow imaging or CFI; color flow mapping or CFM) is an US technology for visualizing vascular structures. It is based on recording the blood flow velocity and using color encoding to superimpose this velocity onto the gray-scale image (Fig. 2.4). This option is incorporated into most modern scanners.

CDI is especially valuable for diagnosing thyroid malignancy. However, some authors consider it to be of limited academic interest and of minor importance for the differential diagnosis of thyroid nodules (Hübsch et al. 1992; Klemens et al. 1997).

The vascular architectonics of the parenchyma (parenchymal blood flow) of the thyroid is usually characterized by the following:

- Vascular pattern intensity
- Symmetry (between the lobes and the segments)
- Regularity of vascular structures within the thyroid parenchyma
- Deformations of the architectonics

The condition of the parenchymal blood flow is an important US indicator of the thyroid status. The vascular pattern in diffuse thyroid diseases is sometimes characterized by the number and the density of color pixels within the parenchyma using the following methods:

1. The color pixel density (CPD) is numerically expressed as the ratio of the area covered by color pixels to the total area of the image (in parts or percent) (Fig. 2.5). Similar calculations can be carried out in three-dimensional US (ratio of volumes). The CPD of a normal thyroid is about 3–15% (Fein et al. 1995; Lelyuk et al. 2007). The CPD is considered to be "increased" if it exceeds 15%, and "decreased" if it is less than 5%.
2. Scoring the number of color cartograms in area units. This is usually performed manually after

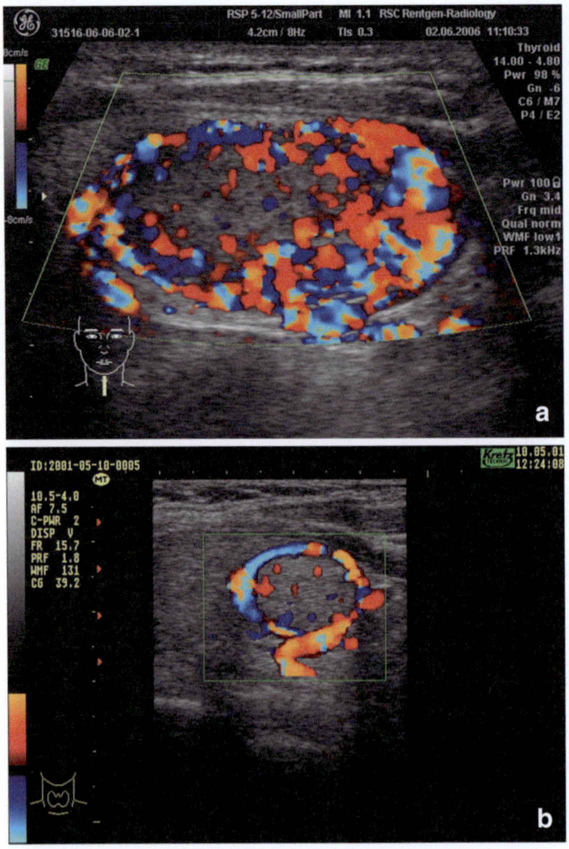

Fig. 2.4 (**a**, **b**) Thyroid sonograms. CDI (**a**) hypervascular thyroid nodule in CDI (**b**) thyroid nodule with peripheral blood flow pattern

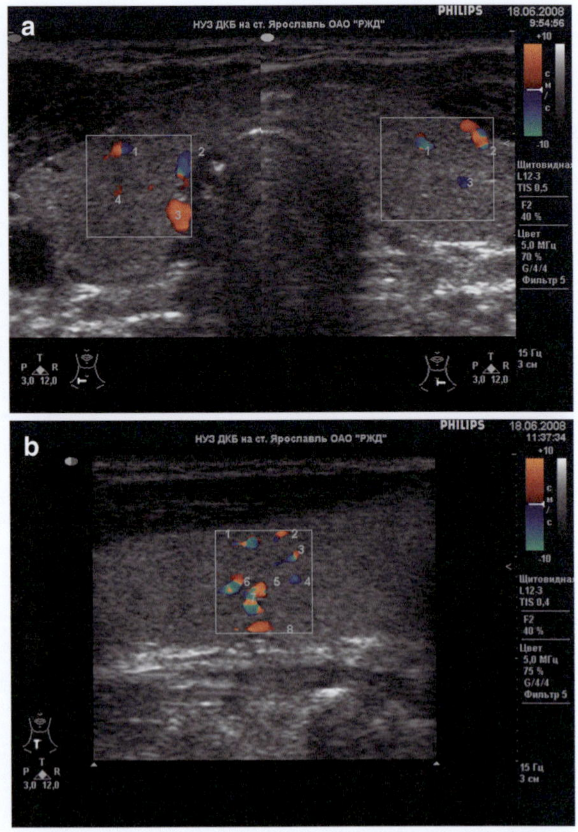

Fig. 2.6 (**a**, **b**) Measurement of the number of color cartograms in a unit area (1 cm^2) (**a**) transverse scan (**b**) longitudinal scan

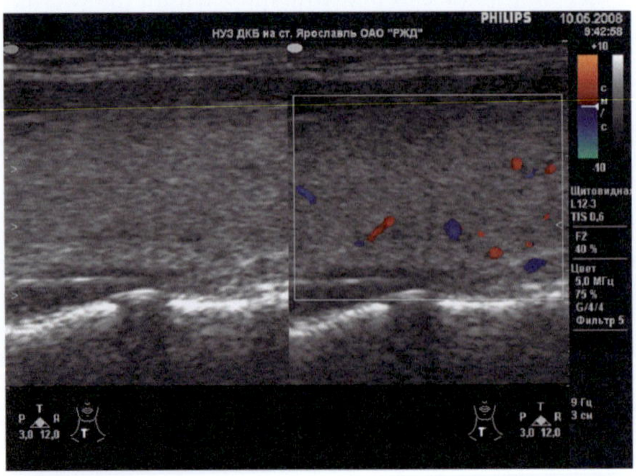

Fig. 2.5 CPD measurement

dividing the image into uniform squares with sides of 1 cm (Fig. 2.6). Color spots from different vessels are recorded in every square. The calculation is approximate, because interstitial vessels are not straight; they can appear in various scanning planes, resulting in separate visualization of the fragments. High scanning frequency and high averaging are utilized for accurate calculation. The proposed reference range for vessel density in a normal thyroid is between 0.4 and 2.5 vessels per 1 cm^2 of thyroid tissue (Fein et al. 1995; Lelyuk et al. 2007).

3. Scoring the amount of color cartograms within the lobe (Fig. 2.7). Only color spots from different vessels are counted. The accepted reference range for a normal thyroid is between five and ten vessels within the lobe (Fein et al. 1995; Lelyuk et al. 2007). The occurrence of more than ten vessels within the lobe at once is interpreted as an increase in parenchymal blood flow. A decrease is characterized by fewer than five vessels within the thyroid lobe.

Sekach et al. (1997) and Laszlo et al. (1998) suggest that the following three vascular patterns can occur in thyroid lesions:

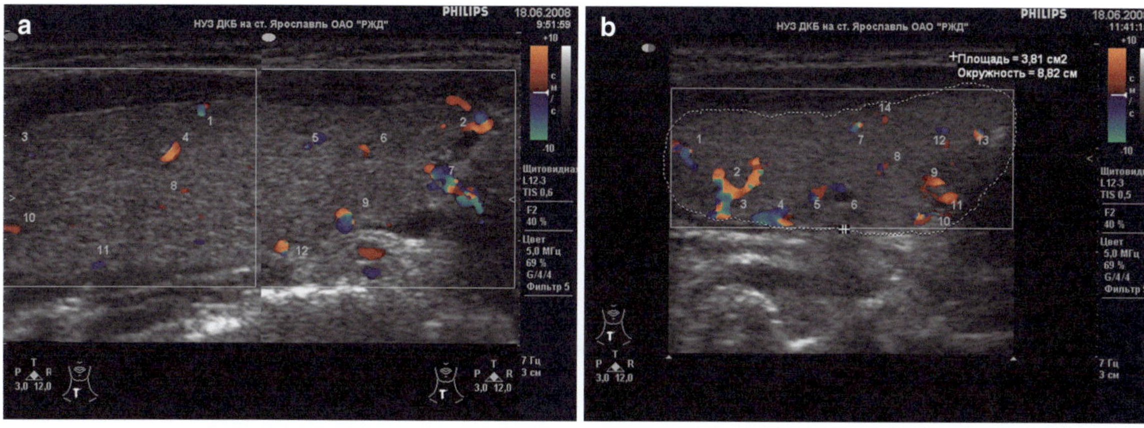

Fig. 2.7 (**a**, **b**) Measurement of the number of color cartograms within the thyroid lobe (**a**) combining two scans in case of large thyroid (**b**) measurement in one scan, the lobe contour is marked with dotts

1. Absence of blood flow both within the nodule and around it
2. Blood flow around the nodule
3. Blood flow both within the nodule and around it

Some authors (Messina et al. 1996; Morozov 1997; Abdulhalimova et al. 1999) additionally describe an intranodular type of vascular pattern, where individual or multiple color signals are registered within the lesion.

Zubarev et al. (2000) suggest that the following three vascular patterns of thyroid nodules should be used in daily practice:

1. Perinodular: the blood flow is mainly in the periphery of the nodule
2. Mixed: vascularization occurs in the periphery of and within the nodule
3. Avascular: there is no sonographically discernible blood flow.

The thyroid nodules can also be divided into the following groups according to the blood flow intensity:

1. Hypervascular nodules show a peripheral rim and multiple arterial and venous vessels within (the sign of a "color crown")
2. Nodules with a medium degree of vascularization have 5–6 color spots within the nodule
3. Hypovascular nodules show 2–3 color spots
4. Avascular nodules have no inner color spots and no peripheral rim

CDI has some disadvantages, such as table distortions of the Doppler spectrum (aliasing artifact), baseline noise, and dependence on the angle of the US beam.

Power Doppler imaging (PDI) permits images of smaller vessels with sharper contours to be obtained. This increases the diagnostic value of US (Fig. 2.8). PDI demonstrates a decreased dependence on the angle between the US beam and the blood flow, shows no aliasing artifact, and has a lower noise level. Therefore, PDI is three- to fivefold more sensitive than CDI (Lagalla et al. 1994, Adler et al. 1995; Spiezia et al. 1996). According to Zubarev (1997), PDI increases diagnostic sensitivity to thyroid pathology from 36 to 79% and specificity from 58 to 62% as compared with CDI.

PDI has some disadvantages, such as its high dependence on the motions of surrounding structures (leading to "motion artifacts") and the staining of perivascular areas.

Fast computer processing of US images permits the *three-dimensional (3D) reconstruction* of the thyroid structure, lesions, the vascular tree, and surrounding tissues (Fig. 2.9). This option may be incorporated into ordinary US scanners as additional software. Data acquisition is achieved by a freehand scan with a usual 2D probe. Such cases demand subsequent computational processing of the data obtained. Some scanners can be equipped with special probes for mechanical 3D scanning. 3D imaging confers many advantages, such as the possibility of viewing planes that are usually inaccessible, and improved accuracy of volume estimation. It is useful for archiving US data in an objective form suitable for delayed analysis and digital transfer.

In comparison with 2D PDI, *3D reconstruction of vascular structures* (3D power Doppler imaging or 3DPD) enables more specific diagnoses of neoplasms based on the objective visual data for the structure

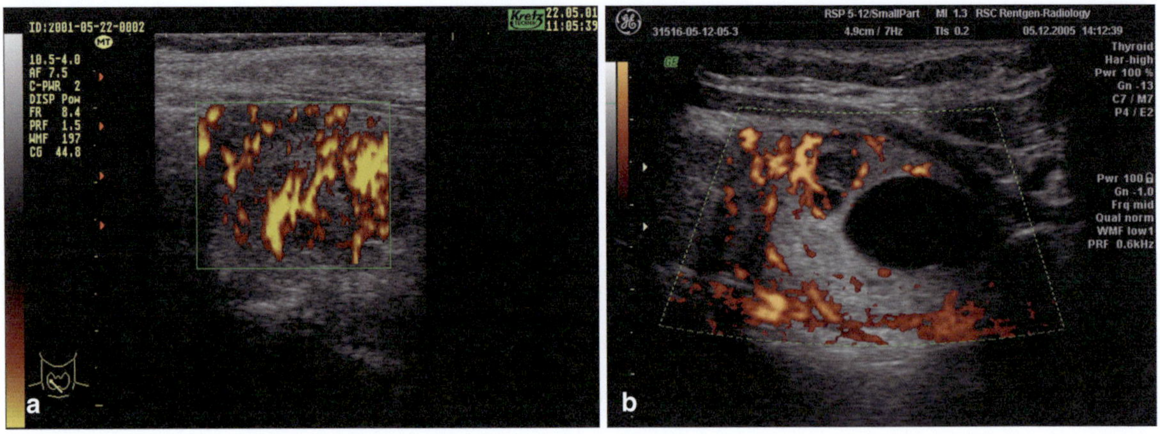

Fig. 2.8 (**a**, **b**) Thyroid sonograms. PDI (**a**) hypervascular thyroid structure (**b**) avascular thyroid nodules

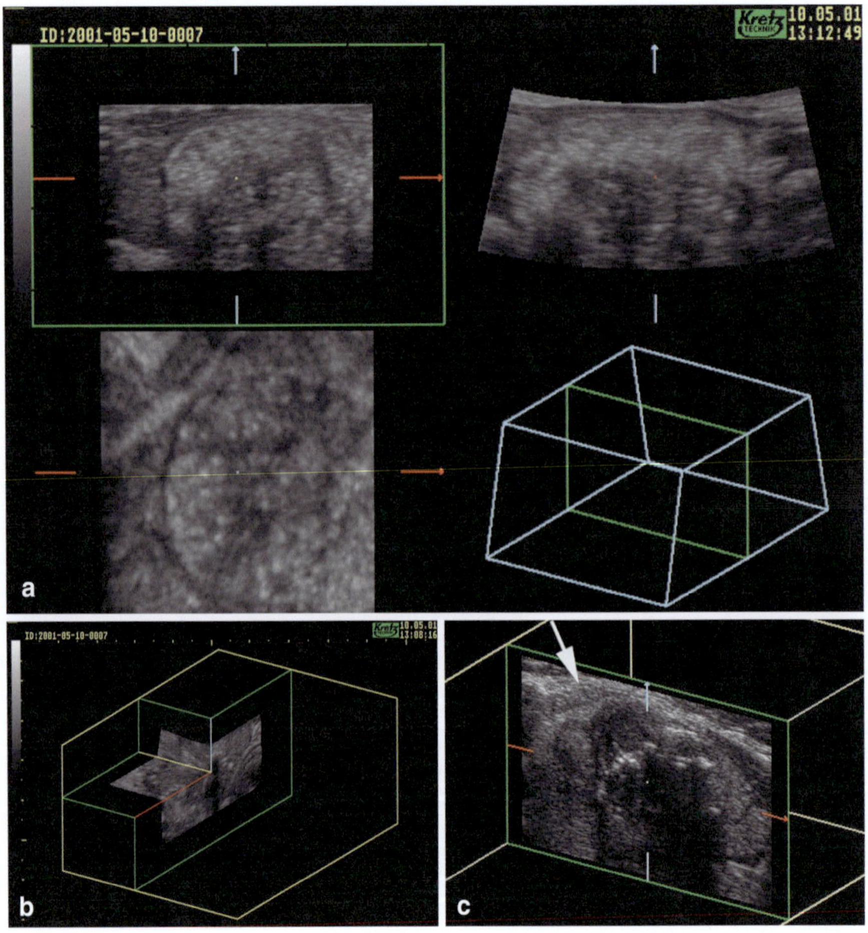

Fig. 2.9 Thyroid sonograms. 3D reconstruction

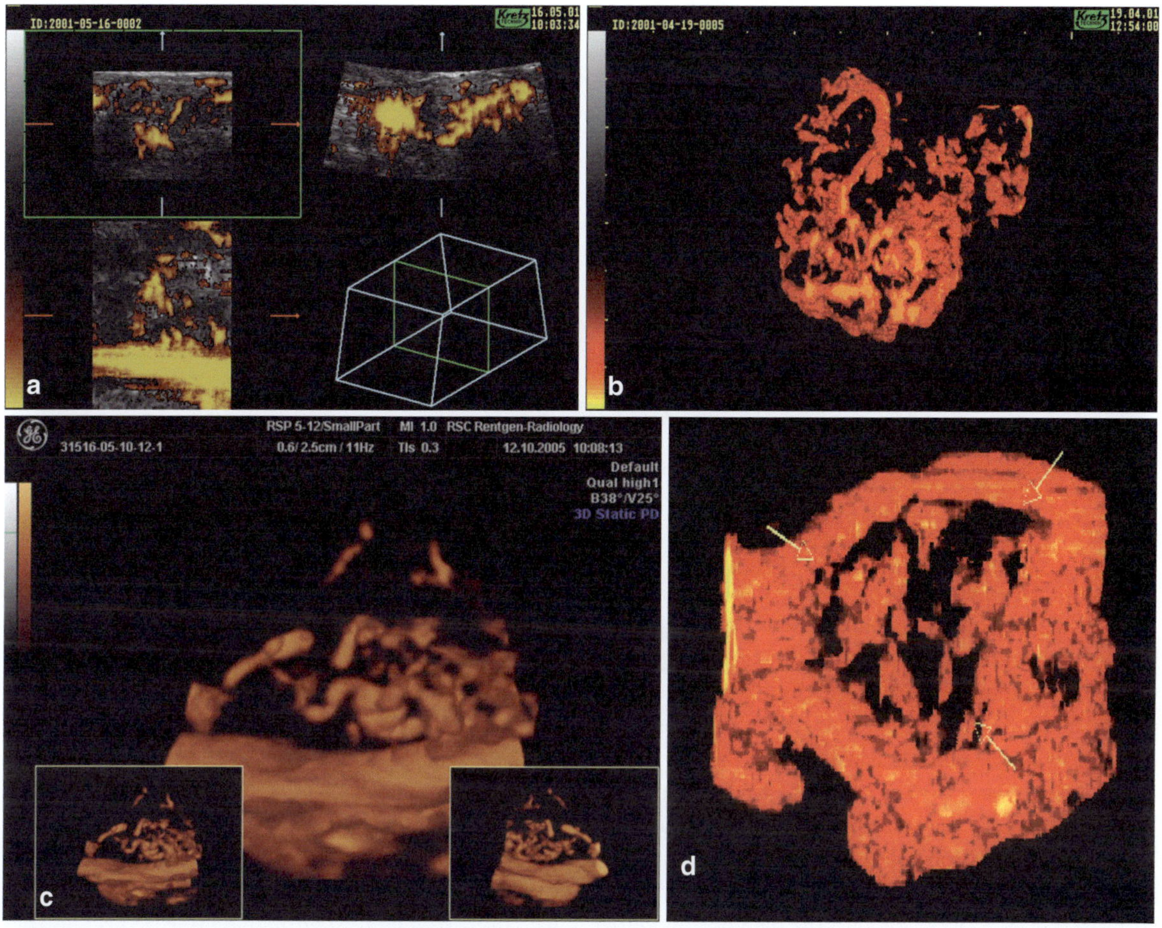

Fig. 2.10 Thyroid sonograms. 3DPD vessels within thyroid nodules

and the intensity of lesion vascularity, and the spatial relationships of different vascular structures of the neck (Fig. 2.10). According to Markova (2004), 3DPD is helpful when assessing the type of lesion vascularity, and it increases the sensitivity of US for the detection and categorization of thyroid lesions from 46 to 80%, and the specificity from 72 to 84%.

4D (real-time 3D) has reportedly been utilized to examine the thyroid gland. The 4D mode is a 3D scanning in real time using special US probes and high-class equipment. 3D image acquisition and reconstruction are performed quickly enough to allow real-time 3D visualization. 4D allows the spatial features of the thyroid to be defined more precisely, with a smaller dependence on noise artifacts. This is especially valuable for thyroid lesions.

In *pulsed-wave (PW) Doppler*, a curve resulting from the Doppler shift is produced via computer processing. This permits the analysis of the velocity and spectral parameters of the blood flow as well as the calculation of some indices (Fig. 2.11).

Markova (2001) suggests the following normal values for various blood flow parameters: the average peak systolic velocity (PSV) in the upper thyroid artery (UTA) is 16.8 ± 0.94 cm/s; in the inferior thyroid artery (ITA) it is 15.8 ± 0.77 cm/s; the end-diastolic velocity (EDV) in UTA is 7 ± 1.2 cm/s; in the ITA it is 6.36 ± 0.29 cm/s; the resistance index (RI) in UTA is 0.56 ± 0.01; in the ITA it is 0.58 ± 0.01. Struchkova (2003) also suggests nominal blood flow data for all thyroid arteries: PSV is 10.4–28.1 cm/s; EDV is 3.1–9.6 cm/s; RI is 0.5–0.75; and the pulsatility index (PI) is 0.7–1.2. RI and PI have been reported to be the most informative.

PW Doppler can confirm an increase in blood flow within the nodule as compared to that in the surrounding parenchyma (much more rarely, the vascularity is

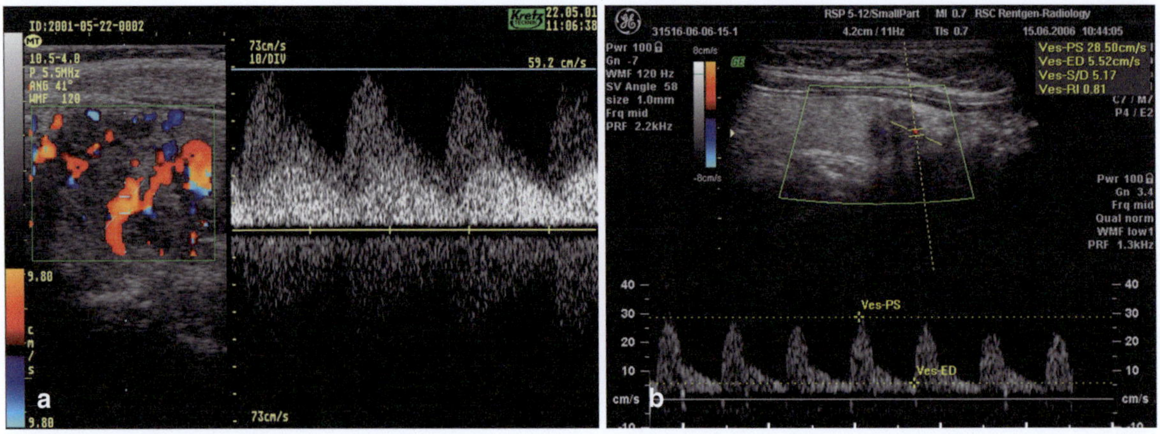

Fig. 2.11 (**a**, **b**) Thyroid sonograms. PW Doppler (**a**) high velocity arterial blood flow (**b**) arterial blood flow with high resistance index

identical). Blood flow data within one nodule may vary substantially, which complicates the interpretation. The vascularity of a nodule was shown to be defined by both its morphological structure and its size. The bigger the nodule, the greater the observed increase in blood flow in one or several vessels.

Argalia et al. (1995) consider that PSV and RI are important for the differential diagnosis of thyroid nodules, and that they help to define the nodules that should be subjected to biopsy. According to Pinsky et al. (1999), blood flow data are undoubtedly higher in the vessels of the lobe that contains a tumor in comparison with the other lobe and the norm. Thus, PW Doppler allows thyroid tumors to be classified without separating them into benign or malignant. According to Kharchenko et al. (1994), malignant tumors are characterized by decreased PSV (39 ± 11 cm/s on the average) compared to those in adenomas.

Delorme et al. (1995) indicate that PW Doppler is subjective in assessments of blood flow changes. This may influence the examination and result in diagnostic errors. The value of the assessment of blood flow in UTA and ITA in the case of thyroid nodules is doubtful. Our own research revealed no regularity in blood flow parameters. PW Doppler data in thyroid nodules show a wide dispersion and do not carry significant additional information. This precludes PW Doppler from being used for the differential diagnosis of thyroid nodules, although it may be used as an accessory feature.

Panoramic scan is an option that permits an extended field of view, thus simplifying the visualization and measurement of long structures. This helps when attempting to assess the precise dimensions of the thyroid and to calculate the volume of the lobes and the whole gland (Fig. 2.12).

The sensitivity of CDI and PDI can be significantly increased by intravenously introducing ultrasound contrast agents in a manner similar to contrast enhancement for CT and MRI. Lacocita et al. (2005) report that *contrast-enhanced ultrasound* (CEUS) is valuable for the diagnosis of thyroid diseases. They used SonoVue as a contrast medium for thyroid nodules. Nikolaeva et al. (2000) and Argalia et al. (2002) note the improvement in visualization of nodules of 0.5–1 cm in size with the use of Levovist. Fukunari et al. (2000) used Levovist to monitor the changes in thyroid nodules after PEI (858 observations).

Ultrasound elastography refers to a number of techniques that assist in the assessment of tissue softness (Fig. 2.13). The examined tissue is periodically exposed to pressure in order to create some form of displacement. The response is measured and processed to form an image. The tissue softness is color coded and observed superimposed on a grayscale image. Different colors correspond to different tissue elasticities. The best application of this modality is for the investigation of stiff tumors in soft tissues. It may be useful for both detection and categorization purposes. Moreover, it allows malignant tumor invasion to be defined more precisely, and small cancers to be

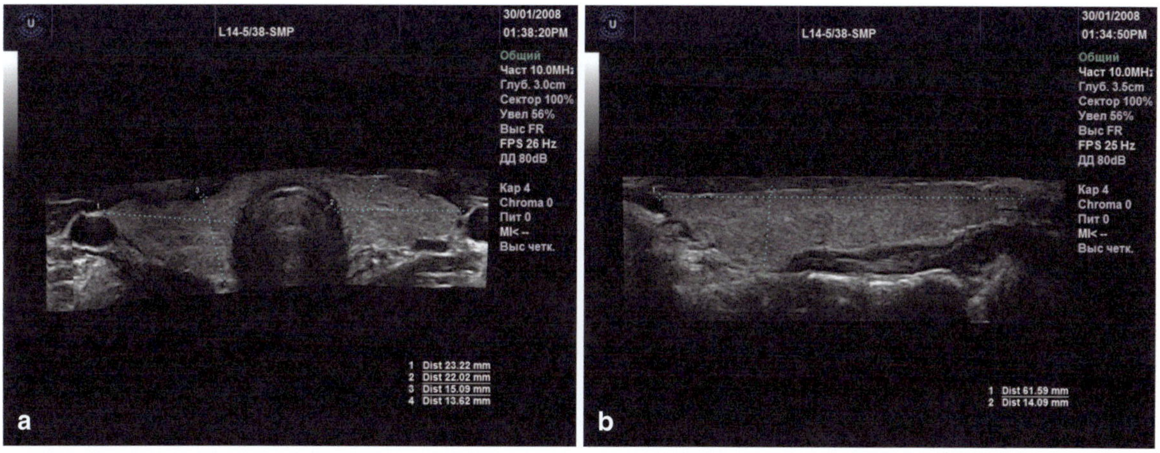

Fig. 2.12 Thyroid sonogram. Panoramic scan. (**a**) Transverse scan. (**b**) Longitudinal scan

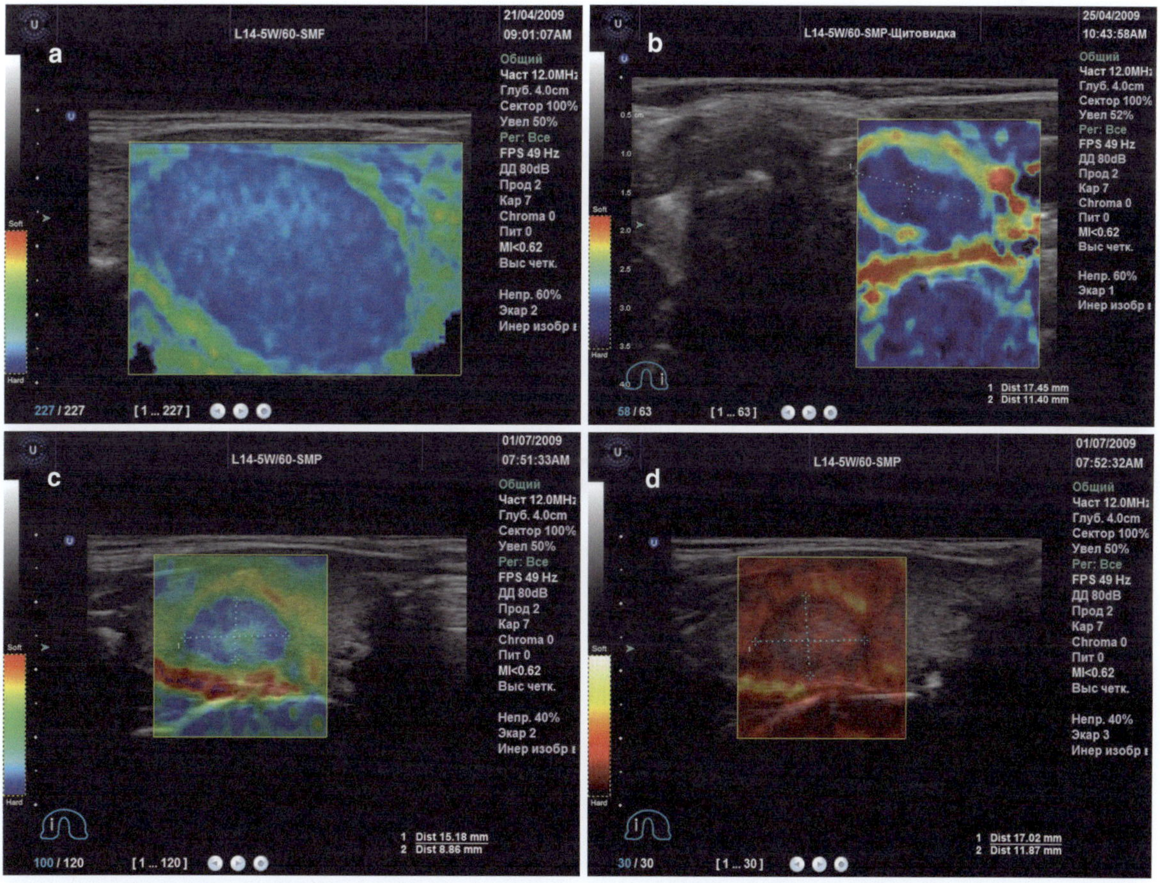

Fig. 2.13 Thyroid sonogram. US elastography

diagnosed (Ophir 1999; Doyley 2000; Lindop et al. 2006). Tanaka et al. (2006) reported a high efficacy of ultrasound elastography for the differential diagnosis of abnormal lymph nodes of the neck.

In *multislice viewing*, a 3D US image is converted into a series of consecutive sections corresponding to intervals of 0.5–5 mm in any plane, similar to CT representations. This aids in the analysis of thyroid images, and makes it objective.

Enhancements to traditional procedures and advances in new technologies are leading to continual improvements in the accuracy and value of diagnostic ultrasound.

2.2 Technology Used in Ultrasound Examinations of the Thyroid Gland

Special preparation of the patient for thyroid US is not required. The patient is positioned supine, with the head thrown back and a bolster under the shoulders (Fig. 2.14). Seriously ill patients may sometimes be examined in a sitting position with the head thrown back.

Thyroid US is performed using a linear probe with a frequency of 5–17 MHz (most often 7.5–12 MHz). A 3.5–5 MHz convex probe is sometimes more convenient for measurements of large thyroids. A sector probe with a frequency of 2.5–5 MHz may be required for the substernal thyroid.

An outline of an US examination is provided below:

(a) The thyroid as a whole
- Location (typical, dystopia, ectopia)
- Dimensions and volume (also in comparison with the norm)
- Margins (regular/irregular, accurate/indistinct)
- Shape (typical; congenital anomalies: lobed constitution, aplasia, hypoplasia; goiter)
- Echodensity (normal, increase, decrease)
- Echostructure (homogeneous, heterogeneous)
- Blood vessels of the thyroid parenchyma (intensity, symmetry)

(b) Thyroid abnormalities
- Character of changes (diffuse, focal, mixed)
- Location (in lobes and segments)
- Number of lesions
- Contours (sharpness)
- Borders (smoothness)
- Dimensions (in three mutually perpendicular planes)
- Echodensity, echostructure of focal lesions
- Vascularity

(c) Mutual relations of the thyroid with the surrounding structures

(d) The status of regional lymph nodes

The US probe is positioned on the front surface of the neck and moved from the breastbone to the hyoid bone. The probe should produce minimal compression in order to avoid shape distortion of the thyroid gland.

The location and the parts of the thyroid are defined by measuring its dimensions and calculating its volume. At least five scanning planes should be evaluated to assess the dimensions of the thyroid: transverse, longitudinal, and oblique for the right and the left lobes (Fig. 2.15).

Thyroid size assessment is based on the linear dimensions and the volumes of the lobes. It is important to measure the linear dimensions only in the transverse or longitudinal sections of the thyroid lobes that show the

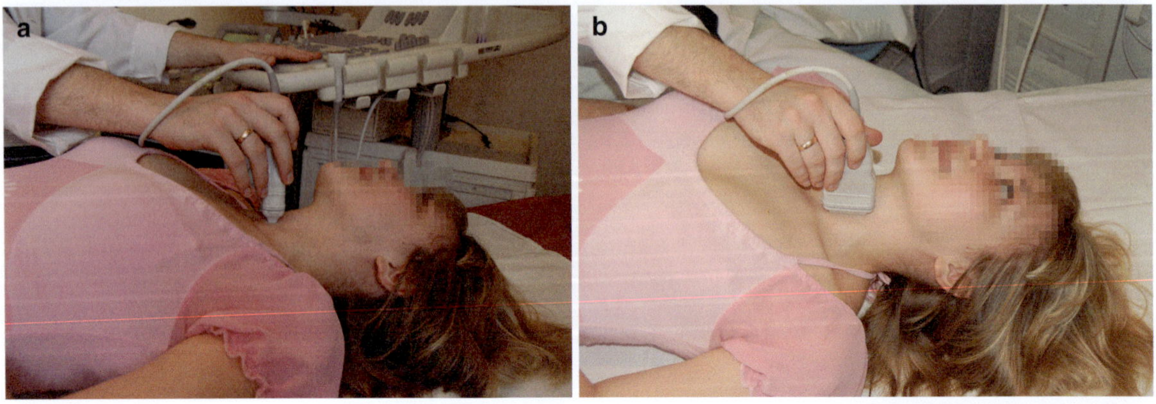

Fig. 2.14 (**a**, **b**) Thyroid US. The position of the patient (**a**) transverse thyroid scan, (**b**) longitudinal thyroid scan

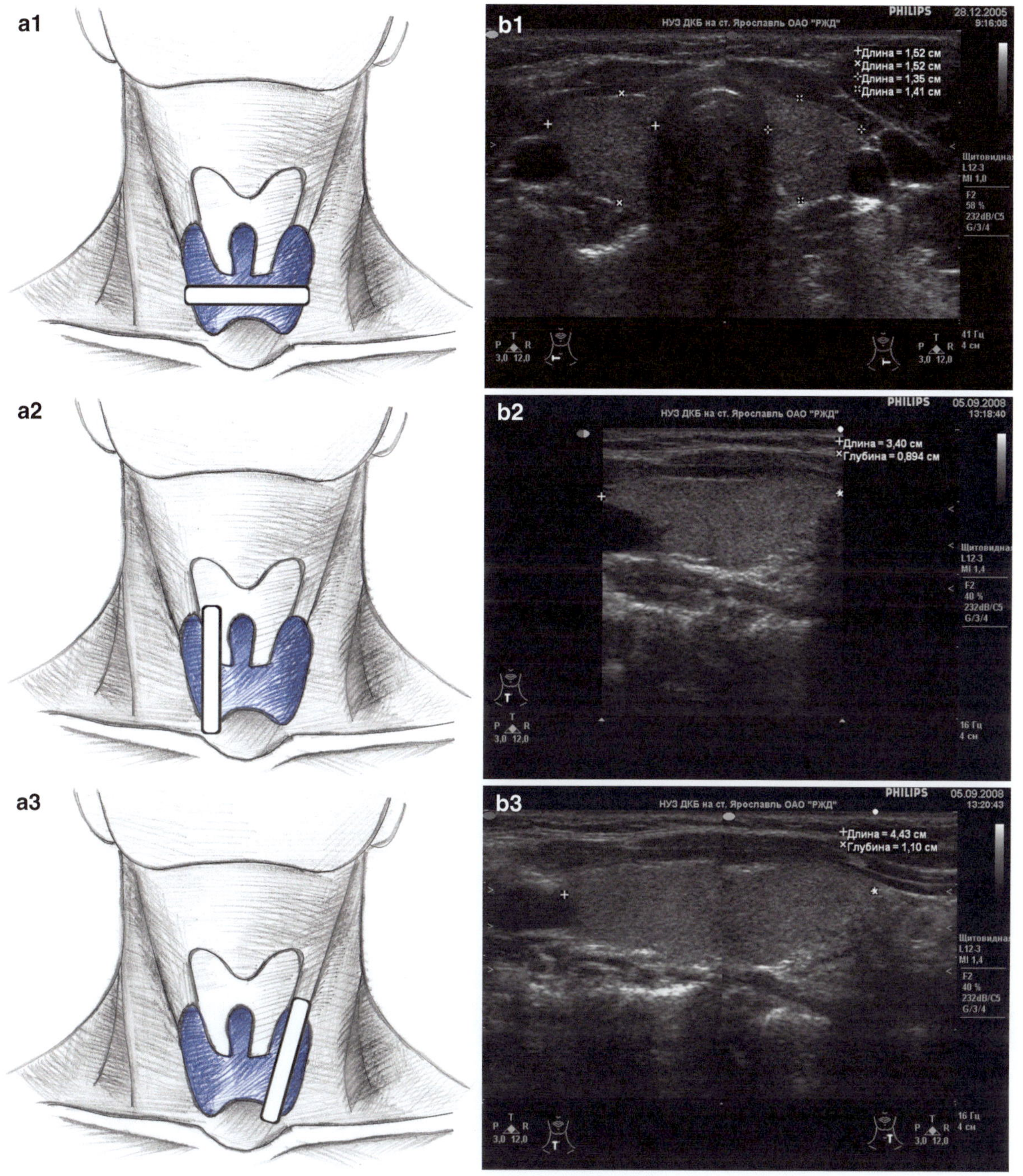

Fig. 2.15 Thyroid US. Basic scanning planes. (**a1–b1**) Transverse. (**a2–b2**) Longitudinal. (**a3–b3**) Oblique

maximum value (Fig. 2.16). When choosing the cross-section, it is necessary to follow the anatomical transverse plane and position the probe perpendicular to the skin with no angle. The longitudinal lobe dimension (the length or height of the lobes) is the largest size of the lobe. It is actually obtained in the plane that deviates from the anatomical longitudinal plane of the neck. The optimal position of the probe is close to parallel with the inner edge of the sternomastoid. Since the length of the lobe usually exceeds the length of a linear probe, it is preferable to measure it with a convex probe adjusted to the maximum possible frequency. The time expended and the reliability of this method of measurement are comparable with panoramic reconstruction of the image.

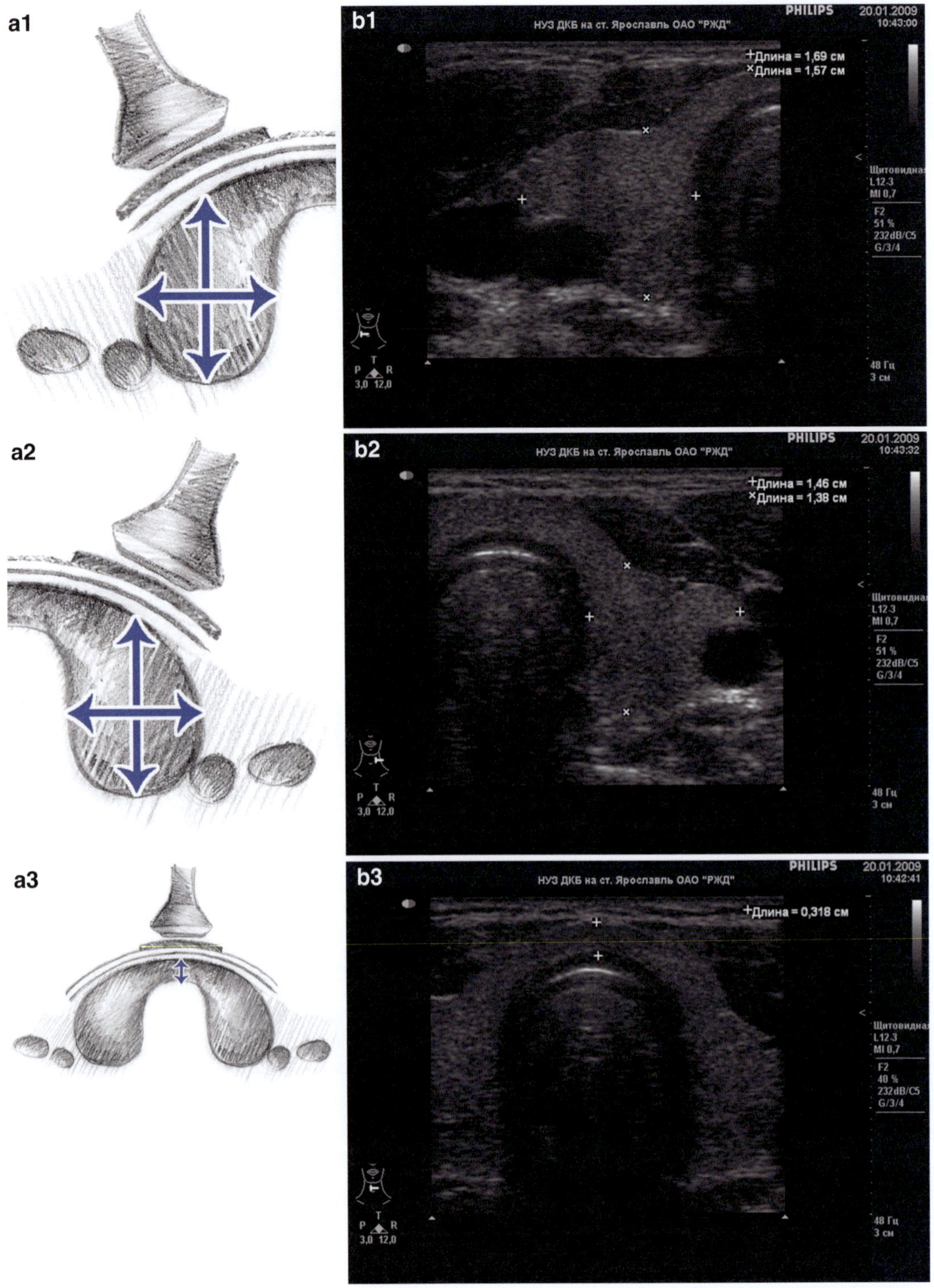

Fig. 2.16 (**a1–a5**, **b1–b5**) Thyroid US. Measurements of the widths, the depths, and the lengths of thyroid lobes, as well as the thickness of the isthmus (**a1–b1**) the depth and the width of the right lobe, (**a2–b2**) the depth and the width of the left lobe, (**a3–b3**) the isthmus (**a4–b4**) measurement of the lobe length in one view (**a5–b5**) combination of two measurements to calycu-late the lobe length

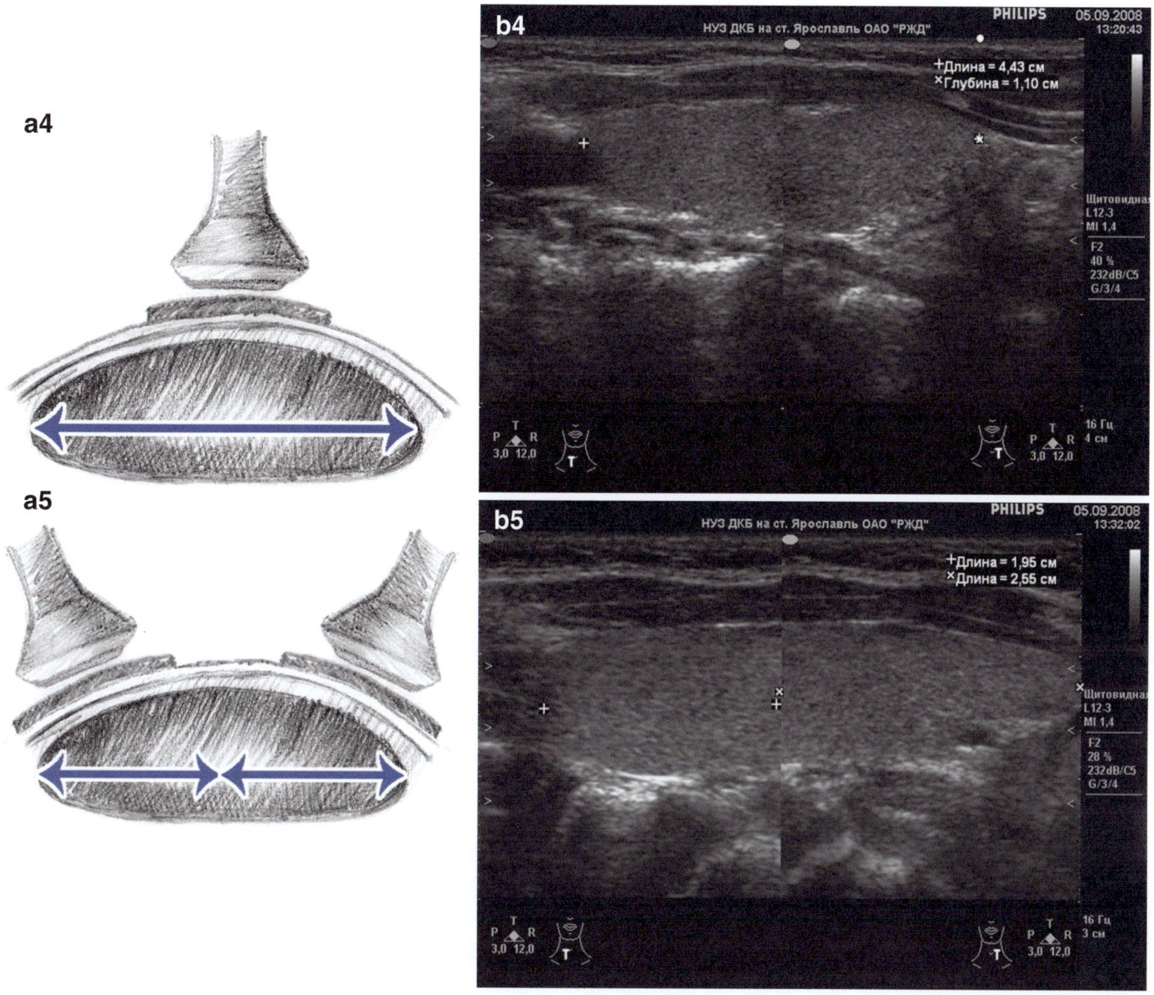

Fig. 2.16 (continued)

The normal US dimensions of an adult thyroid can vary. A thyroid lobe is about 13–18 mm wide, 16–18 mm deep, and 45–60 mm long, while the isthmus is 2–6 mm deep; the thyroid has a volume of 7.7–22.6 cm^3 in men and 4.55–19.32 cm^3 in women Ilyin 1995). The literature does not report any significant difference in US dimensions between the right and left thyroid lobes. Hence, separately defined linear parameters are of no value. It is important to note that the size of the organ is characterized only by the total volume of the glandular tissue.

The volume of a thyroid lobe is calculated by the formula $A \times B \times C \times 0.479$, where A is the length, B is the width, and C is the thickness (depth) of the lobe, while 0.479 (0.524) is the correction factor for the ellipsoidal shape of the lobe (Brunn et al. 1981). The total thyroid volume encompasses the volumes of the right and left lobes. The volume of the isthmus (if thinner than 10 mm) is omitted.

The volume of a normal thyroid in both adults and children is still the source of debate (see Chap. 3). The World Health Organization suggests a normal volume in men of 7.7–25 cm^3 and in women of 4.4–18 cm^3. The calculated thyroid volume in adults can be compared with recommended standards that depend on age, height, weight, and body surface area (Parshin 1994; Ilyin 1995).

The optimal volume of the thyroid and criteria for its enlargement are currently being studied. No unified classification of thyroid enlargement based on sonographic data is being utilized yet. The classifications available are not accepted by the professional societies for general use.

They anchor the US data to the degree of enlargement of the thyroid gland based on imperfect palpation and visual assessment (for example the 1994 WHO scale).

At the same time, only one aspect is important in most cases: whether the patient's thyroid volume differs from the norm. Many authors suggest that presenting the degree of deviation as a percentage may be of benefit for the dynamic assessment of changes in thyroid volume during treatment.

2.3 Basic Mistakes in Thyroid Ultrasound

Factors that result in inaccurate US assessment of the status of the thyroid gland can be divided into the following groups:

1. Objective
   - Anatomical, physiological, and constitutional features of the patient leading to a decrease in visualization
   - Limitations of the equipment (the quality of the scanner, the characteristics of the probes, etc.)
2. Subjective
   - Insufficient US specialist experience
   - Faulty thyroid US technique

High intra- and interobserver variations in thyroid sonography are largely due to the quality of the equipment and the skill level of the operator. According to Bataeva et al. (2006), an expert fails to reproduce the results of the 2D thyroid volume calculation in 8.7% of cases; assessments performed by different experts differ by 12.8%. Measurements taken in 3D methods of surface reconstruction and segmentation show differences of 4 and 4.8%, respectively. One disadvantage of using US in some cases is a low detection efficacy for thyroid dystopia and ectopia. Retrosternal location of the thyroid below the tracheal bifurcation significantly limits the possibility of ultrasonography (see Chap. 10).

High-resolution US equipment allows several thyroid pathologies to be detected, which used to be considered the norm. For example, medium- and large-sized cellular patterns (multiple fine hypo- and anechoic lesions 2–4 mm in size) that were interpreted as the norm years ago are now considered abnormal. This kind of sonogram is widely seen for people living in iodine-deficient regions, and precedes a diffuse endemic goiter. It corresponds to colloid cystic change with dilation of the follicles due to extra colloid accumulation. The hyperechoic points within such follicles are a consequence of the dense consistency of the colloid. Another type of small change is inflammatory foci during the initial stages of autoimmune thyroid disease (AITD). These relate to a tendency for a decrease in echodensity and a slight heterogeneity of thyroid tissue resulting from small foci of lymphoplasmacytic infiltration and edema.

Alternatively, there are hyperdiagnostic cases when normal thyroid structures are interpreted as nodules. This especially concerns structures behind the left lobe or along the posterior margin of the inferior compartment of the right lobe. This type of error can be caused by the proximity of the esophagus, which may be reported as a nodule if imaged only with a transverse scan. The normal vascular pattern of the inferior thyroid artery (ITA) can result in hyperdiagnostics of thyroid nodules. In some cases, the ITA trunk does not split into fine branches when entering the inferior pole of the thyroid lobe. It may be traced within the lobe, where it borders a roundish region of healthy tissue that imitates a nodule.

Lymph nodes adjacent to the isthmus frequently complicate the diagnosis. The enlarged lymph nodes present in AITD are often located close to the upper or inferior part of the isthmus and can be interpreted as thyroid nodules. Differential diagnosis may benefit from the use of the highest probe frequency, as it permits a more detailed image. It is necessary to pay attention to specific features of lymph nodes, such as form, echostructure with differentiation of the cortical and central parts, and type of blood flow. The opposite type of error, where nodules of the thyroid isthmus are interpreted as neck lymph nodes, are quite rare.

Differential diagnosis of thyroid nodules and inflammatory foci in AITD is rather difficult (see Chap. 5). In this case, it is necessary to consider the sharpness and regularity of the contours of the lesion, its form, and the blood flow pattern. Nevertheless, the correct diagnosis sometimes requires long observations or the use of other diagnostic modalities.

Rare neck pathologies may be misdiagnosed due to insufficient experience of the US operator. In many cases, adenomas and hyperplasia of the parathyroid glands are interpreted as thyroid nodules. This pathology is relatively rare, so general practitioners or US specialists who do not practice at a specialized endocrinology center are not aware of it and have little experience in its diagnosis (see Chap. 11). The same can be said about the diverticulum of the esophagus (see Chap. 12). In most cases, sonographers have a mental image of "typical" thyroid nodules based on their own experience, so any lesion differing from this typical image should be interpreted with extra caution.

Special opportunities for differential diagnosis are provided by auxiliary methods, such as turning the patient's head, compression of the neck tissues with fingers, swallowing, and others.

Note that modern equipment permits accurate US visualization of solid thyroid nodules larger than 2–3 mm in size. The presence of smaller lesions is preferably reported without the term "nodule." Drawing a conclusion about the lesion is expedient only when it can be clearly visualized in at least two mutually perpendicular scans.

It is very important to adhere to the correct examination technique. Thyroid structure including small parts can be estimated only with linear probes at frequencies of 7.5 MHz and higher. Convex abdominal probes may be used to measure the lengths of thyroid lobes or for large thyroids. The use of a convex probe alone for thyroid examination results in multiple severe errors and discredits the field of sonography.

Rational timescales for thyroid US are as follows:

- Normal thyroid: once every two years for preventive purposes
- Benign diffuse or nodular thyroid pathology: 1–2 times a year to monitor the dynamics of the disease
- Inoperable thyroid malignancy: once every two months to define the stage.

3 Ultrasound Examination of the Thyroid Gland in Children

The thyroid gland affects the development of a child at any age. Adequate thyroid function is necessary for the development of the brain and other organs and systems, including the immune system and sexual development. Much attention is paid to examining the thyroid gland in children, taking into account the influences of numerous negative factors. The most significant factors are iodine deficiency, an unfavorable ecological situation, urbanization, and an intense rhythm of life with stressful influences. In this regard, regular screening has become a medical standard, especially in children suspected of having a thyroid pathology.

The technique of thyroid US in children actually does not differ from that in adults, except for special demands in relation to the accuracy of the volume calculation. A change in gland volume accompanies almost all thyroid pathologies in children. Inspection and palpation fail to assess the thyroid volume correctly in about 35% of cases (Kasatkina et al. 1993). This demonstrates the high value of US.

The issue of correctly interpreting the US measurements obtained in children and teenagers is a pertinent one. Several ways of addressing this problem have been introduced in different countries over the last three decades, such as the following:

- 1974: the first description of the volume calculation (Hegedus et al.)
- 1981: the updated formula for volume calculation (Brunn et al.)
- 1991–1993: the norms by Gutekunst and Martin-Teichert
- 1997: the norms by Delange et al., adapted by the WHO

Thyroid volume in children can be assessed in several ways: in relation to body surface area (Delange 1997), age (Delange 1997; Panunszi et al. 1998), average group values (Parshin 1994), etc. (see Tables 3.1 and 3.2).

The norms listed above for the thyroid volume with respect to age or BSA have been simplified and adapted for US screening. They do not take into account the physical development of a child and puberty in a teenager. Kasatkina et al. (1998) suggested a method of defining thyroid hyperplasia and hypoplasia in children which is linked to anthropometric parameters that depend on age and the presence of puberty. The volume calculation was based on the standard formula (Brunn et al. 1981): vol = ([length × width × depth] of the left lobe + [length × width × depth] of the right lobe) × 0.479. Depending on the child's age and the presence of puberty, the following anthropometric parameters were measured: thoracic circumference at maximal expiration at the ages of 4–6 years, leg length (distance between the greater trochanter and the sole) at 7–9 years of age and in children over ten years of age who are yet to enter puberty, and body weight in children undergoing puberty. Table 3.3 is used to interpret the obtained data.

In cases of obvious enlargement of the total volume of thyroid lobes, the isthmus depth is usually neglected. The thickness of the isthmus can be taken into account indirectly if the thyroid volume appears close to the upper limit. The boundary volume of the thyroid gland is reported to be normal if the isthmus thickness is normal. If the isthmus is enlarged (thicker than 3 mm in children under ten years of age, and more than 5 mm in teenagers), the thyroid is reported to be enlarged.

The reliability of palpation in children is low, so the staging of thyroid hyperplasia based on the WHO recommendations is subjective. Classifications of thyroid enlargement based on US data usually assess the ratio of the current volume of the child's thyroid to the

V.P. Kharchenko et al., *Ultrasound Diagnostics of Thyroid Diseases*,
DOI: 10.1007/978-3-642-12387-0_3, © Springer-Verlag Berlin Heidelberg 2010

Table 3.1 Upper limits on normal thyroid volume in children as a function of age (Gutekunst 1991)

	Age (years)									
	6	7	8	9	10	11	12	13	14	15
Thyroid volume (mL)	3.5	4.0	4.5	5.0	6.0	7.0	8.0	9.0	10.5	12.0

Table 3.2 Upper limits on normal thyroid volume in children as a function of age and gender

Age	Gutekunst et al. (1986)		Panunszi et al. (1998)		Delange et al. (1997)		Sasakawa (Ashizava et al.) 1997	
	Boys ($n=297$)	Girls ($n=322$)	Boys ($n=517$)	Girls ($n=523$)	Boys ($n=3{,}758$)	Girls ($n=3{,}841$)	Boys ($n=57{,}529$)	Girls ($n=61{,}649$)
5							4.2	4.1
6	1.8	1.9	2.06	2.48	3.2	3.3	5.0	5.1
7	2.7	3.1	2.47	2.46	3.2	3.1	5.6	5.9
8	3.1	2.9	3.04	3.00	3.4	3.8	6.8	6.7
9	3.8	5.2	3.10	3.41	4.0	4.3	7.2	7.6
10	3.2	4.2	3.62	3.75	4.2	5.0	8.4	8.4
11	4.2	4.3	3.81	4.76	4.8	5.2	8.9	9.6
12	5.2	6.3	4.27	5.46	5.2	6.0	10.1	11.0
13	7.1	9.8	5.39	5.83	6.0	6.3	11.0	12.1
14	8.1	9.0	6.01	6.04	6.8	7.2	13.0	13.2
15	10.5	10.0			7.1	8.0	13.8	13.7
16	10	3	9.8				14.6	14.3

Table 3.3 Limits on normal thyroid volume in children as a function of age, anthropometric parameters and puberty (Kasatkina et al. 1998)

Prior to puberty						During puberty		
4–6 years			7–9 years			13–15 years		
TC (cm)	LL (mL)	UL (mL)	Leg length (cm)	LL (mL)	UL (mL)	Weight (kg)	LL (mL)	UL (mL)
46	0.42	2.12	46	0.43	2.93	30	0.42	7.34
47	0.48	2.18	47	0.43	3.01	31	0.43	7.41
48	0.53	2.23	48	0.50	3.08	32	0.43	7.49
49	0.59	2.29	49	0.58	3.16	33	0.50	7.56
50	0.64	2.34	50	0.65	3.23	34	0.58	7.64
51	0.70	2.40	51	0.73	3.31	35	0.65	7.71
52	0.76	2.46	52	0.81	3.39	36	0.73	7.79
53	0.81	2.51	53	0.88	3.46	37	0.80	7.86
54	0.87	2.57	54	0.96	3.54	38	0.88	7.94
55	0.92	2.62	55	1.03	3.61	39	0.95	8.01
56	0.98	2.68	56	1.11	3.69	40	1.03	8.09
57	1.04	2.74	57	1.19	3.77	41	1.10	8.16
58	1.09	2.79	58	1.26	3.84	42	1.18	8.24

Table 3.3 (continued)

Prior to puberty						During puberty		
4–6 years			7–9 years			13–15 years		
TC (cm)	LL (mL)	UL (mL)	Leg length (cm)	LL (mL)	UL (mL)	Weight (kg)	LL (mL)	UL (mL)
59	1.15	2.85	59	1.34	3.92	43	1.25	8.31
60	1.20	2.90	60	1.41	3.99	44	1.33	8.39
61	1.26	2.96	61	1.49	4.07	45	1.40	8.46
62	1.32	3.02	62	1.57	4.15	46	1.48	8.54
63	1.37	3.07	63	1.64	4.22	47	1.55	8.61
64	1.43	3.13	64	1.72	4.30	48	1.63	8.69
65	1.48	3.18	65	1.79	4.37	49	1.70	8.76
66	1.54	3.24	66	1.87	4.45	50	1.78	8.84
67	1.60	3.30	67	1.95	4.53	51	1.85	8.91
68	1.65	3.35	68	2.02	4.60	52	1.93	8.99
69	1.71	3.41	69	2.10	4.68	53	2.00	9.06
70	1.76	3.46	70	2.17	4.75	54	2.08	9.14
71	1.82	3.52	71	2.25	4.83	55	2.15	9.21
72	1.88	3.58	72	2.33	4.91	56	2.23	9.29
73	1.93	3.63	73	2.40	4.98	57	2.30	9.36
74	1.99	3.69	74	2.48	5.06	58	2.38	9.44
75	2.04	3.74	75	2.55	5.13	59	2.45	9.51
76	2.10	3.80	76	2.63	5.21	60	2.53	9.59
77	2.16	3.86	77	2.71	5.29	61	2.60	9.66
78	2.21	3.91	78	2.78	5.36	62	2.68	9.74
79	2.27	3.97	79	2.86	5.44	63	2.75	9.81
80	2.32	4.02	80	2.94	5.51	64	2.83	9.89
81	2.38	4.08	81	3.01	5.59	65	2.90	9.96
82	2.44	4.14	82	3.09	5.67	66	2.97	10.04
83	2.49	4.19	83	3.16	5.74	67	3.05	10.11
84	2.55	4.25	84	3.24	5.82	68	3.12	10.19
85	2.60	4.30	85	3.32	5.89	69	3.20	10.26
86	2.66	4.36	86	3.39	5.97	70	3.27	10.34
87	2.72	4.42	87	3.47	6.05	71	3.35	10.41
88	2.77	4.47	88	3.54	6.12	72	3.42	10.49
89	2.83	4.53	89	3.62	6.20	73	3.50	10.56
90	2.89	4.58	90	3.70	6.27	74	3.57	10.46

TC, thoracic circumference at maximal expiration; *LL*, lower limit on thyroid volume; *UL*, upper limit on thyroid volume. For children of 10–12 years in the absence of puberty, the columns for children of 7–9 years are used (anthropometric parameter: leg length); in the presence of puberty, the columns for children of 13–15 years are used (anthropometric parameter: weight). At adiposity during puberty (13–15 years), it is necessary to use not the actual body weight value but the upper limit on the normal weight taken from standard height–weight tables norm and express it in percent. However, the steps between the stages differ (from 30 to 150%). Such staging is of low value for determining the algorithm of further diagnostics and treatment of thyroid pathology. The ratio of the actual thyroid volume to the upper limit of the norm, expressed in percent, is more informative.

The echodensity of thyroid tissue in children, as well as in adults, is compared to that of the salivary gland (Figs. 3.1 and 3.2). Normal thyroid tissue shows homogeneous echostructure. However, in rare cases, the homogeneity of the tissue does not exclude initial stages of sporadic or endemic diffuse euthyroid goiter.

CDI and PDI of the thyroid gland in children are difficult to standardize due to their variability according to the type of equipment used. Nevertheless, CDI and PDI allow changes in the functional activity of both the thyroid gland and nodules to be gauged, and several pathologic conditions to be differentiated based on the vascularization features (Fig. 3.3).

Attempts at quantitative assessment using PW Doppler are even more subjective, especially for the vessels of the parenchyma. This is mainly due to the inability to perform proper angle correction and the limitations of control volume adjustments. In practice, a PSV of more than 45 cm/s is worrisome for diffuse thyroid changes.

3D reconstruction of the image permits a more accurate definition of thyroid margins, a precise calculation of the volume, and allows lesions to be analyzed and characterized for vascularity and invasiveness.

Thyroid pathology is widespread in children and teenagers. It is most often observed in girls. Morbidity increases distinctly with age and reaches its peak in puberty.

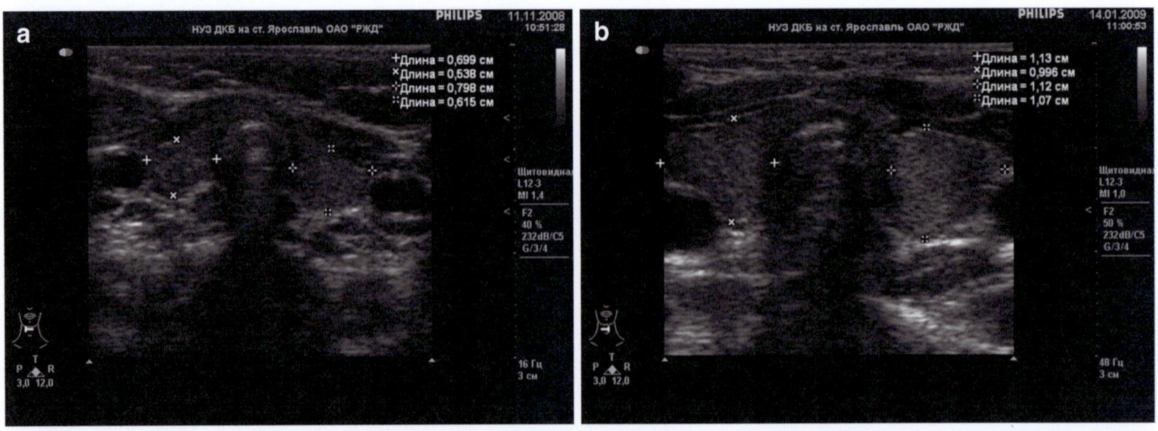

Fig. 3.1 Sonogram of a normal thyroid gland. B-scale. (**a**) A one year old. (**b**) A five year old child

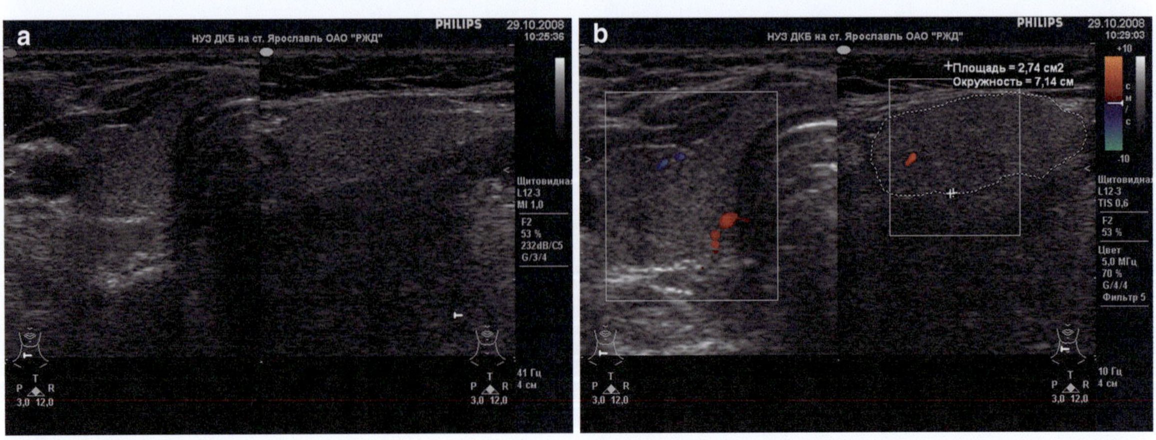

Fig. 3.2 (**a**, **b**) Sonograms of the thyroid and the submandibular salivary gland. The age of the child is 14 years. (**a**) B-scale and (**b**) CDI

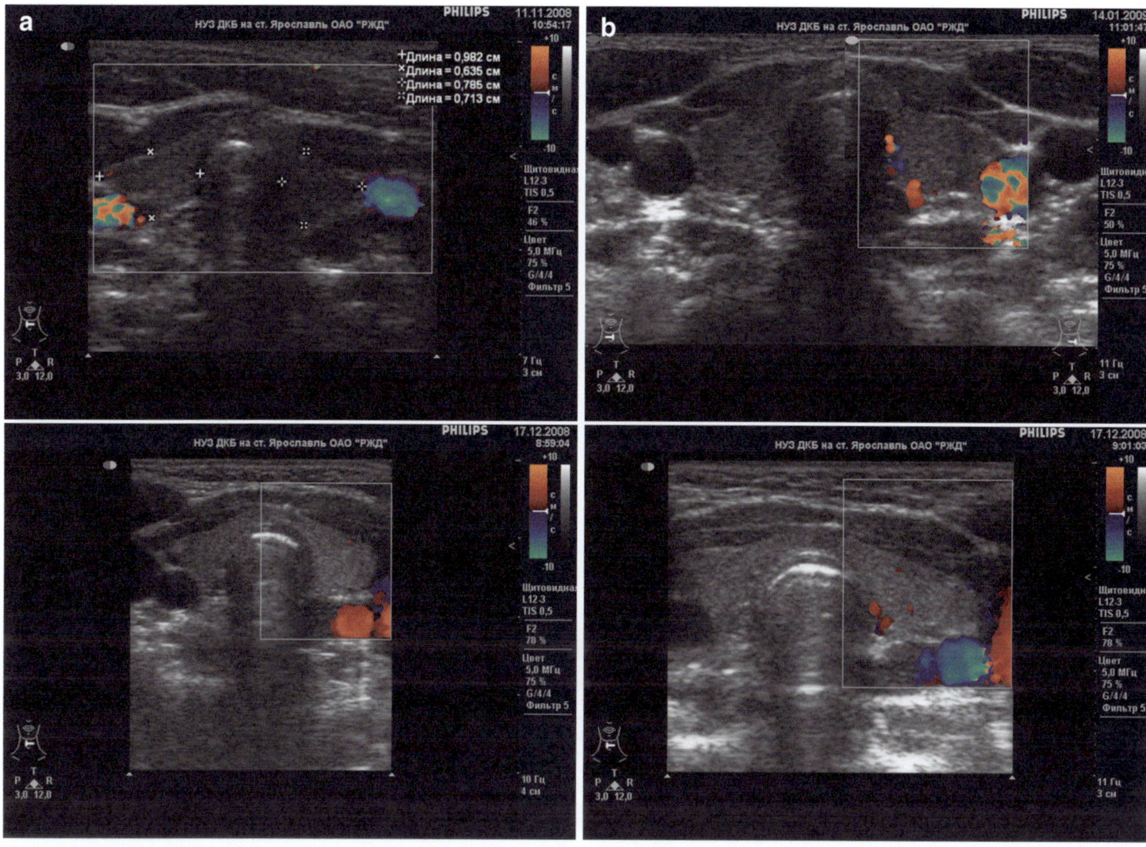

Fig. 3.3 Sonogram of a normal thyroid gland. CDI. (**a**) A one year old child. (**b**) A five year old child

3.1 Congenital Anomalies of the Thyroid

Congenital anomalies of the thyroid do not occur in more than 0.3–0.5% of the population. They appear at the stage of prenatal development. The embryonic primordium of the gland descends between weeks 3 and 5 of gestation as a median diverticulum from the floor of the pharynx, which makes its appearance at the level of the second pair of pharyngeal pouches. It evaginates, migrating caudally to the level of the III–IV pairs of pharyngeal pouches, and retains its connection with the pharynx only by a narrow thyroglossal duct at the root of the tongue. It is contributed to by the primordia, which arise laterally from the fourth pharyngeal pouches. The thyroglossal duct obliterates and the germs of lateral lobes grow quickly and migrate caudally to the inferior part of the fetal neck. The first signs of independent function in the fetal thyroid are observed at week 8 of gestation. Thyroid function becomes apparent between weeks 12 and 14 of gestation.

At the stage of embryogenesis, the thyroid germ migrates from the level of the stomatopharynx to the inferior part of the neck. Various congenital anomalies of the thyroid gland can be formed in cases where the embryo experiences disturbances during histo- or organogenesis resulting in pathology of the thyroid primordium, or the thyroid germ fails to successfully migrate. Thus, thyroid anomalies may be divided into size and position anomalies.

Thyroid size anomalies include the following:

- Aplasia (agenesia)
- Hemiagenesia
- Hypoplasia

Thyroid aplasia is the complete absence of thyroid tissue (athyrosis). This is a widespread cause of congenital hypothyrosis, which has been recorded to occur in one in every 3000–5000 newborns. Here, the thyroid tissue cannot be sonographically visualized in its typical position or higher up.

Congenital hypoplasia of the thyroid is the second cause of congenital hypothyrosis. Here, sonography reveals a low thyroid volume (Fig. 3.4). The gland tissue appears echogenic and heterogeneous with irregular margins.

Thyroid hemiagenesia is usually a purely sonographic finding, and is not accompanied by thyroid disorders. Here, only one thyroid lobe can be detected at its typical site (Fig. 3.5). Its volume, as a rule, does not exceed the standard limits for the total volume of a normal thyroid gland. The second lobe cannot be visualized.

Thyroid gland position anomalies are as follows:

- Dystopia
- Ectopia

Thyroid dystopia and ectopia are sonographically characterized by an absence of thyroid tissue at its typical location. Dystopia refers to the localization of thyroid tissue close to the typical site along the route of natural migration during embryogenesis (within the neck, along the thyroglossal duct). If thyroid tissue is found at an atypical site outside the path of the thyroglossal duct, it is known as thyroid ectopia. An ectopic thyroid gland is at an increased risk of malignant transformation compared to either dystopic or normal thyroid glands.

Thyroid dystopia can take the form of the following variants, depending on the height of location:

- Lingual (goiter of the tongue root)
- Intralingual (lingual goiter)
- Sublingual
- Thyroglossal
- Pre- and intratracheal
- Intraesophageal
- Intrathoracic (truly retrosternal, in cases with an entirely retrosternal location)

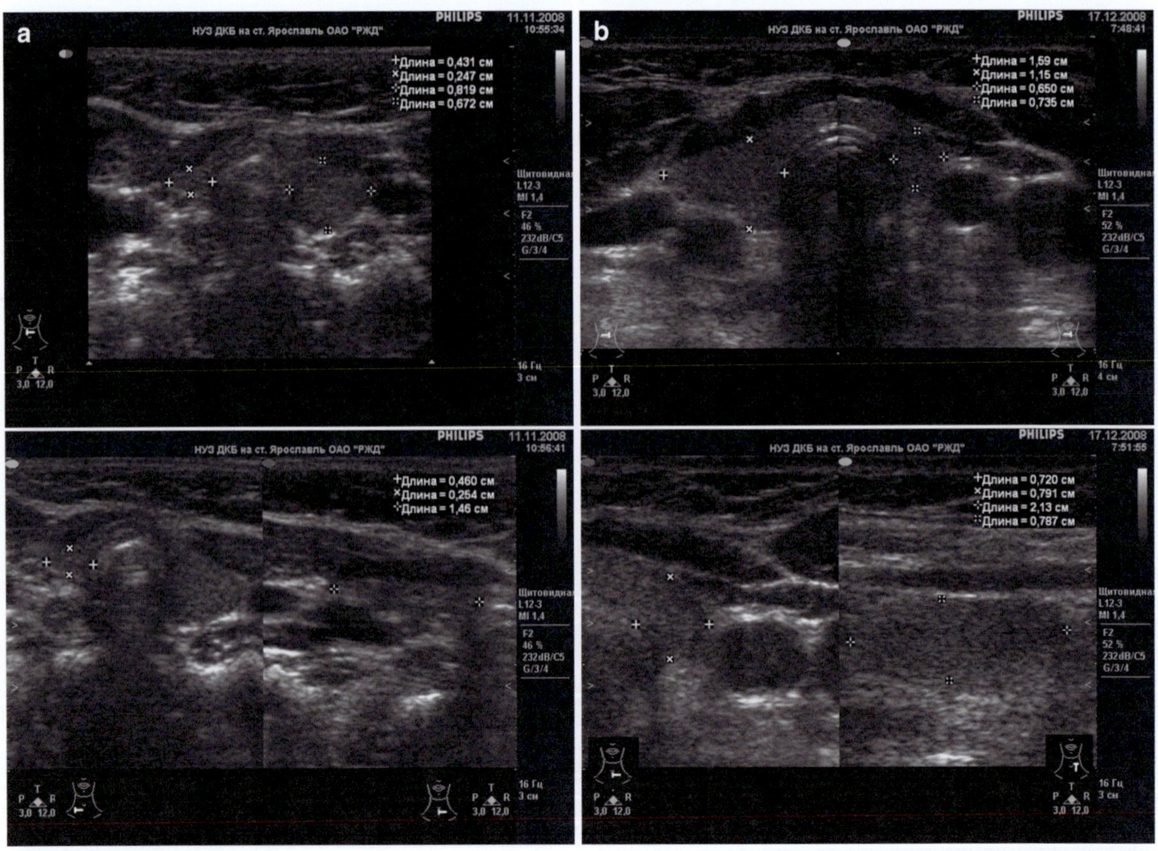

Fig. 3.4 Thyroid sonograms. B-mode. (**a**) Hypoplasia of the right thyroid lobe. The age of the child is nine months. (**b**) Hypoplasia of the left thyroid lobe. The age of the child is twelve years

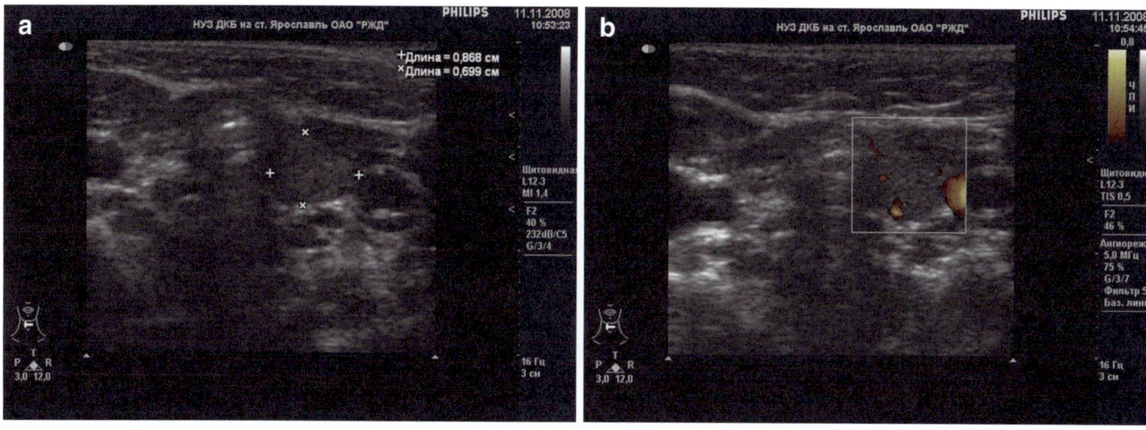

Fig. 3.5 (**a**, **b**) Thyroid sonograms. Hemiagenesia of the right lobe of the thyroid gland. The age of the child is six months. (**a**) B-mode and (**b**) PDI

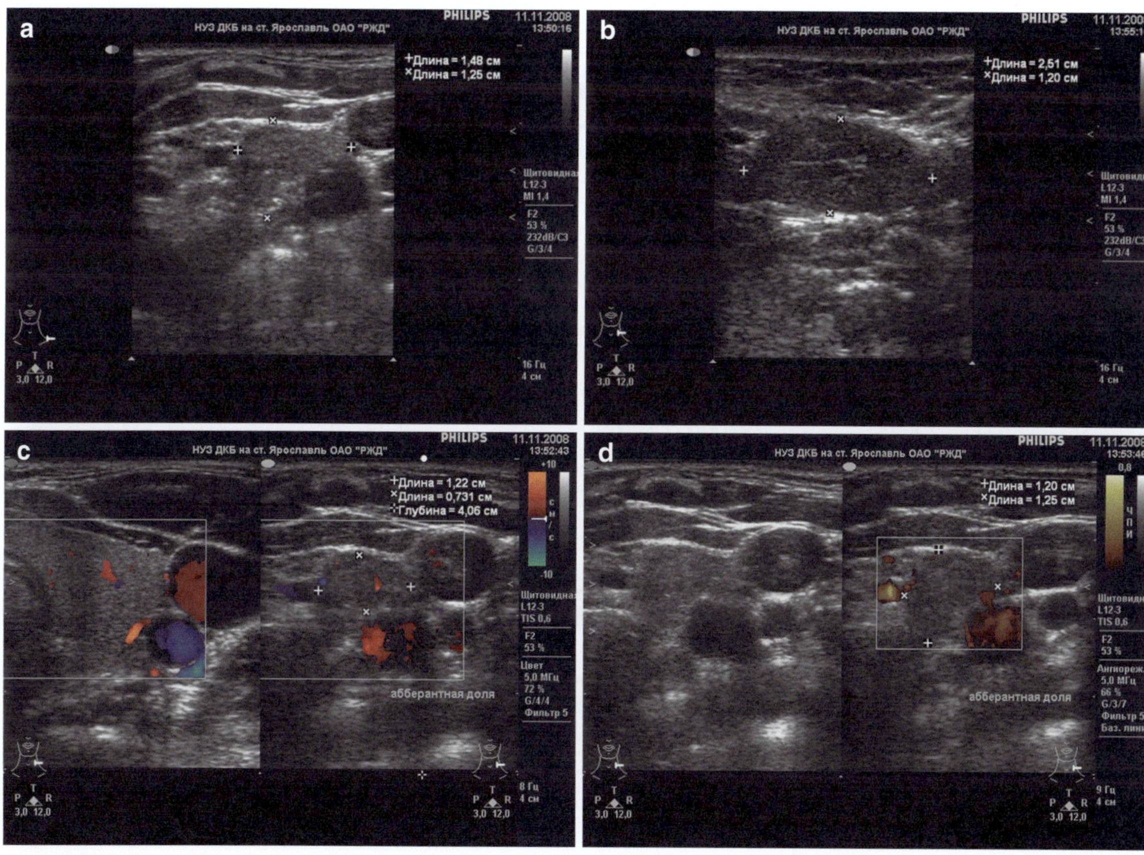

Fig. 3.6 (**a–d**) Sonogram. Aberrant thyroid gland in the left supraclavicular area. The age of the child is 13 years. (**a, b**) B-mode, (**c**) CDI and (**d**) PDI

Thyroid ectopy can often be found in the lateral neck (Fig. 3.6), in an ovary (struma ovarii), in a testicle (struma testis), in pericardium (struma pericardii), etc.

Median cysts of the neck are similar to dystopia in their pathogenesis. Failed obliteration of the thyroglossal duct during fetal thyroid migration results in the formation of an epithelial cavity with subsequent fluid accumulation. US detects the normal thyroid gland at its typical site. A cystic lesion of variable size may be identified cranial to the gland (see Chap. 12).

3.2 Diffuse Thyroid Diseases in Children

Diffuse thyroid diseases in children include pathologic processes characterized by hypertrophy and/or hyperplasia of glandular tissue with thyroid enlargement, or by its atrophy with an decrease in thyroid size. Different variants of diffuse euthyroid goiter dominate among diffuse thyroid diseases in children. Diffuse goiter is a universal pathologic sign of several diseases, such as the following:

- Endemic goiter
- Simple nontoxic (juvenile) goiter
- Iodine-induced goiter
- Idiopathic goiter
- Autoimmune thyroid disease
- Graves' disease
- Pendred syndrome
- Congenital nontoxic goiter

Children and teenagers contribute 5–40% of the cases of *diffuse endemic goiter* that occur in different regions (Kasatkina 1999). This disease is sonographically characterized by normal thyroid tissue. The echostructure remains homogeneous and isoechoic with unchanged tissue vascularity according to CDI, PDI, and 3DPD (Fig. 3.7). The only sign of the disease is an increase in thyroid volume, which thus differentiates it from the norm.

Autoimmune thyroid disease in children under 15 years of age reaches 20–25 cases per 100,000. 17–100 cases have been recorded per 100,000 schoolchildren (Nelson 1989; Levit 1991). AITD accounts for 20–60% of the cases of diffuse goiter in children (Ryumin 1997). The features of AITD in children are related to the short duration of the disease and minimal changes in the thyroid tissue. Hence, the disease is more difficult to diagnose than it is in adults. The US image is characterized by the heterogeneity of thyroid tissue due to hypoechoic foci, which contrast with the normal or hypoechoic surrounding tissue.

AITD quite often leads to subclinical hypothyrosis in early age. A high rate (up to 60%) of seronegative cases during the initial stages of the disease is a peculiarity of the humoral immune response in children (Shilin et al. 1995). Such cases of AITD are verified by puncture biopsy and cytology.

Expressed autoimmune changes during the initial stages of AITD do not lead to a very big goiter, unlike in adults. The thyroid gland is more often enlarged to the II–III degree. The majority of children with AITD, as well as those with endemic goiters, demonstrate thyroid volumes that are enlarged by 50–60% compared to the norm (Kasatkina et al. 1998). The ultrasound image may show decreased echodensity and heterogeneous echostructure of the gland (Fig. 3.8).

Graves' disease is a serious endocrine pathology. The annual morbidity is 2–4 cases per 100,000 children. The disease disproportionately affects girls 10–15 years of age. The clinical symptoms of Graves' disease in children are variable, but they do not develop as quickly as in adults. Organ compression symptoms may arise in cases with a retrosternal thyroid location. However, the degree of thyroid enlargement does not define the severity of thyrotoxicosis. The results of treatment depend on the accuracy and the timeliness of diagnosis.

Sonography usually reveals an enlarged thyroid with regular, well-defined margins, and relatively homogeneous and significantly hypoechoic parenchyma. The blood flow velocity in the main arteries is significantly increased. "Thyroid inferno," which was first described in adults (see Chap. 5), is most often observed in CDI, PDI, and 3DPD (Ralls et al. 1988). Wide veins and arteriovenous shunts have also been recorded.

Thyroid nodules in children and teenagers are noted less often than in the adult population. The incidence of thyroid nodules in children does not exceed 0.5–1% (Jaksic 1994; Wang 1997; Aghini-Lombardi 1999). More than half of the nodules (63.4%) are detected with US screening, and they are more prevalent in elder children. Solitary nodules are detected in about 88.6% of cases (Kiyaev 2008). Nodule size, as a rule, does not correlate with age. Thyroid nodules in children do not show specific US features, and are similar to such lesions in adults. This presents similar difficulties in the diagnosis of thyroid malignancy (Fig. 3.9).

Thyroid cancer is the most widespread tumor of the endocrine system in children (Danese et al. 1997; Shishkov et al. 2000; Niedziela 2006). Thyroid malignancy is observed in one in every two million children

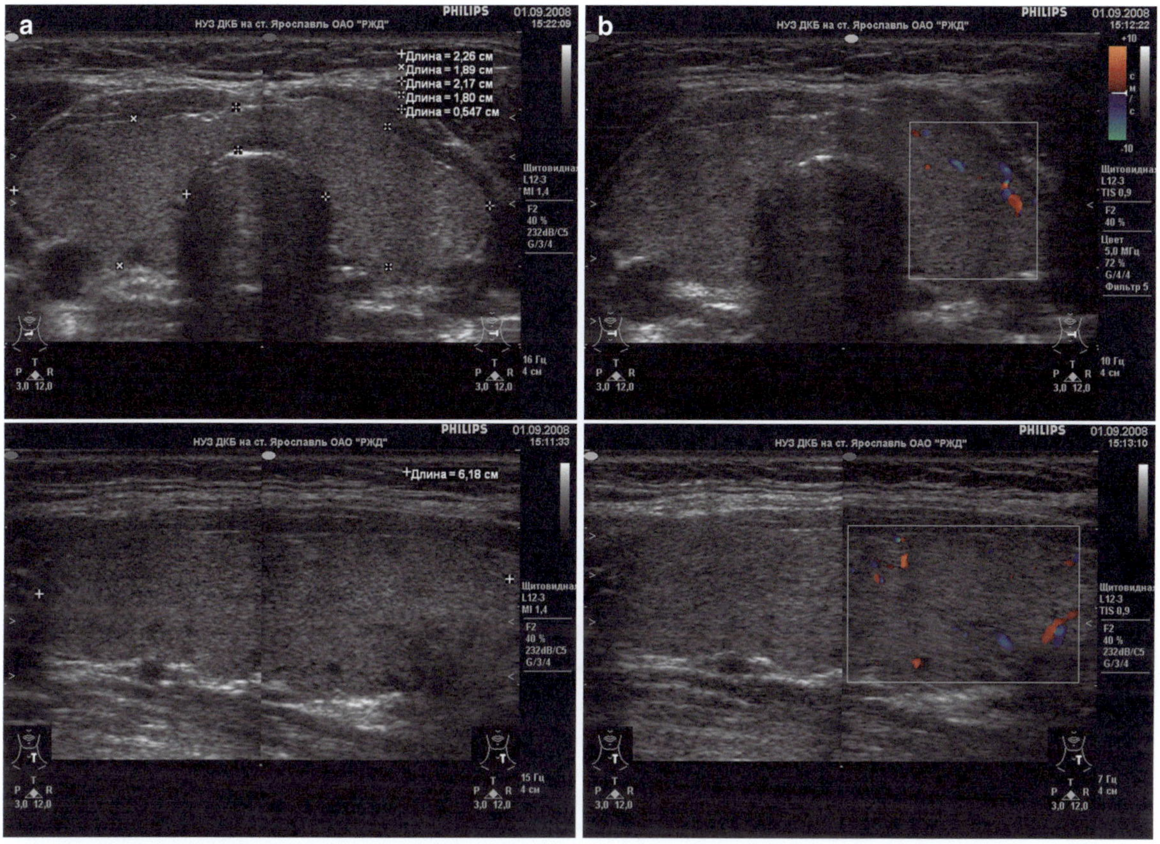

Fig. 3.7 Sonograms. Diffuse hyperplasia of the thyroid gland. The age of the child is 13 years. (**a**) B-mode. (**b**) CDI

per year. According to Kiyaev (2008), thyroid cancer in children is detected in 11.5% of suspicious thyroid nodules subject to puncture biopsy. Children 8–14 years of age show the disease more often, with the peak occurring during puberty (Durnov 1993; Lebedinsky 1993). The ratio of boys to girls with thyroid malignancy is about 1:1.6 (Polyakov et al. 1998). Papillary cancer dominates among all thyroid malignancies in children, as well as in adults (Polyakov 1998). The disease is more aggressive in children than in adults (Durnov 1997; Dinauer et al. 1998), and is characterized by a high frequency of intra- and extrathyroidal invasion. It also shows a high frequency of lymph node metastases, reaching 40–60%. Demidchik et al. (1996) reports that in children who underwent surgery for thyroid cancer, bilateral cervical metastases were found in 31.4%, metastases to the paratracheal lymph nodes in 40%, and remote metastases in 2.1% of cases. Thyroid cancer recurrence occurs more often in children than in adults, and constitutes 19–39% (Sweeney et al. 1995).

Precise sonography with all accessible options in children with thyroid malignancy before and after surgery permits improved management of thyroid cancer.

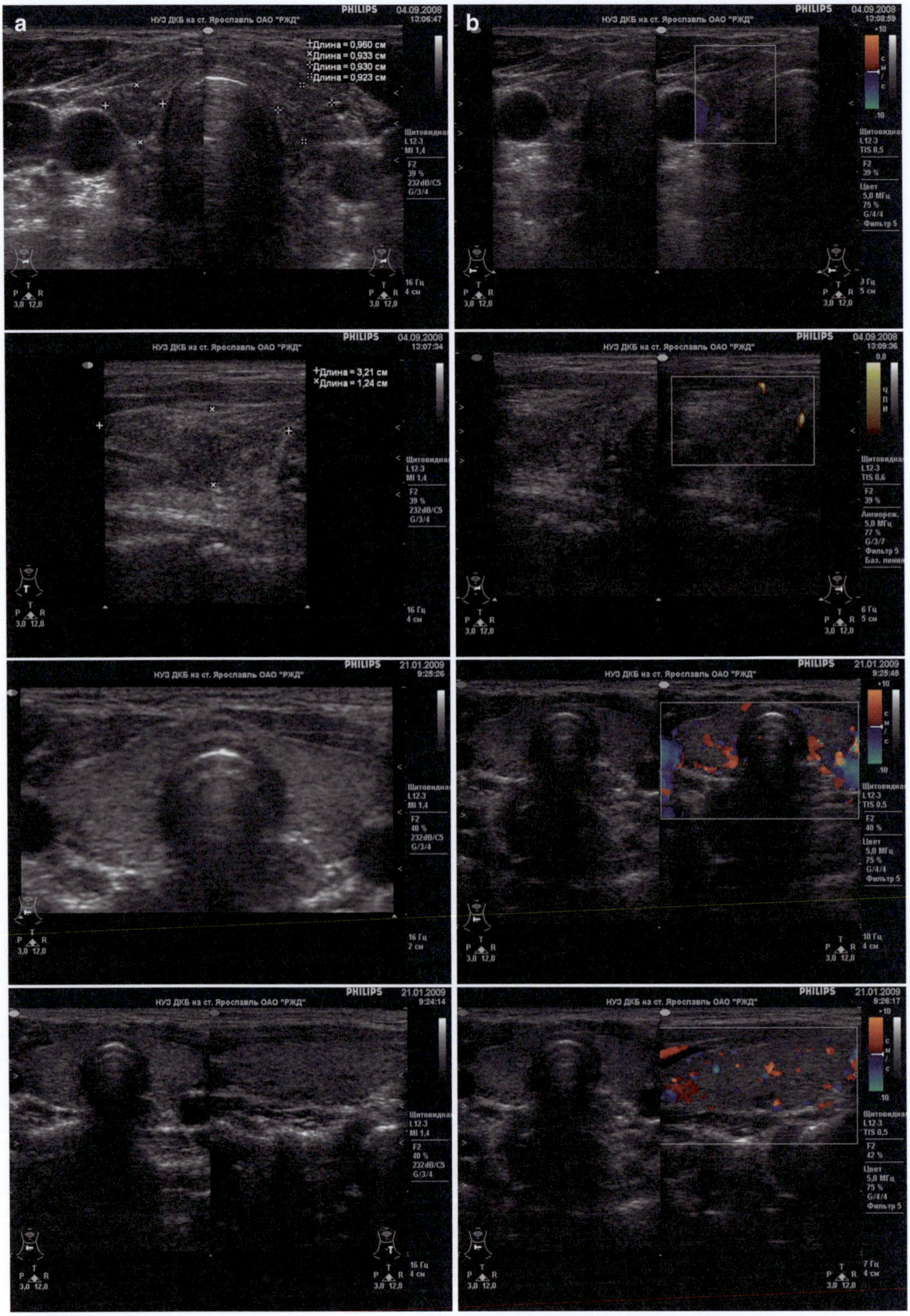

Fig. 3.8 Sonograms. AITD. The age of the child is ten years. (**a**) B-mode. (**b**) CDI and PDI

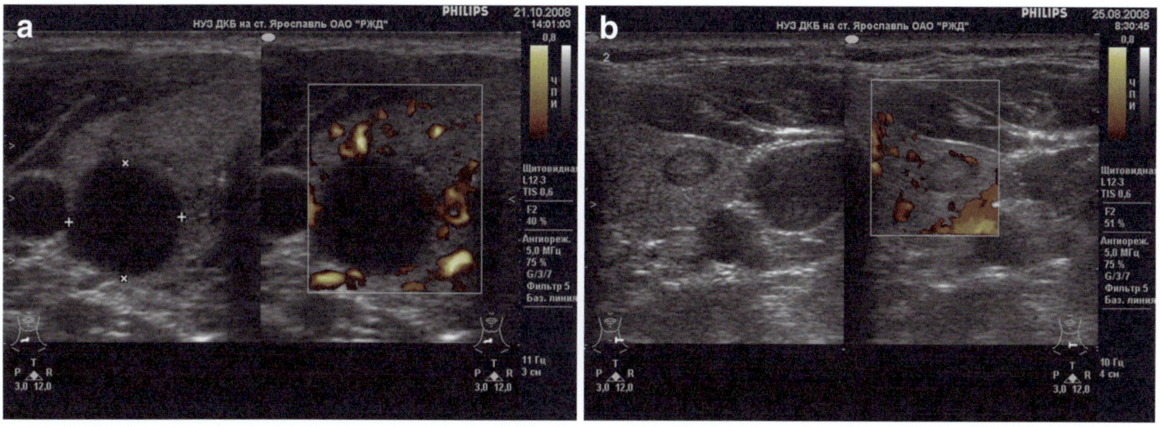

Fig. 3.9 Sonograms. Thyroid nodules. The age of the child is 11 years. B-mode and PDI

Normal Thyroid

4

The thyroid gland is normally located in the midline of the neck about 1–3 cm above the breastbone and clavicle. It consists of right and left lobes and the isthmus (Fig. 4.1). A pyramidal lobe arising cranially from the isthmus (more often from the left part) towards the hyoid bone may sometimes be observed. The thyroid is usually a butterfly-shaped gland. It can sometimes take a different shape, depending on individual features.

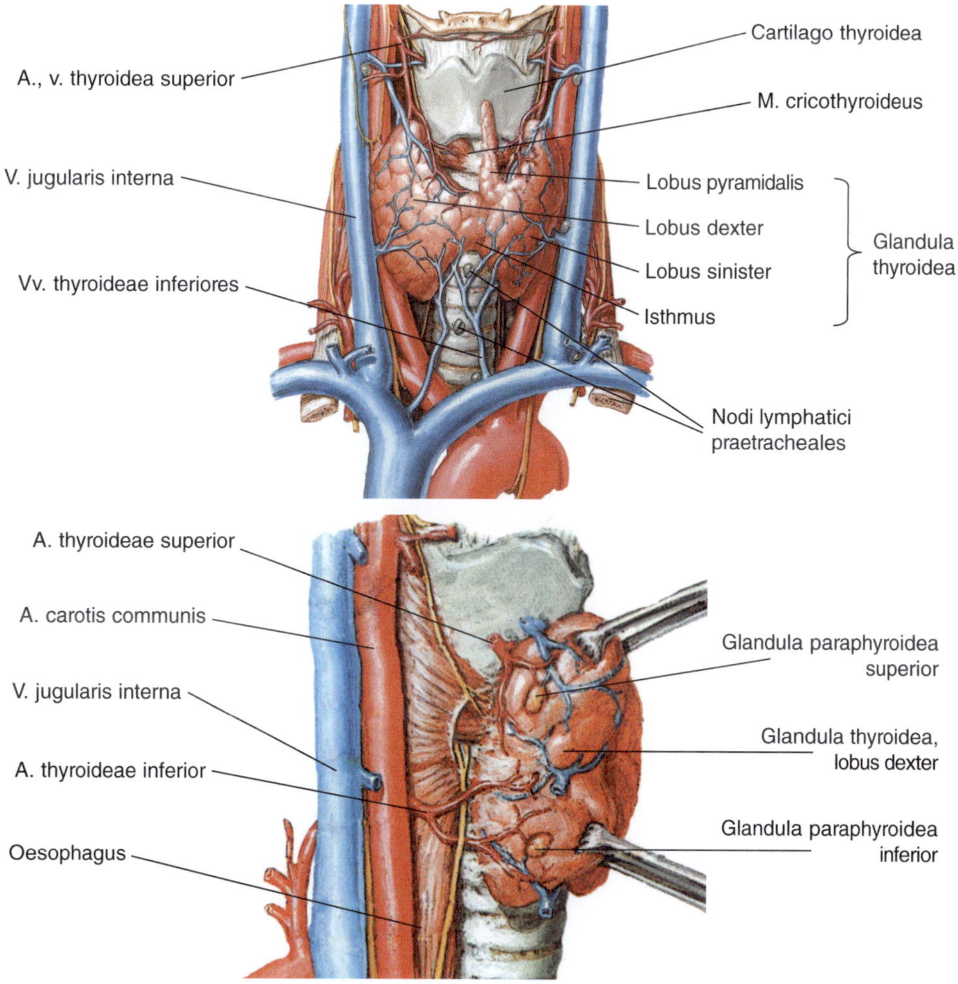

Fig. 4.1 (**a**, **b**) Thyroid location (Netter 2003)

V.P. Kharchenko et al., *Ultrasound Diagnostics of Thyroid Diseases*,
DOI: 10.1007/978-3-642-12387-0_4, © Springer-Verlag Berlin Heidelberg 2010

The thyroid surrounds the larynx and trachea, which are situated in the central part of the neck dorsally from the isthmus and medially from the thyroid lobes. The gland is covered ventrally and laterally by the symmetric prethyroid muscles (sternothyroid, sternohyoid, the superior belly of the omohyoid, and partially by the sternocleidomastoid), subcutaneous fat, and skin.

The vascular bundles of the neck are represented by the symmetric common carotid arteries (CCA) and internal jugular veins (IJV) (Fig. 4.2). The CCA is sonographically detected as a large incompressible vessel laterally adjacent to the thyroid lobes. It shows an arterial spectrum upon PW Doppler interrogation. IJV exhibits venous blood flow, has thinner walls, and can be completely compressed with the US probe. It is located laterally to the CCA.

The esophagus is usually observed neighboring the dorsal and medial margins of the left thyroid lobe. It looks like a pipe-shaped stricture with differentiation of the wall layers and a rough inner contour (Fig. 4.3). Swallowing can help to differentiate it from neck lesions. Peristalsis is easily discerned when hyperechoic masses pass caudally through its lumen.

According to the WHO, the normal volume of the thyroid gland is 7.7–25 cm^3 in men and 4.4–18 cm^3 in women. The width of the thyroid lobe in adults is about 13–18 mm, its depth is 16–18 mm, its length is

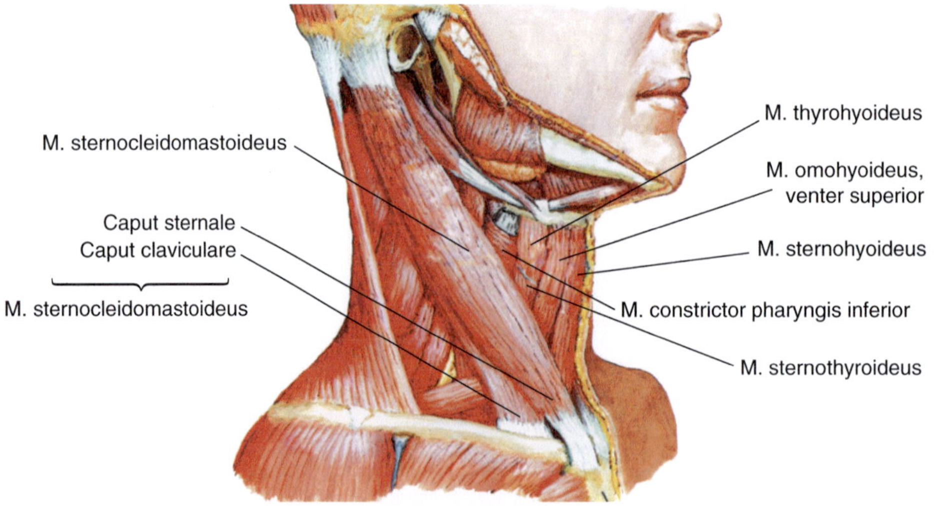

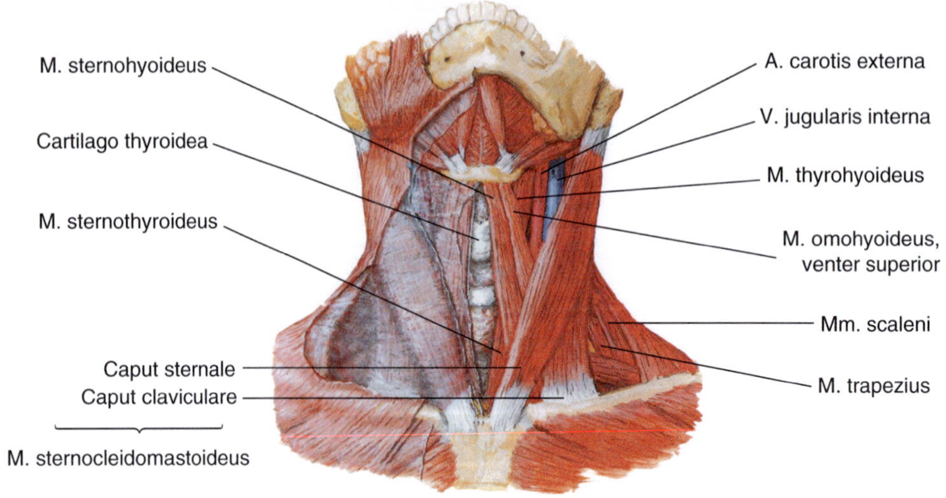

Fig. 4.2 (**a**, **b**) Thyroid location. Muscular layers (Netter 2003)

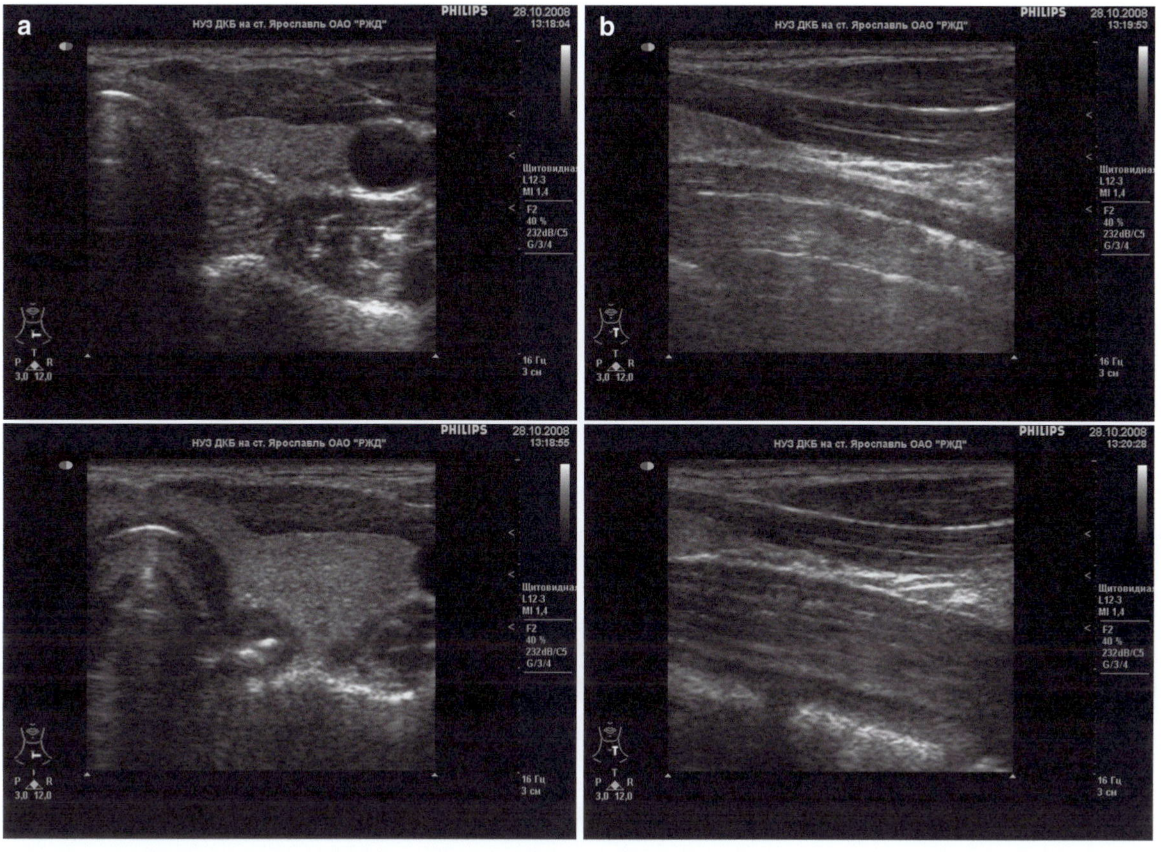

Fig. 4.3 US view of the esophagus. (a) Transverse scan. (b) Longitudinal scan

45–60 mm, and the depth of the isthmus is 2–6 mm (Ilyin 1995).

Sonographically, normal thyroid shows isoechoic homogeneous echostructure, accurate regular margins, and an echogenic capsule (Figs. 4.4, 4.5, and 4.10). The structure of the glandular tissue is considered homogeneous in cases with fine granularity that does not exceed 1 mm. The presence of areas that differ in echodensity from the normal background is interpreted as heterogeneous echostructure. This may correspond to diffuse or nodular thyroid pathology.

An anatomical classification that divides the thyroid into segments has been suggested (Parshin et al. 1999). However, it is reasonable to describe the upper, middle, and inferior segments that correspond to one-third of the length of each lobe in daily sonographic practice. The front (ventral) and back (dorsal) surfaces, paratracheal and paravasal sites, and the right, left, superior, and inferior segments of the isthmus may be described to specify the locations of lesions.

The thyroid gland has a pyramidal lobe in about 75% of cases. This arises from the upper part of the isthmus or from the adjacent portion of either lobe. However, thyroid US reveals it in only 10–15% of cases. This lobe most often appears similar in echodensity, homogeneity, and vascularity to the isthmus and lobes (Fig. 4.6).

The thyroid is supplied with blood from two paired upper thyroid arteries (UTA) and inferior thyroid arteries (ITA). The fifth artery, the thyroid ima, which supplies the isthmus with blood, is sometimes defined. The average gauge of the arteries does not exceed 1–2 mm. The UTA form the first branch of the external carotid artery. In rare cases they depart from the common carotid artery. The UTA split off at the level of the upper poles of the thyroid lobes into three branches: anterior, inferior, and internal (the isthmus branch). The ITA usually form a branch of the thyrocervical trunk, which emerges from the proximal part of the subclavian artery. The ITA divide into three

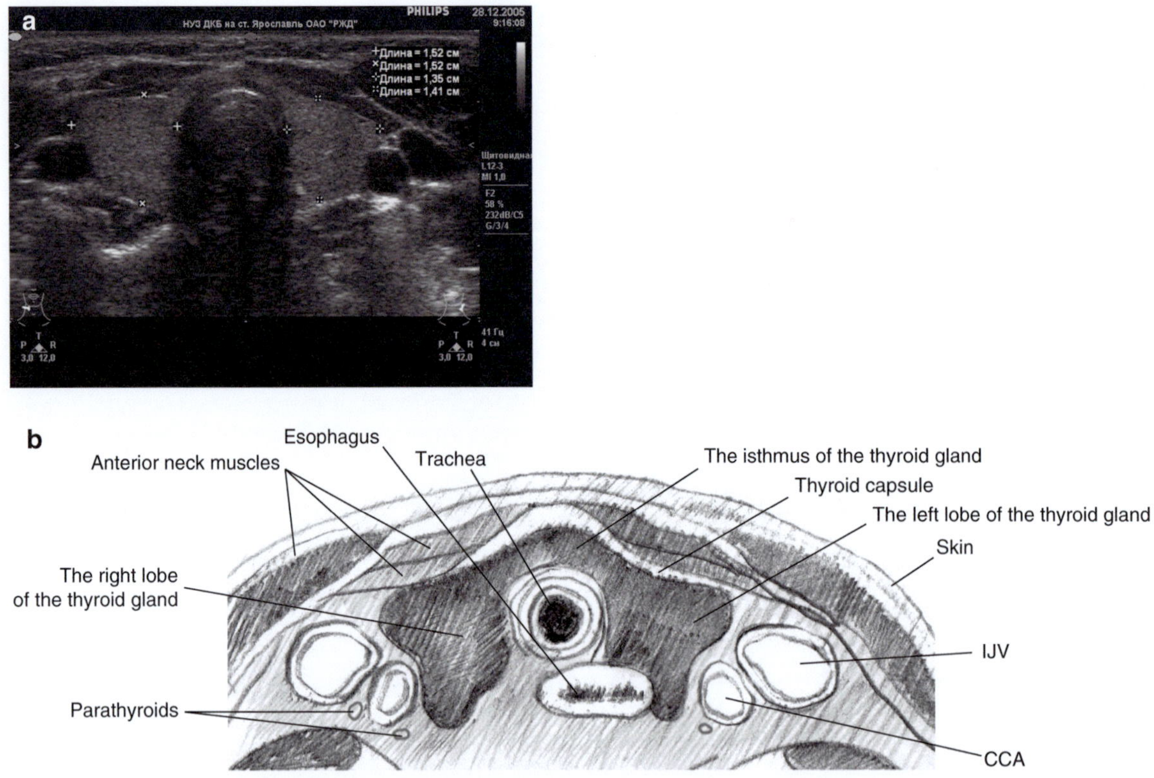

Fig. 4.4 US image of the thyroid. (**a**) Transverse scan. (**b**) Scheme

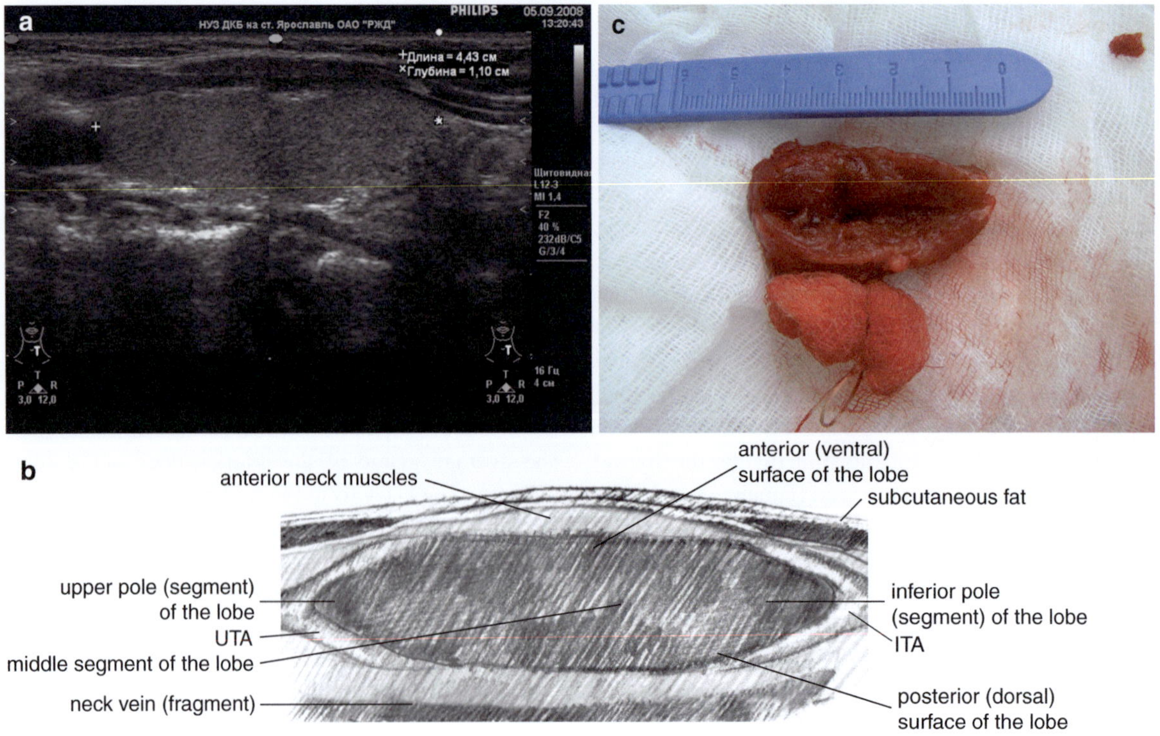

Fig. 4.5 US image of the thyroid. (**a**) Longitudinal scan. (**b**) Scheme. (**c**) Macroscopic view

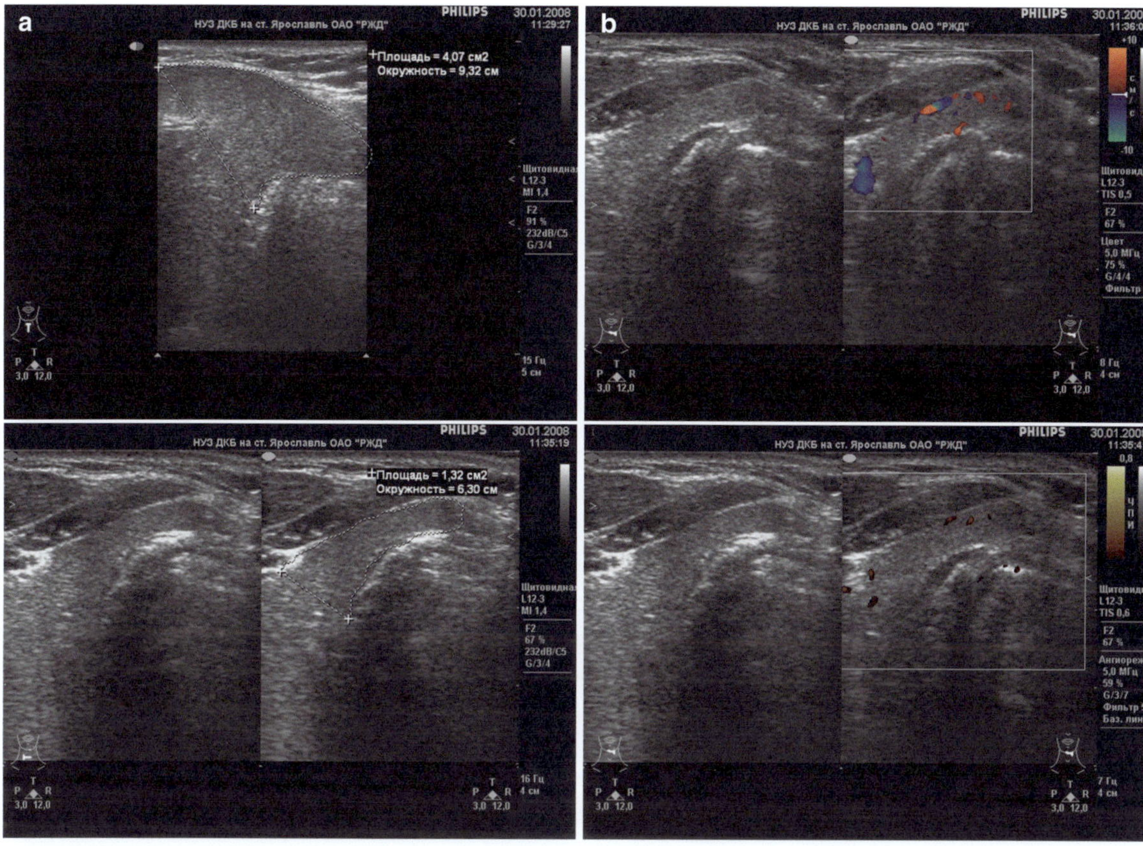

Fig. 4.6 Sonogram. Pyramidal lobe of the thyroid. (**a**) Grayscale. (**b**) CDI and PDI

branches (inferior, superior, and deep) close to the back surface of the inferior segments or the inferior poles of the thyroid lobes. Congenital anomalies, including anomalies in the number and location of the arteries, may be observed in rare cases. Thyroid arteries, as a rule, are sufficiently well-defined sonographically in both grayscale and color mapping (Fig. 4.7).

Statistically significant differences in blood flow velocity with PW Doppler in the UTA and ITA in men and women have not been discerned. The following parameters for blood flow in the thyroid arteries are normally defined: PSV in the UTA, 16.8±0.94 to 23.98±5.71 cm/s; in the ITA, 15.8±0.77 to 22.74±7.37 cm/s; EDV in the UTA, 7±1.2 to 8.03±2.79 cm/s; in the ITA, 6.36±0.29 to 9.53±3.16 cm/s; RI in the ITA, 0.58±0.1; in the UTA, 0.56±0.01 to 0.66±0.05; PI in the UTA, 0.96±0.34 to 1.06±0.54; in the ITA, 0.85±0.24 to 0.88±0.26 (Markova 2001; Lelyuk et al. 2007).

Struchkova (2003) defines the following norms for blood flow in all four arteries: PSV, 10.4–28.1 cm/s; EDV, 3.1–9.6 cm/s; RI, 0.5–0.75; PI, 0.7–1.2.

The venous blood from the thyroid is drained via the twin upper, middle, and inferior thyroid veins. As a rule, they emerge from the venous plexus of the thyroid, accompany the corresponding arteries, and drain into the IJV. The diameters of the thyroid veins do not usually exceed 2–2.5 mm. The blood flow in the thyroid veins is related to breathing. The velocity of the blood flow does not show significant any difference between the left and the right sides. The average blood flow velocity in the thyroid veins registered with PW Doppler ranges from 1.0 to 36.0 cm/s (Lelyuk et al. 2007).

Individual color spots in thyroid parenchyma are normally detected with CDI and PDI. They may be of various sizes, and are usually rather symmetric with a relatively uniform distribution (Figs. 4.8 and 4.9). The average color pixel density (CPD) in a normal thyroid is 5–15%. The average number of color cartograms of various vessels is 0.4–2.5 in 1 cm^2, and the number of color pixels within the normal thyroid lobe ranges from 5 to 10 (Fein et al. 1995; Lelyuk et al. 2007).

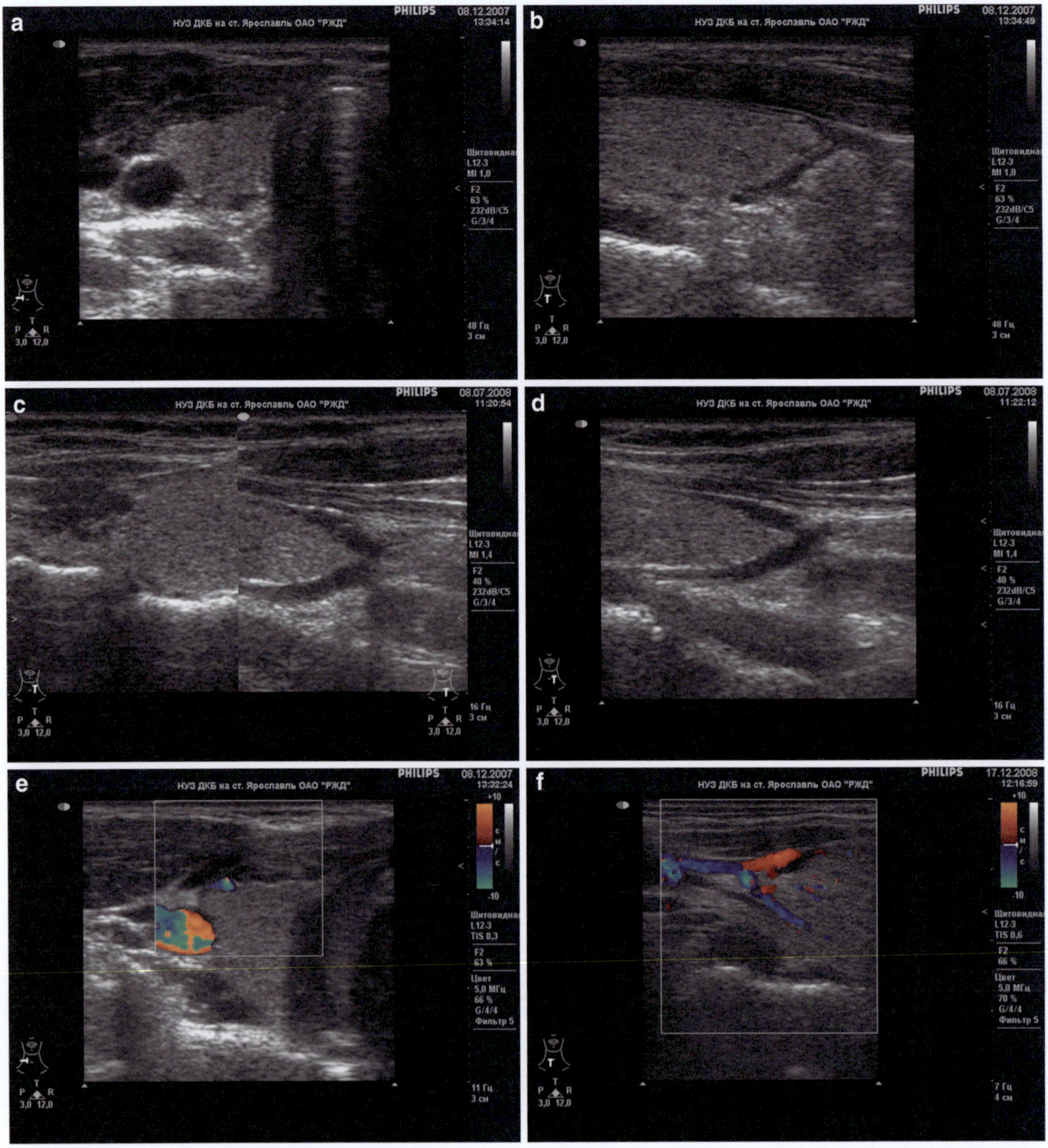

Fig. 4.7 (**a–j**) Thyroid arteries. Grayscale and CDI

The average gauge of arteries and veins within the thyroid parenchyma does not, as a rule, exceed 1–2 mm in CDI, PDI, and 3DPD.

3D reconstruction gives more detailed information on the location of the thyroid, its structure and margins, and its relations with surrounding organs and tissues (Fig. 4.10).

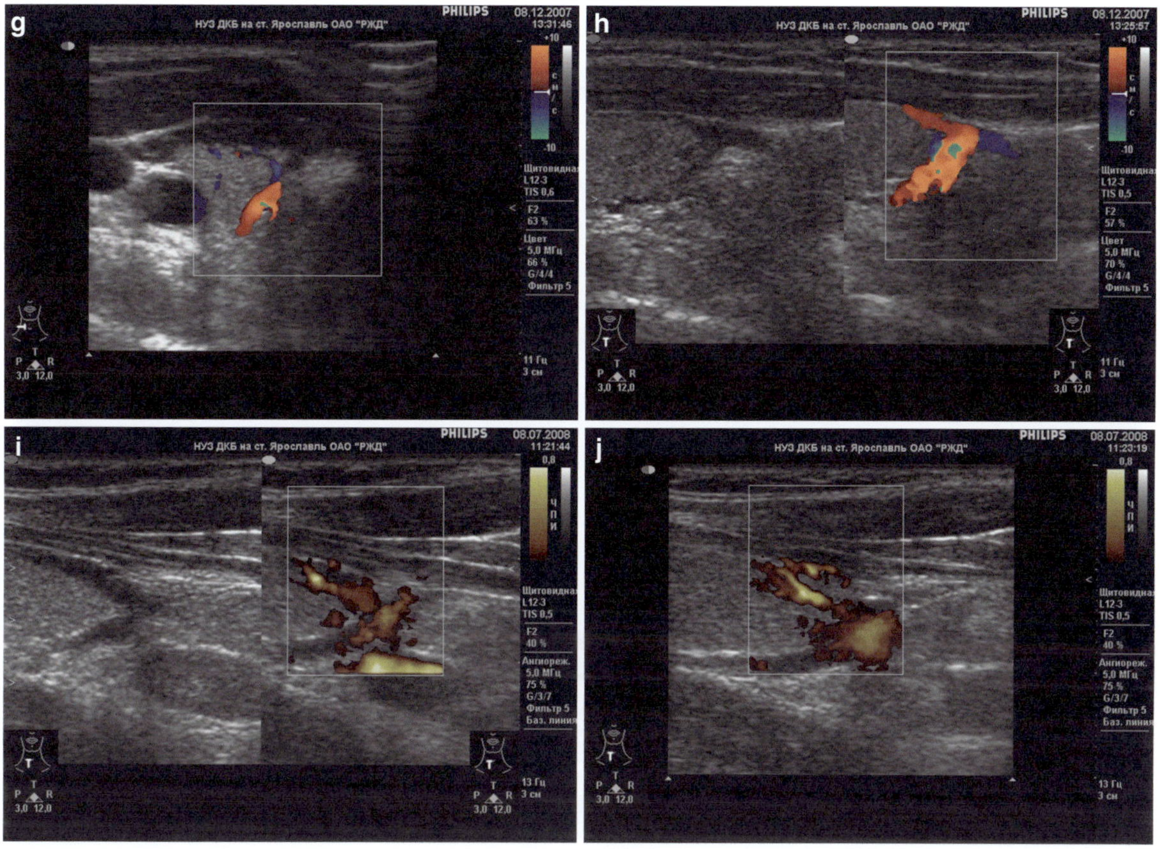

Fig. 4.7 (continued)

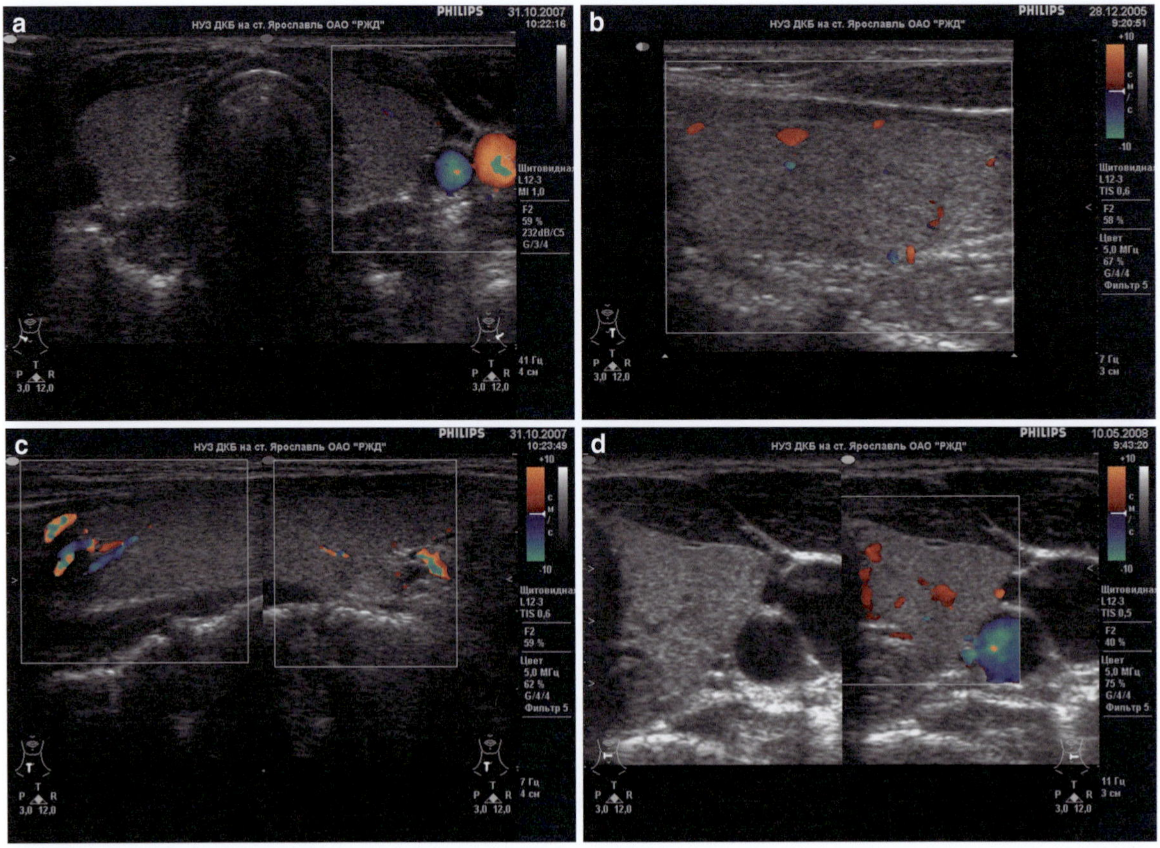

Fig. 4.8 (**a–d**) Thyroid US. CDI. Normal vascular pattern

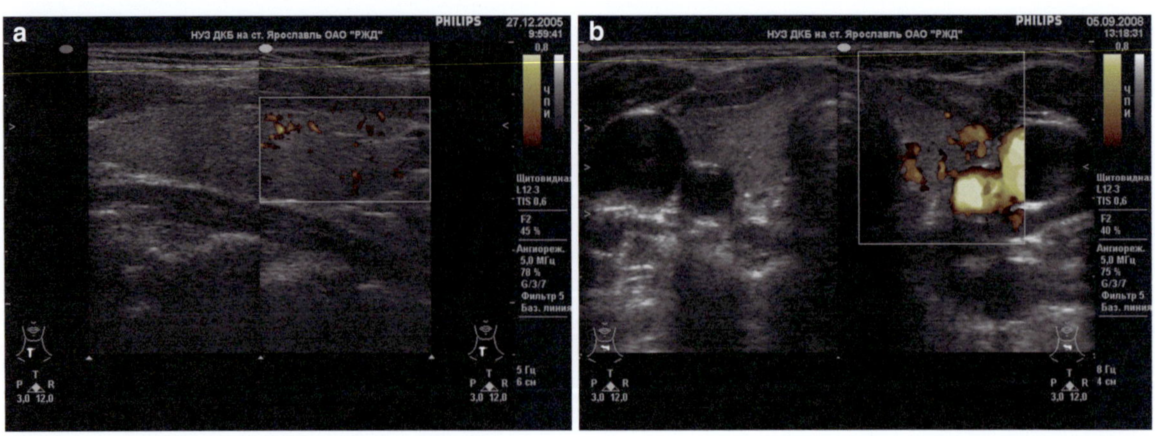

Fig. 4.9 (**a**, **b**) Thyroid US. PDI. Normal vascular pattern

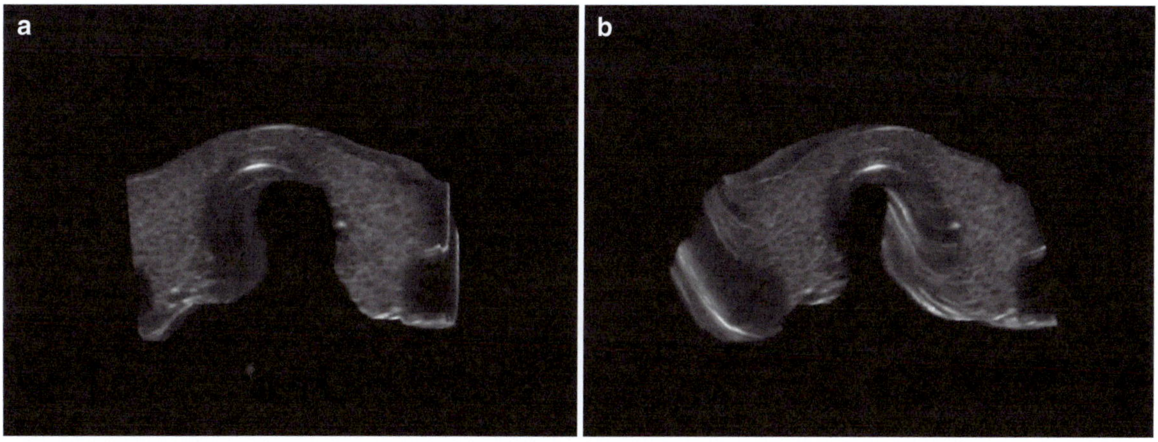

Fig. 4.10 (**a**, **b**) The US image of normal thyroid. 3D reconstruction

The example of US report in diffuse thyroid hyperplasia

First name, middle initial, last name:
Age:
Date:
The number of case history:
US scanner:
The thyroid gland is typically located with regular well-defined margins and homogeneous isoechoic structure. The capsule is uniform and continuous on all extent. Cystic and solid lesions are not detected.

The depth of the isthmus - 7 mm	
Right lobe	**Left lobe**
Depth 27 mm Width 20 mm Length 55 mm	Depth 14 mm Width 14 mm Length 47 mm
Volume 6.1 cm^3	Volume 4.6 cm^3

The total volume 10.7 cm^3 does not exceed the upper limit for the endemic region and the WHO recommendations.
The vascular pattern of the parenchyma of the gland is normal and symmetric in CDI, PDI, and 3DPD. CPD is up to 10 %.
The average number of color cartograms of vessels is 2 in 1 cm^2 and up to 10 color pixels within the structure of each lobe.
The topographic relation of the thyroid gland with the muscles and neck organs is typical.
The lymph nodes in the neck and supraclavicular areas are not enlarged.
CONCLUSION: Normal thyroid.
US specialist:

5 Diffuse Changes of the Thyroid Gland

There are various forms of thyroid pathology (ICD-10, 2007):

1. Congenital iodine-deficiency syndrome, including neurological, myxedematous, mixed types, and unspecified congenital iodine-deficiency syndrome
2. Iodine-deficiency-related thyroid disorders and allied conditions, including diffuse (endemic) goiter, multinodular (endemic) goiter, unspecified (endemic) goiter, and other iodine-deficiency-related thyroid disorders and allied conditions
3. Subclinical iodine-deficiency hypothyroidism
4. Other forms of hypothyroidism, including congenital hypothyroidism with diffuse goiter or without goiter, hypothyroidism due to medicaments and other exogenous substances, postinfectious hypothyroidism, acquired atrophy of the thyroid, myxedema coma, and other specified and unspecified forms of hypothyroidism
5. Other nontoxic goiters, including nontoxic diffuse goiter, single thyroid nodule, multinodular goiter, and other specified and unspecified nontoxic goiters
6. Thyrotoxicosis, including thyrotoxicosis with diffuse goiter, with a toxic single thyroid nodule, with a toxic multinodular goiter, from ectopic thyroid tissue, factitia, crisis or storm, and other specified and unspecified thyrotoxicoses
7. Thyroiditis, including acute, subacute, chronic thyroiditis with transient thyrotoxicosis, autoimmune thyroiditis, drug-induced thyroiditis, and other chronic specified and unspecified forms of thyroiditis
8. Other disorders of the thyroid, including hypersecretion of calcitonin, dyshormogenetic goiter, and other specified and unspecified disorders of the thyroid.

All thyroid abnormalities that can be detected sonographically are divided into diffuse and nodular changes.

Diffuse changes confer the following pathologies:

- Diffuse hyperplasia
- Thyroiditis
- Diffuse toxic goiter (Graves' disease)

5.1 Diffuse Hyperplasia

Diffuse hyperplasia of the thyroid gland is observed in 1–5% of the population and accounts for 80–85% of all thyroid abnormalities.

Diffuse hyperplasia is characterized by the following US features (Figs. 5.1–5.4):

- Increase in thyroid volume.
- Homogeneous isoechoic echostructure with a middle- or fine-grained pattern.
- Regular accurate margins. The contours of the poles may sometimes appear rounded.
- A very big thyroid may cause difficulties in visualizing the adjacent organs (vessels, esophagus, etc.) due to their dislocation dorsally or laterally.
- CDI, PDI, and 3DPD may reveal a negligible symmetric increase in the number of vessels within thyroid lobes with a uniform distribution. A normal color pattern is usually observed.

It is not entirely clear whether staging of thyroid enlargement is necessary (see Chap. 2). Nevertheless, Zabolotskaya et al. (1994) suggested a way to subcategorize thyroid enlargement in the US report. The authors stage the thyroid hyperplasia as follows: I–II degree if the thyroid volume appears to be increased by less than 30%; III degree if it is increased by 30 to 50%; and IV degree if it is increased by over 50%.

V.P. Kharchenko et al., *Ultrasound Diagnostics of Thyroid Diseases*,
DOI: 10.1007/978-3-642-12387-0_5, © Springer-Verlag Berlin Heidelberg 2010

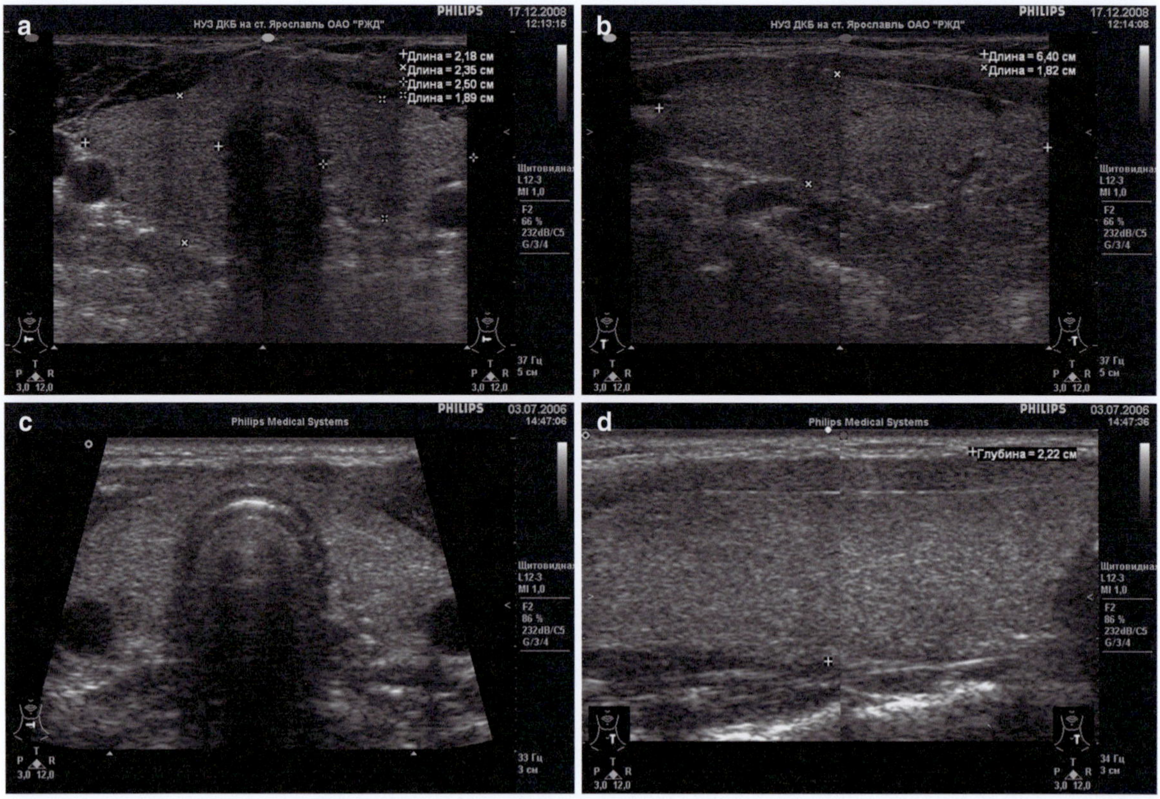

Fig. 5.1 (**a–d**) Diffuse thyroid hyperplasia. Grayscale image

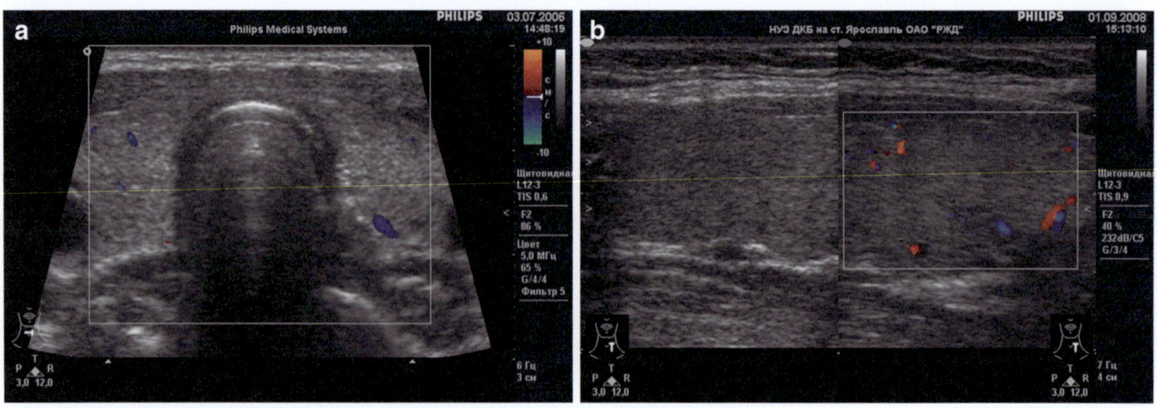

Fig. 5.2 (**a**, **b**) Diffuse thyroid hyperplasia. CDI

Doppler modalities do not add any significant data to that afforded by grayscale sonography in most cases. The intensity and pattern of color mapping do not differ from the norm in the majority of patients (Lelyuk et al. 2007).

Big thyroids cause difficulties in assessing the lengths of thyroid lobes. This is a consequence of them being much longer than the length of the US probe, meaning that the whole lobe cannot be viewed in one scanning range. The following techniques can be employed to solve this problem:

- Combining two scanning ranges (Fig. 5.5a)
- Use a "virtual convex" or trapezoid mode (Fig. 5.5b)
- Utilizing a convex probe (Fig. 5.5c; see Chap. 2)
- Panoramic scan (Fig. 5.5d)

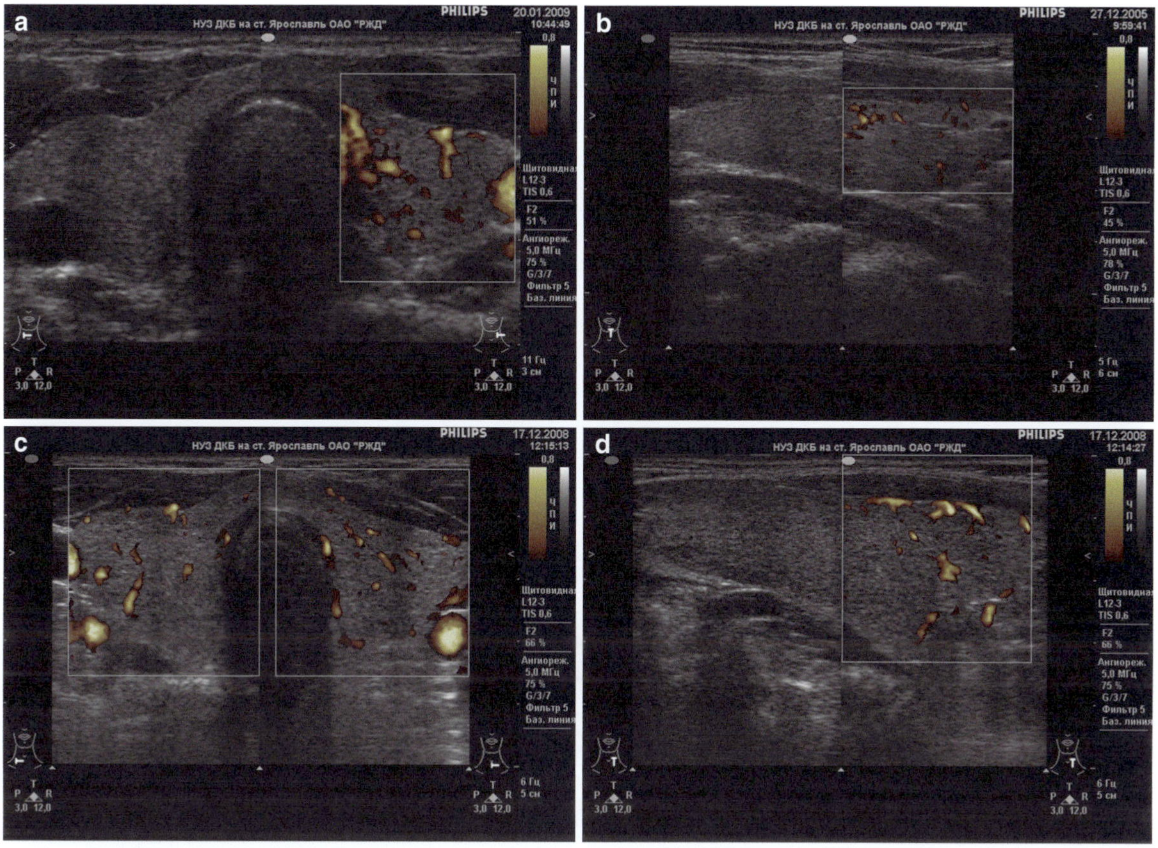

Fig. 5.3 (**a–d**) Diffuse thyroid hyperplasia. PDI

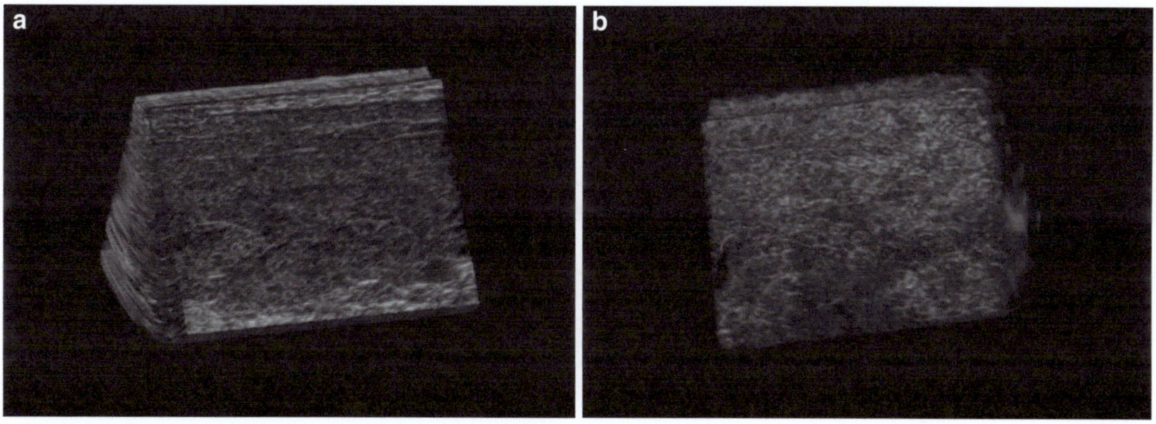

Fig. 5.4 (**a**, **b**) Diffuse thyroid hyperplasia. 3D reconstruction

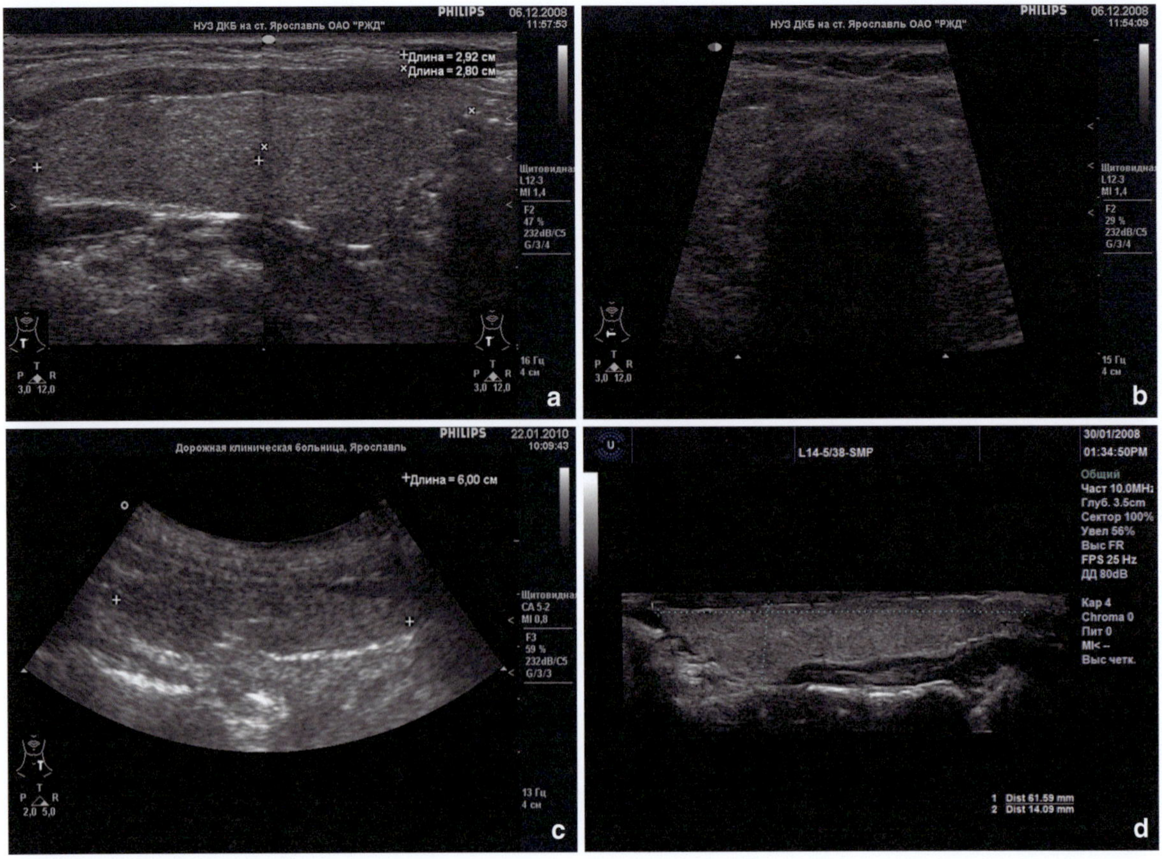

Fig. 5.5 (**a–d**) Sonograms. Measurements of the thyroid. Grayscale (**a**) combining two scanning ranges, (**b**) trapezoid mode, (**c**) utilizing a convex probe, (**d**) panoramic scan

The example of US report in diffuse thyroid hyperplasia

First name, middle initial, last name:
Age:
Date:
The number of case history:
US scanner:
The thyroid gland is typically located with regular well-defined margins and homogeneous isoechoic structure. The capsule is uniform and continuous on all extent. Cystic and solid lesions are not detected.

The depth of the isthmus - 7 mm					
Right lobe			**Left lobe**		
Depth	27	mm	Depth	25	mm
Width	20	mm	Width	19	mm
Length	55	mm	Length	52	mm
Volume	14.8	cm^3	Volume	12.4	cm^3

The total volume 27.2 cm^3 exceeds the upper limit for endemic region and the WHO recommendations.
The vascular pattern of the parenchyma is symmetric in CDI and PDI. The intensity of blood flow is insignificantly increased. CPD is 15-20 %. The topographic relation of the thyroid gland with the muscles and neck organs is typical.
The lymph nodes in the neck and supraclavicular areas are not enlarged.
CONCLUSION: US signs of the 2 degree of diffuse thyroid hyperplasia.
US specialist:

5.2 Thyroiditis

All types of thyroiditis are associated with either inflammatory or autoimmune cytotoxic processes in thyroid tissue. If the inflammation arises in a diffuse goiter with a significantly enlarged thyroid, the term "strumitis" may be used instead of "thyroiditis."

ICD-10 (2007) defines the following types of thyroiditis:

1. Acute thyroiditis
2. Subacute thyroiditis
3. Chronic thyroiditis with transient thyrotoxicosis
4. Autoimmune thyroiditis
5. Drug-induced thyroiditis
6. Other chronic thyroiditis
7. Thyroiditis, unspecified

5.2.1 Acute Thyroiditis

Acute thyroiditis (AT) is a relatively rare disease. Women suffer four times more often than men. The mean age of presentation is 30–40 years old. AT may be purulent or nonpurulent and further distinguished based on the diffuse or focal involvement of the thyroid parenchyma.

Purulent AT is a consequence of the penetration of bacterial coccal flora into thyroid tissue from sites of infection (abscess, tonsillitis, pneumonia, etc.), mediated by lymphogenous or hematogenous extension. The inflammatory process seldom involves the whole thyroid gland due to structural features (isolation of lobes with the connective tissue septa). Typically, only one lobe is affected. Purulent AT can be complicated by abscess formation, the development of a fistula or mediastinitis. In rare cases, the extensive destruction of thyroid parenchyma can result in hypothyroidism.

Nonpurulent AT is associated with aseptic inflammation of thyroid tissue after closed trauma, radiation therapy, or radioiodine therapy in patients with Grave's disease.

The principal US features of AT are as follows (Figs. 5.6–5.9):

1. Asymmetric enlargement of the thyroid, mainly at the expense of one lobe
2. Local or diffuse decrease in echodensity
3. Heterogeneous structure with hypoechoic fields of various sizes and shapes
4. Pain upon the compression of the lobe by the US probe, limited mobility of the thyroid

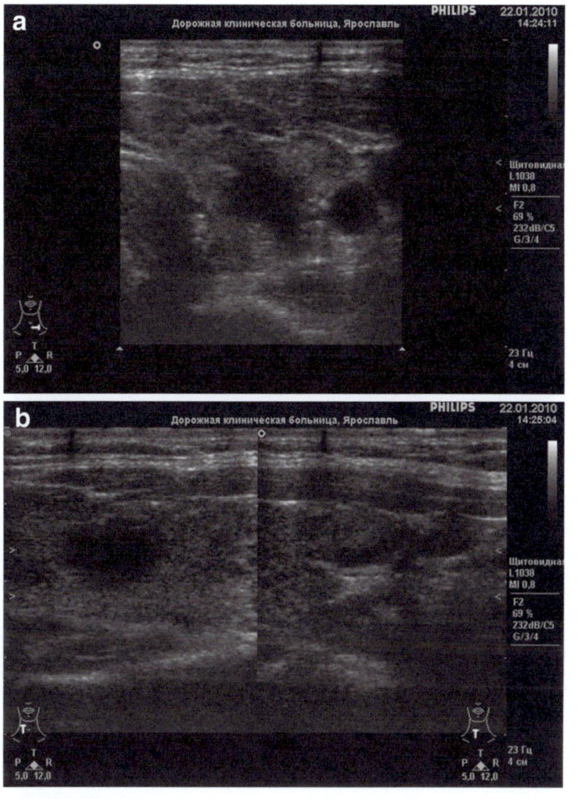

Fig. 5.6 (**a**, **b**) Acute thyroiditis. Grayscale image

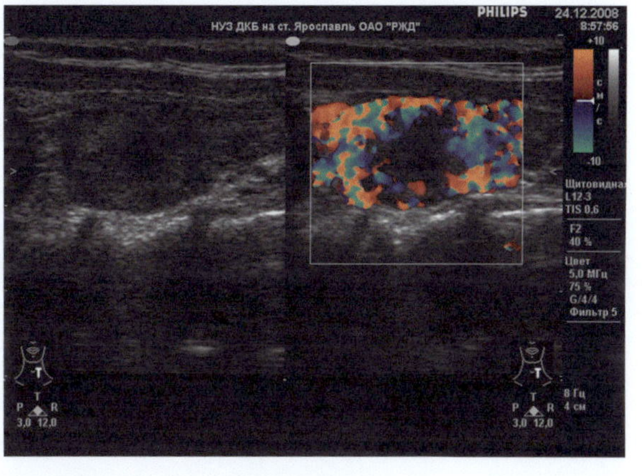

Fig. 5.7 Acute thyroiditis. CDI

5. Decrease in the vascularity of the affected area in CDI, PDI, and 3DPD
6. Cervical lymphadenitis

In rare cases, AT may result in a thyroid abscess. In such cases, sonography shows a hypoechoic heterogeneous lesion with an echogenic capsule along with

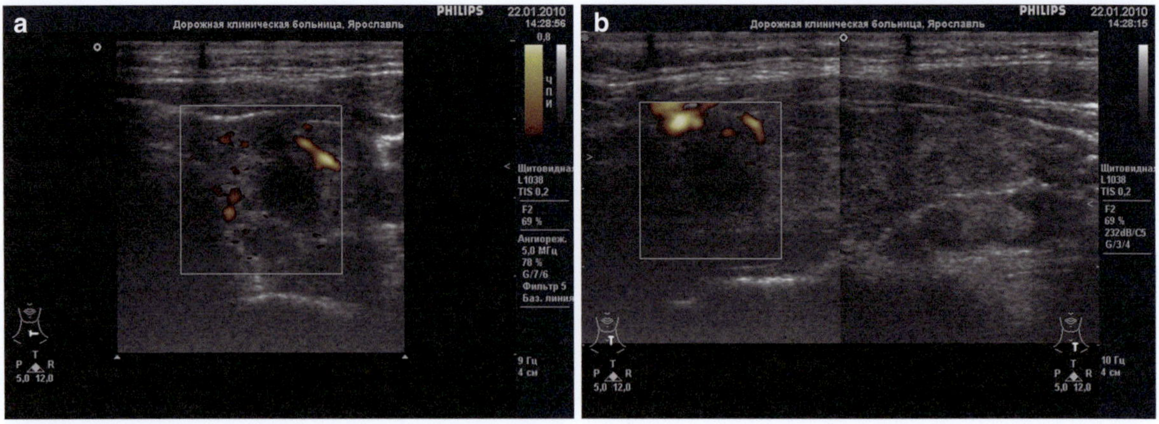

Fig. 5.8 (a, b) Acute thyroiditis. PDI

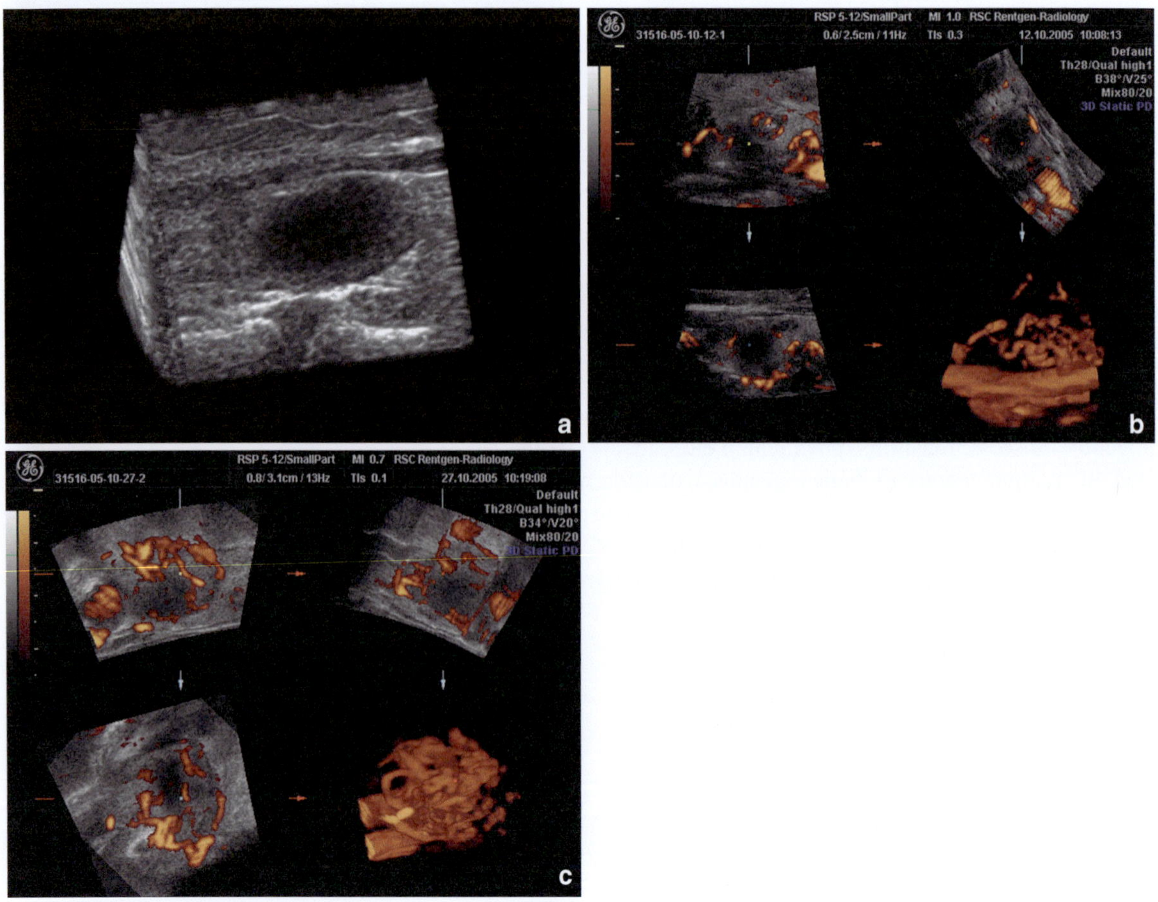

Fig. 5.9 (a–c) Acute thyroiditis. 3D reconstruction and 3DPD

diffuse changes in the thyroid parenchyma. The abscess contains fluid collections with an echogenic suspension, and is characterized by fast changes in US features (Fig. 5.10). Liquefaction of the fluid component of the thyroid abscess may result in a cyst. Alternatively, the organization of the abscess may result in a heterogeneous hypoechoic thyroid nodule with echogenic inclusions.

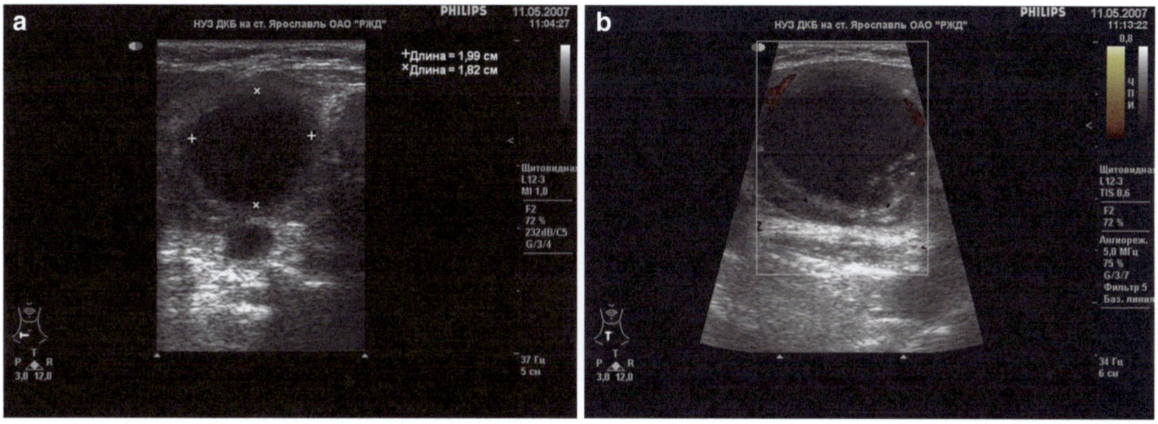

Fig. 5.10 (**a**, **b**) Thyroid abscess. (**a**) Grayscale and (**b**) PDI

The example of US report in acute thyroiditis

First name, middle initial, last name:
Age:
Date:
The number of case history:
US scanner:
The thyroid gland is typically located with regular well-defined margins and homogeneous isoechoic structure. The capsule is uniform and continuous on all extent.

The depth of the **isthmus** - 4 mm	
Right lobe	**Left lobe**
Depth 15 mm Width 16 mm Length 50 mm	Depth 21 mm Width 23 mm Length 57 mm
Volume 6.0 cm^3	Volume 13.8 cm^3
The total volume 19.8cm^3 exceeds the upper limit for endemic region and the WHO recommendations.	
No lesions detected.	Hypoechoic hypovascular areas of different size and shape with irregular blurred margins and small fluid collections containing homogenous suspension, painful with compression are located within the middle and inferior segments.

Vascular pattern of the parenchyma out of described areas in CDI and PDI is unchanged. CPD is 10 %.
The topographic relation of the thyroid gland with the muscles and neck organs is typical.
The lymph nodes along vascular bundles of the neck are enlarged up to 0.8-2.0 cm, hypoechoic, heterogeneous with regular well-defined margins, unchanged differentiation, and moderately increased vascularity in hilus and central part. The lymph nodes in supraclavicular areas are not enlarged.
CONCLUSION: The 1 degree of the increase in thyroid volume. Diffuse changes of the left lobe suspicious for acute thyroiditis.
US specialist:

5.2.2 Subacute Thyroiditis

Subacute thyroiditis (SAT) was first described by de Quervain in 1905. Unlike acute thyroiditis, SAT is of viral origin, and is most often preceded by an upper respiratory tract infection. Morbidity relating to SAT corresponds to about 0.16–0.36% of all patients with thyroid pathology (Fomina 2003). As a rule, the patient's age is 20–50 years, and it is much more prevalent in women, with a ratio of 5:1. The disease is characterized by inflammation and lymphocytic infiltration of thyroid tissue.

The clinical classification of SAT is as follows (Balabolkin 1994):

1. SAT with an expressed inflammatory reaction (54.8%)
2. Slowly progressing SAT (28.2%)
3. SAT with clinical hyperthyroidism (14.6%)
4. Pseudoneoplastic SAT (2.4%).

The development of US equipment introduced new possibilities for the diagnosis of SAT.

SAT is characterized by the following basic US features (Fig. 5.11):

1. Thyroid enlargement
2. Local or diffuse decrease in echodensity
3. Hypoechoic areas of various sizes and shapes with indistinct margins
4. Pain upon the compression of the thyroid by the US probe, especially at sites where the echodensity decreases
5. Significant decrease in vascularity in hypoechoic areas with CDI, PDI, and 3DPD
6. Cervical lymphadenitis can be detected in the acute period

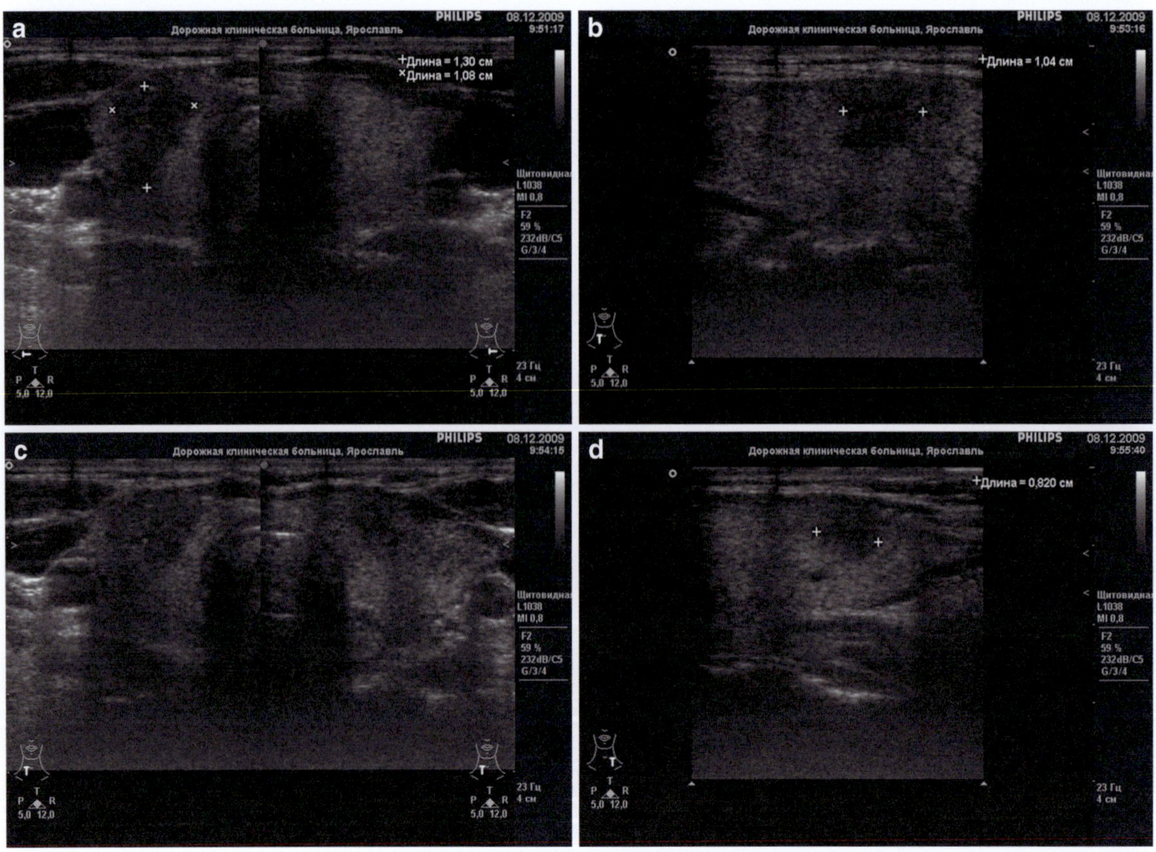

Fig. 5.11 (a–d) Subacute thyroiditis. Grayscale image

Fomina (2003) describes the following three sonographic types of SAT

1. Hypoechoic foci (66.1%). These are often observed in patients with a slowly progressing form of SAT.
2. Cystiform lobes (26.6%). This picture is seen in patients with both an expressed inflammatory reaction and clinical hyperthyroidism.
3. Hypoechoic lobes (7.3%).

Hypoechoic areas appear avascular or significantly hypovascular with CDI and PDI in the acute period of de Quervain's thyroiditis. At the same time, the vascularity of the surrounding parenchyma is usually not affected, or is slightly decreased (Figs. 5.12 and 5.13). According to Fomina (2003), the average blood flow velocities in the arteries within the pathological foci decrease twofold or more (PSV of 9.83±2.42 cm/s, EDV of 4.7±2.05 cm/s, RI of 0.52±0.16, and PI of 0.72±0.23). The blood flow

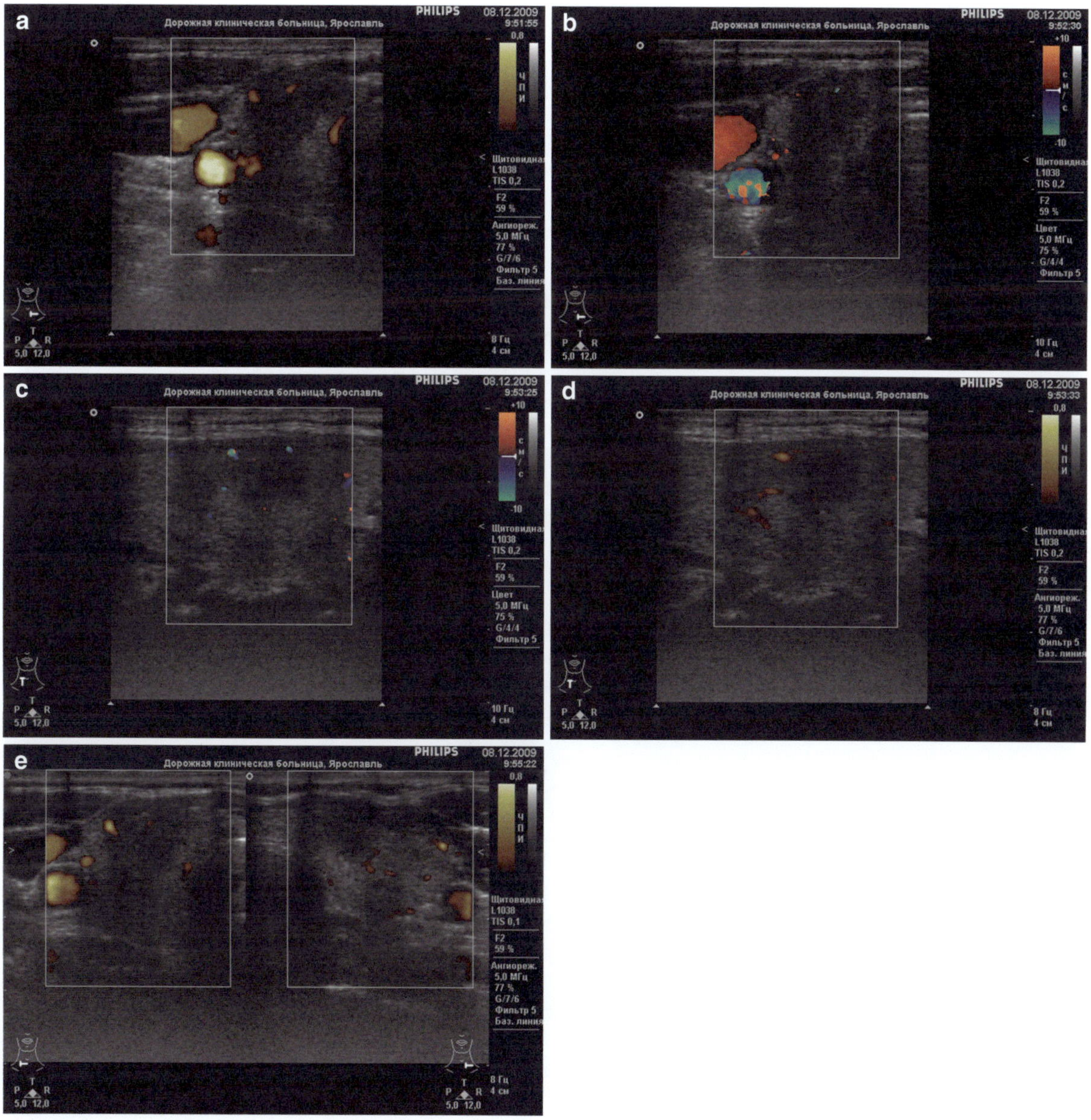

Fig. 5.12 (**a–e**) Subacute thyroiditis. PDI and CDI

velocities and resistance indices observed with PW Doppler in the main thyroid vessels do not differ from the normal thyroid in SAT (Lelyuk et al. 2007).

The stage of reconvalescence is sonographically characterized by a gradual decrease in thyroid volume (on average by 81.5% during the first month of treatment) and the restoration of the normal structure of the thyroid parenchyma (Fig. 5.14). Complete restoration may take from two months up to 1.5 years. The structure becomes normal again in about 75% of patients. Residual changes can thus be observed in 25% of the patients.

SAT recurrence arises in 30–35% of patients, and is easily detected sonographically, even in cases with minimal clinical signs. Slow restoration of normal thyroid echostructure is a predictor of SAT recurrence.

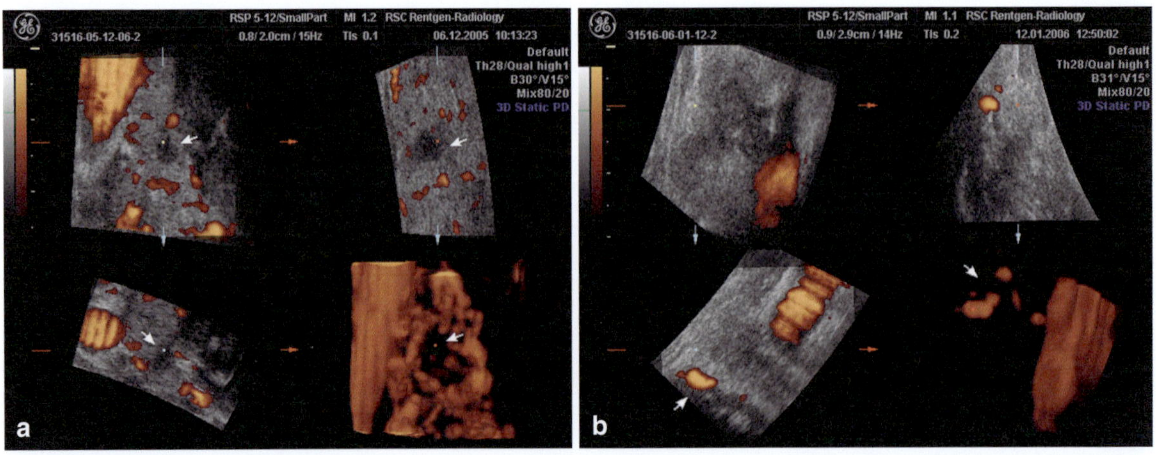

Fig. 5.13 (**a**, **b**) Subacute thyroiditis. 3DPD

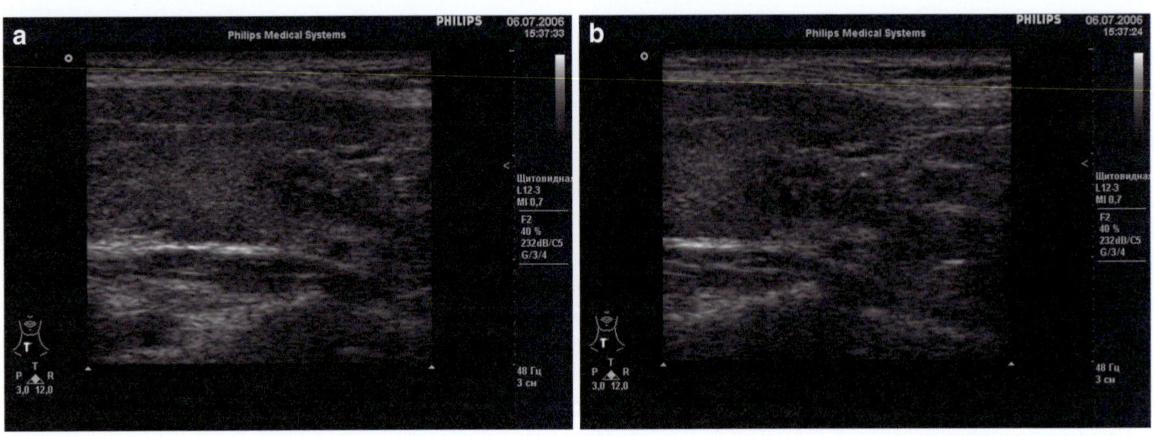

Fig. 5.14 (**a**, **b**) Subacute thyroiditis. The stage of reconvalescence. Grayscale image

The example of US report in subacute thyroiditis

First name, middle initial, last name:
Age:
Date:
The number of case history:
US scanner:
The thyroid gland is typically located with regular well-defined margins and homogeneous isoechoic structure. The capsule is uniform and continuous on all extent.

The depth of the **isthmus** - 6 mm	
Right lobe	**Left lobe**
Depth 22 mm Width 29 mm Length 54 mm	Depth 23 mm Width 24 mm Length 52 mm
Volume 17.2 cm^3	Volume 14.3 cm^3
The total volume 31.5 cm3 exceeds the upper limit for the endemic region and the WHO recommendations.	
The hypoechoic focus of 1.8x2.5x2.0 cm in size with irregular blurred margins, hypovascular, moderately painful with compression is located in the inferior segment.	Hypoechoic heterogeneous avascular areas of different size and shape with irregular blurred margins, moderately painful with compression are located within the middle and inferior segments.

The echodensity of the thyroid parenchyma is moderately diffusely decreased. Vascular pattern of the parenchyma out of described areas in CDI and PDI is unchanged. CPD is 10 %.
The topographic relation of the thyroid gland with the muscles and neck organs is typical.
The lymph nodes along vascular bundles of the neck are enlarged up to 0.8-1.4 cm, hypoechoic, heterogeneous with regular well-defined margins, and unchanged differentiation and vascularity. The lymph nodes in supraclavicular areas are not enlarged.
CONCLUSION: The 3 degree of the increase in thyroid volume. Diffuse and local changes of the thyroid gland suspicious for subacute thyroiditis.
US specialist:

5.2.3 Autoimmune Thyroiditis

Autoimmune thyroiditis (AIT) was first described by Dr. Hashimoto in 1912. It is one of the most widespread diseases of the thyroid. It is present in up to 6–11% of the adult population (Kasatkina et al. 1999). The rate of clinically significant forms of AIT in the general population is about 1%, and among the adult population it is 3–45 per 1,000. The disease disproportionately affects women. The number of women with AIT exceeds the number of men with AIT by 4–8 times. Incidence peaks at 40–60 years of age. The rate of AIT in children from different countries is 0.1–1.2%. AIT is the most frequent form of chronic thyroiditis.

Bronstein (1997) suggests the following three basic histological types of AIT: classical (diffuse and diffuse-nodular), chronic lymphomatous thyroiditis, and chronic lymphomatous strumitis. The classification by Gerasimov and Dedov (1992) divides AIT into hypertrophic (diffuse and pseudo-nodular) and atrophic.

The following US signs are characteristic of AIT (Fig. 5.15):

1. Enlargement of thyroid lobes and isthmus with predominant enlargement of the depth and width of the lobes; the atrophic variant of the disease can present a decreased or unchanged thyroid size.
2. Irregular echodensity decrease with different degrees of manifestation.
3. Diffuse heterogeneity (from fine-grained to coarse-grained) resulting from hypoechoic areas of various sizes distributed within the thyroid tissue sometimes merging into each other.
4. Echogenic inclusions with different shapes (more often linear or point-like) related to the stromal component.
5. Hypovascularity of hypoechoic areas is typical. Diffuse hypervascularization is possible. The blood flow pattern with CDI and PDI depends on the type of AIT.

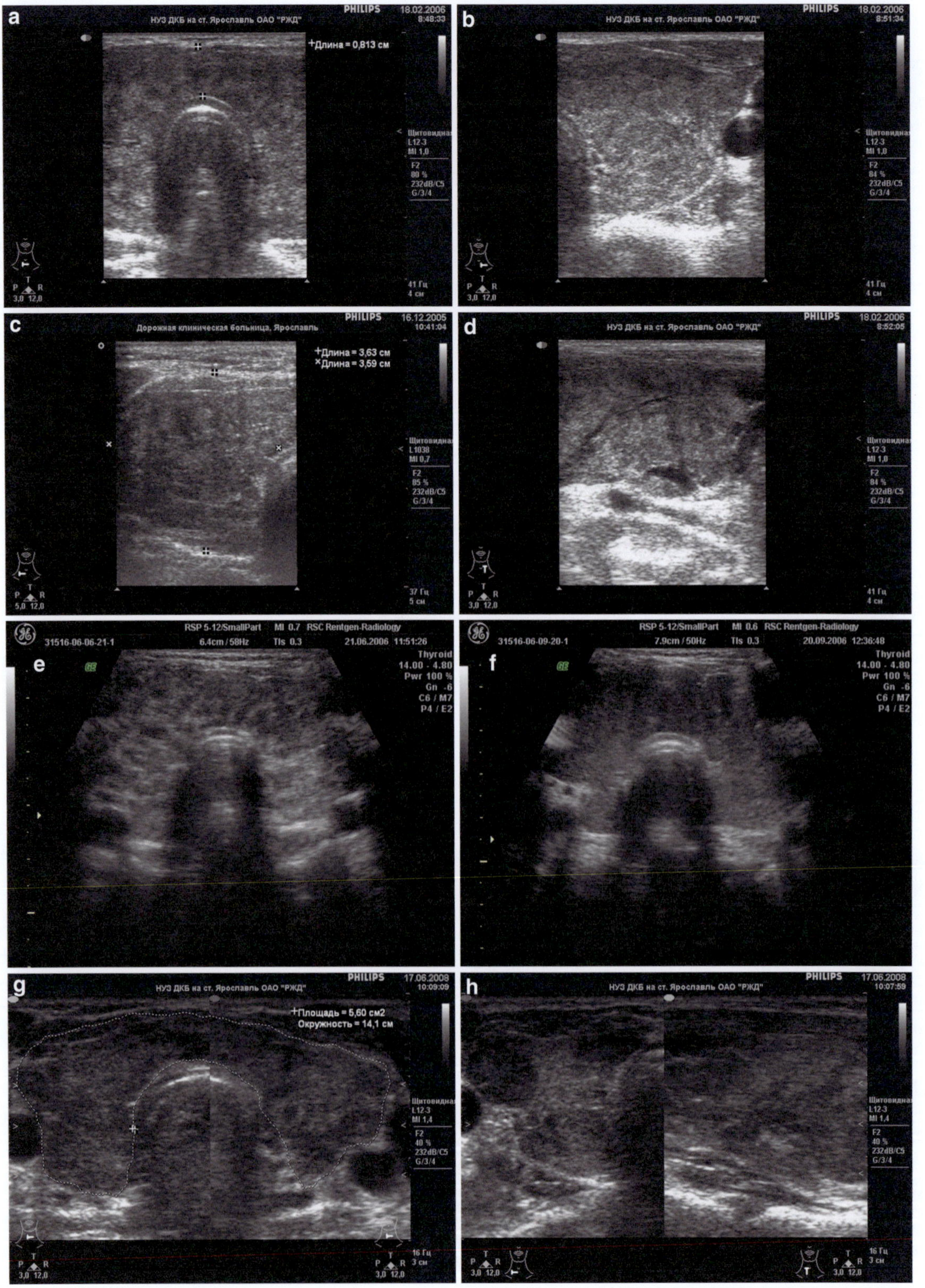

Fig. 5.15 (a–i) AITD. Grayscale

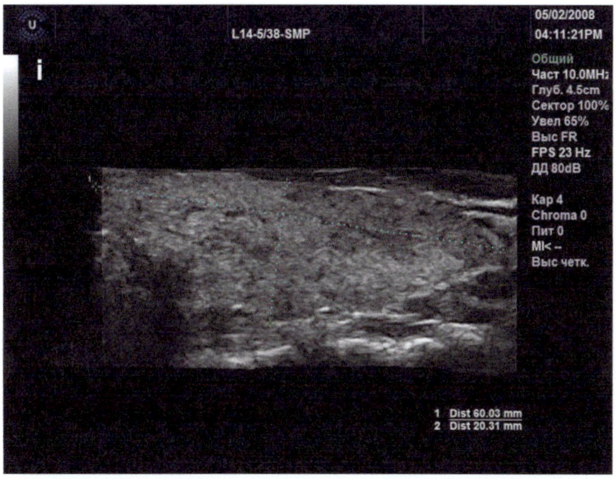

Fig. 5.15 (continued)

The signs of AIT are variable and include tuberosity of the back margin, an indistinct margin between the front surfaces of the thyroid lobes and the neck muscles (Pashchevsky 2004), blurred, rough contours, and regional lymph node enlargement.

Harchenko et al. (1999) proposed the following four types of AIT, based on US features:

1. Diffuse type, characterized by an enlarged thyroid with an ordinary shape, well-defined margins, and diffuse changes in parenchyma.
2. Focal type.
3. Diffuse-nodular type, characterized by a lesion or several lesions along with diffuse changes of the whole gland.
4. Mixed with nodules. This type exhibits true nodules with different echodensities and structures along with AIT.

The atrophic type of AIT shows a decrease in thyroid size and echodensity, structural heterogeneity, hypovascularity in CDI and PDI, and a dense pattern with sonoelastography (Figs. 5.16 and 5.17).

In hypertrophic AIT, the thyroid parenchyma contains small, heterogeneous, hypoechoic areas with inaccurate contours. In cases with intensification of cytotoxic processes, the thyroid gland enlarges with an increase in heterogeneity, a decrease in echodensity, and hypoechoic areas enlarge and tend to merge (Fig. 5.18). US may also detect pseudo-nodules (false nodules) in the autoimmune thyroid. This refers to local hypertrophy of the thyroid parenchyma that imitates a nodule (Figs. 5.17–5.20).

According to Gerasimov et al. (1998), the conclusion of "chronic AIT with the formation of nodules" is incorrect. The authors state that any lesion can occur in the autoimmune thyroid, but this is a different disease that often precedes the occurrence of AITD. According to Pashchevsky et al. (2001), the possibility of differentiating the focal type of AIT from the true nodule by means of US is doubtful (Table 5.1).

According to Bogazzi et al. (1996), the hypervascularity of the thyroid parenchyma and the increase in blood flow velocity in thyroid arteries correspond to the activity of the intrathyroidal autoimmune process. Lelyuk et al. (2007) report that Doppler modalities do not provide any extra value in AITD. The authors did not identify any significant change in blood flow in the afferent arteries with PW Doppler, or changes in the density of color pixels with CDI and PDI.

Markova (2001) reports that AIT is associated with statistically significant increases in blood flow velocities with PW Doppler in the upper thyroid arteries ($PSV = 21.4 \pm 1.2$ cm/s, $EDV = 7.6 \pm 0.47$ cm/s, $RI = 0.64 \pm 0.01$) and in the inferior thyroid arteries ($PSV = 23 \pm 1.13$ cm/s, $EDV = 7.97 \pm 0.49$ cm/s, $RI = 0.64 \pm 0.015$). Hamzina et al. (1999) provide the following data on blood flow in the parenchyma of the autoimmune thyroid: PSV = 0.3–0.75 m/s, RI = 0.44–0.79, PI = 0.7–1.7. The authors show that the PSV in the inferior thyroid artery in hypothyroidism is about 0.17 m/s, in euthyroidism it is 0.4 m/s, and in thyrotoxicosis it is 0.9–1.17 m/s (Fig. 5.21).

According to Ahuja et al. (2000), the parenchyma of the autoimmune thyroid is avascular in CDI. Hypertrophic AIT with hyperthyroidism is characterized by increased blood flow in the parenchyma and the connective tissue septa of the thyroid (Figs. 5.22 and 5.23). According to Kotlyarov et al. (2001), lesions in the diffuse-nodular type of AIT show hypervascularity in CDI, PDI, and 3DPD, with dilated arcade vessels in 85.7% of cases. Hamzina et al. (2007) suggest the following types of blood flow in the autoimmune thyroid, based on CDI:

- Diffuse hypervascularity with prevalence of arterial blood flow (60%)
- Increase in vascularity around the hypoechoic foci with arterial blood flow (20%)
- Moderate vascularity or a decrease in vascularity with prevalence of venous blood flow (20%)

The specificity of US for the diagnosis of AITD in grayscale, CDI, PDI, and 3D image reconstruction is about 68–94.8%; its sensitivity is 54.4–89.2% and its diagnostic accuracy is 92.1% (Markova 2001; Pashchevsky 2004; Miheeva 2007).

FNAB in patients with AIT is reasonable due to the possible combination of the disease with malignant epithelial tumors and lymphomas (Fig. 5.24). The majority of tumors found in combination with AITD correspond morphologically to papillary cancer (87.4%); follicular thyroid carcinoma is recorded less often. The combination of AITD with medullary and anaplastic cancer is extremely rare.

One frequent indirect sign of AITD is enlarged lymph nodes near the inferior poles of the thyroid lobes and isthmus. Lymph nodes can compose either a

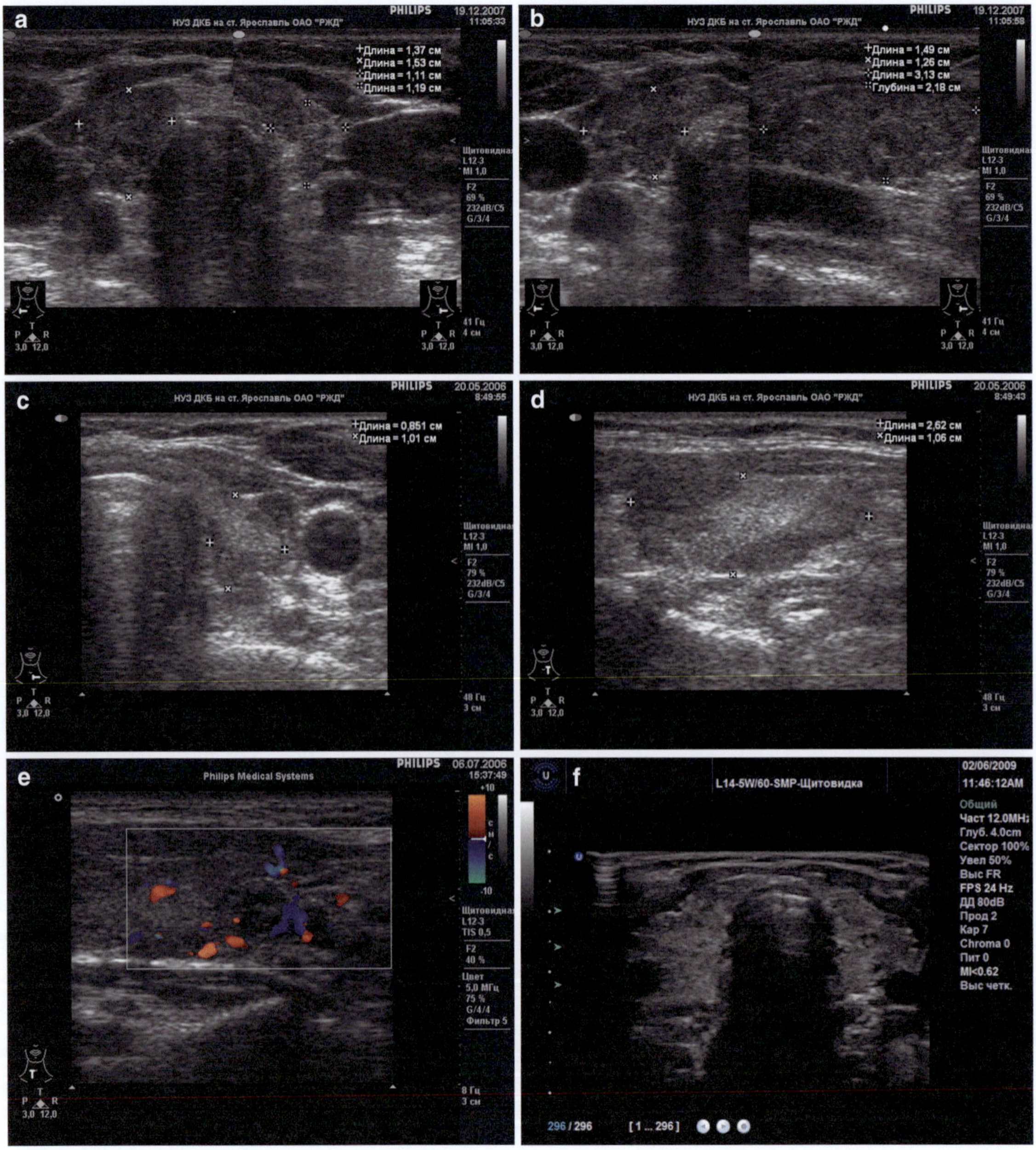

Fig. 5.16 (**a–g**) AITD. Atrophic form. (**a–d, f**) Grayscale, (**e**) CDI, and (**g**) sonoelastography

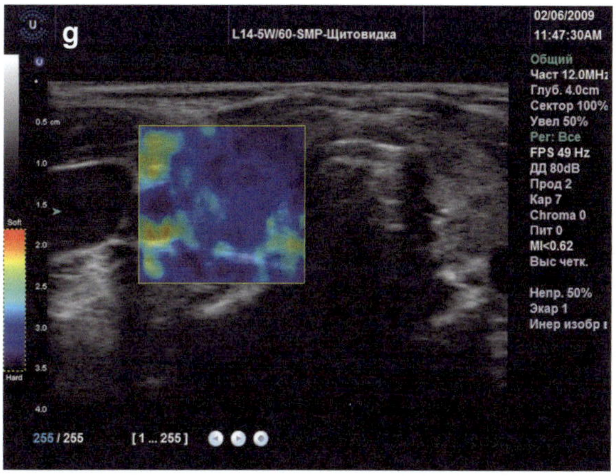

Fig. 5.16 (continued)

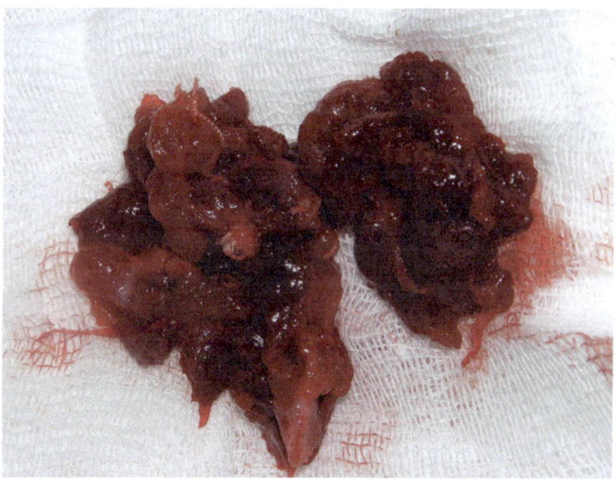

Fig. 5.17 Macroscopic view of the nodules with AIT

"mass" or a "chain" that spreads down to the anterior mediastinum. The nodules can exhibit homogeneous structure and decreased echodensity, or, less often, unchanged differentiation of the hilum, smooth well-defined margins, and oval or roundish shapes. Lymph node vascularization in CDI, PDI, and 3DPD is normally decreased with an unchanged vascular pattern.

5.2.4 Graves' Disease

Toxic diffuse goiter (Graves' disease, thyrotoxicosis with diffuse goiter) is a serious thyroid abnormality of the thyroid gland characterized by thyrotoxicosis. Its incidence is 20–25 in 100,000 people. Women 30–50 years of age suffer more often than other parts of the population (Dedov et al. 2001).

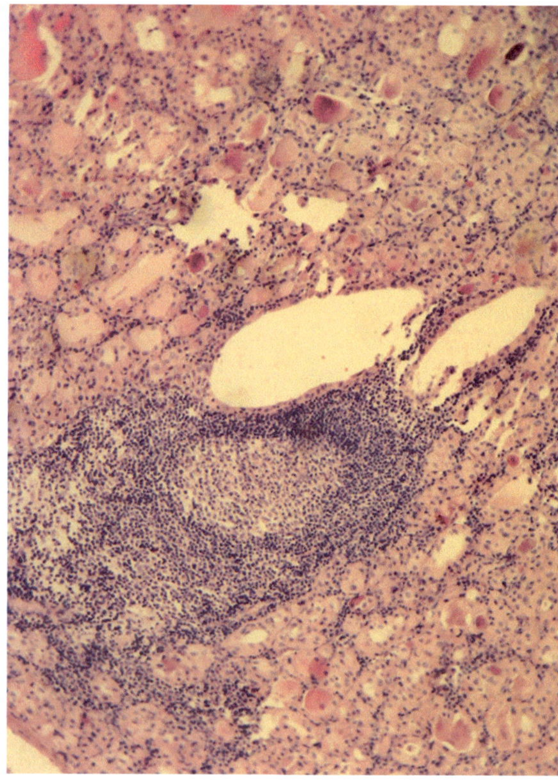

Fig. 5.18 AIT (hematoxylin and eosin stained smears; original magnification, ×200)

The basic US features of Graves'disease are as follows (Figs. 5.25–5.27):

- Volume change (usually symmetric enlargement of the entire thyroid)
- Protrusion of the anterior surfaces of the lobes, enlargement of the isthmus
- Diffuse decrease in echodensity
- Distinct lobular structure of the thyroid with stromal component and linear echogenic inclusions
- Significant symmetric hypervascularity of the parenchyma in CDI, PDI, and 3DPD
- Displacement of vascular bundles of the neck laterally or/and dorsally resulting from the enlargement of the thyroid lobes

PW Doppler in Graves' disease reveals a 8–10-fold increase in the PSV in the thyroid arteries. The PSV in the vessels of the thyroid parenchyma is 136.0 ± 26.4 cm/s,

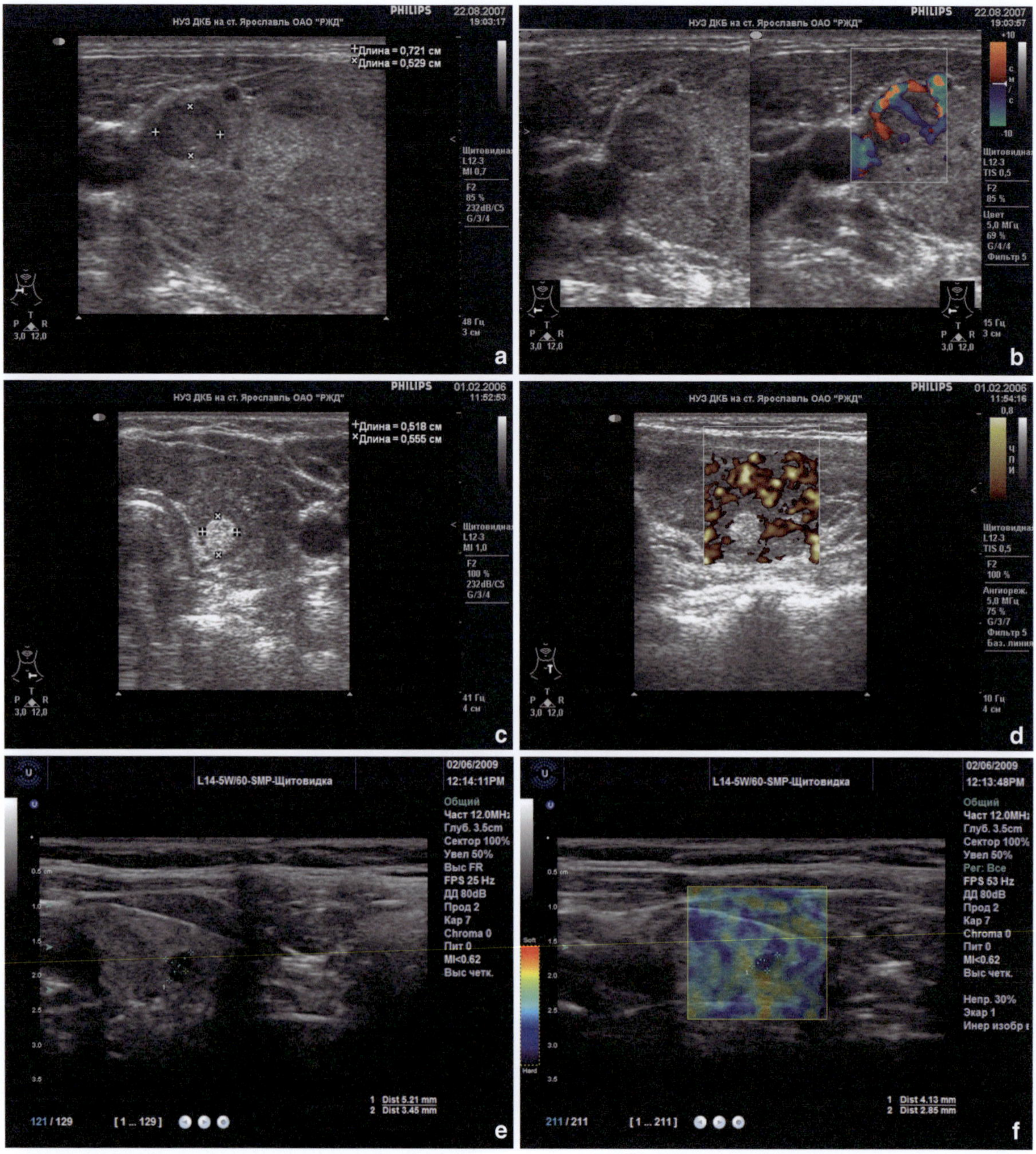

Fig. 5.19 (**a–f**) Thyroid nodule with AIT. Sonogram. (**a, c, e**) Grayscale, (**b**) CDI, (**d**) PDI, and (**e**) sonoelastography

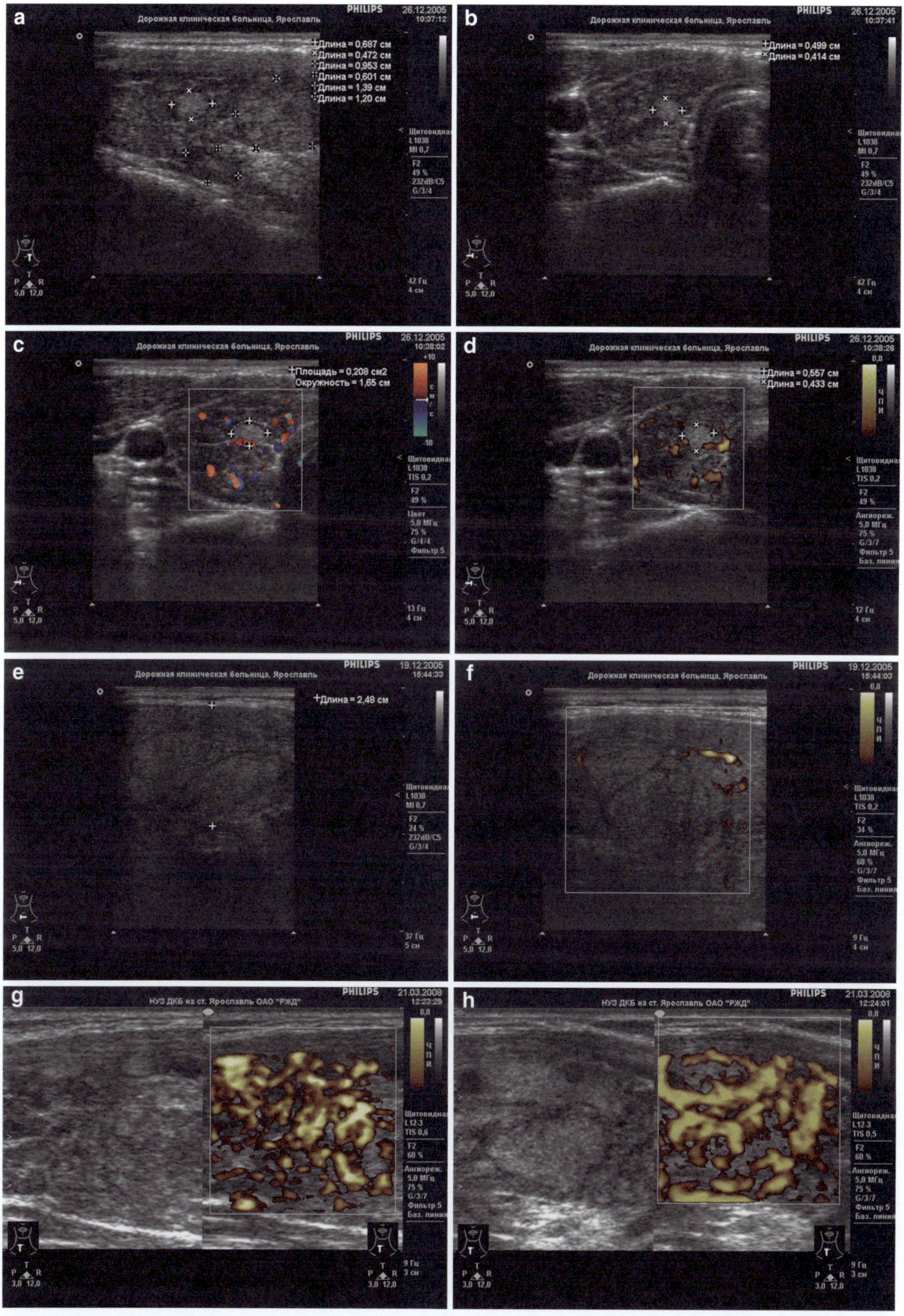

Fig. 5.20 (**a–h**) Pseudo-nodules of an autoimmune thyroid. Sonogram. (**a, b, e**) Grayscale, (**c**) CDI, and (**d, f, g, h**) PDI

Table 5.1 US criteria for nodules with AIT according to different authors

US features	Pripachkina (1997) $n=48$	Kotlyarov et al. (2001) $n=24$	Kurzantseva et al. (2006) $n=7$	Own data $n=300$
Shape:				
Oval	–	20.8		18.0
Spherical	100	62.5		71.3
Irregular	–	16.7		10.7
Margins:				
Smooth	91.7	87.5		91.3
Rough	8.3	12.8		8.7
Contours:				
Well defined	87.5	79.2	71.4	69.3
Indistinct	12.5	20.8	28.6	30.7
Halo:				
Hypoechoic	–	29.2	42.8	25.7
Absent	–	70.8	57.2	74.3
Echodensity:				
Hyper-	75.0	41.6	–	44.7
Iso-	–	29.2	71.4	34.3
Hypo-	18.8	29.2	28.6	21
An-	–	–	–	–
Echostructure:				
Homogeneous	35.4	45.8		52.3
Heterogeneous	64.6	54.2		47.7
Calcifications:				
Present	2.1	12.5		11.3
Absent	–	87.5		88.7
Posterior enhancement:				
Present	–	12.5		9.3
Absent	–	87.5		90.7
Thyroid capsule:				
Unchanged				99.3
Irregular				0.7
Vascularity:				
Avascular	–	–	28.5	–
Perinodular	–	100	71.5	100
Among them:	–	85.7	–	76.3
Hypervascular	–	14.3	–	23.7
Hypovascular				

a b

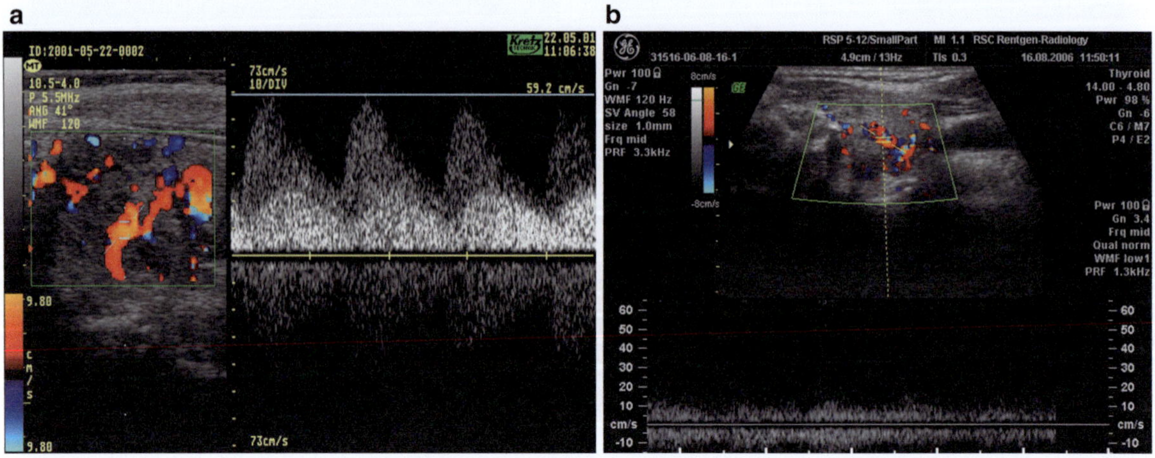

Fig. 5.21 (**a, b**) AITD. PW Doppler

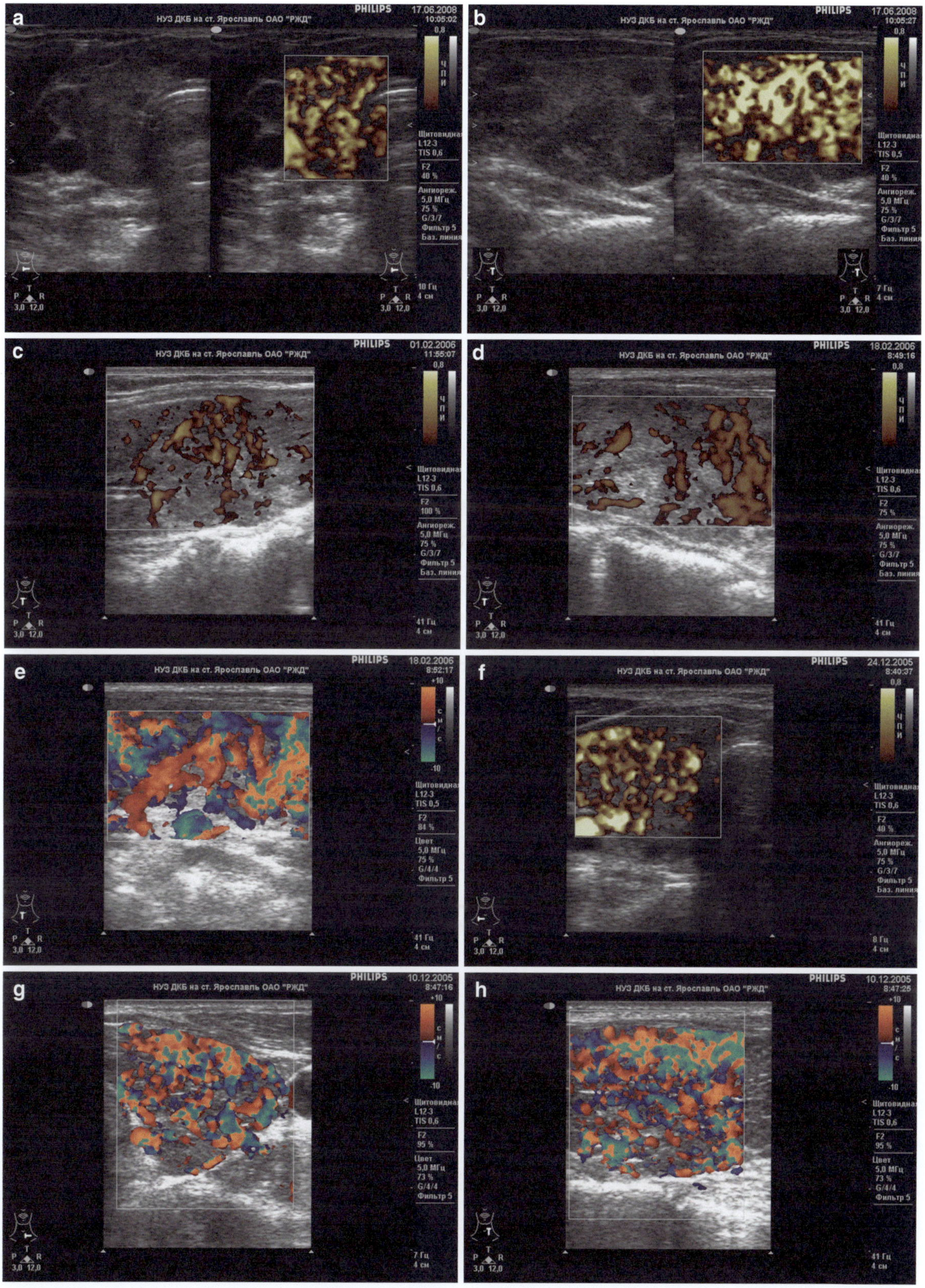

Fig. 5.22 (**a–n**) AITD. Diffuse hypervascularity. CDI and PDI

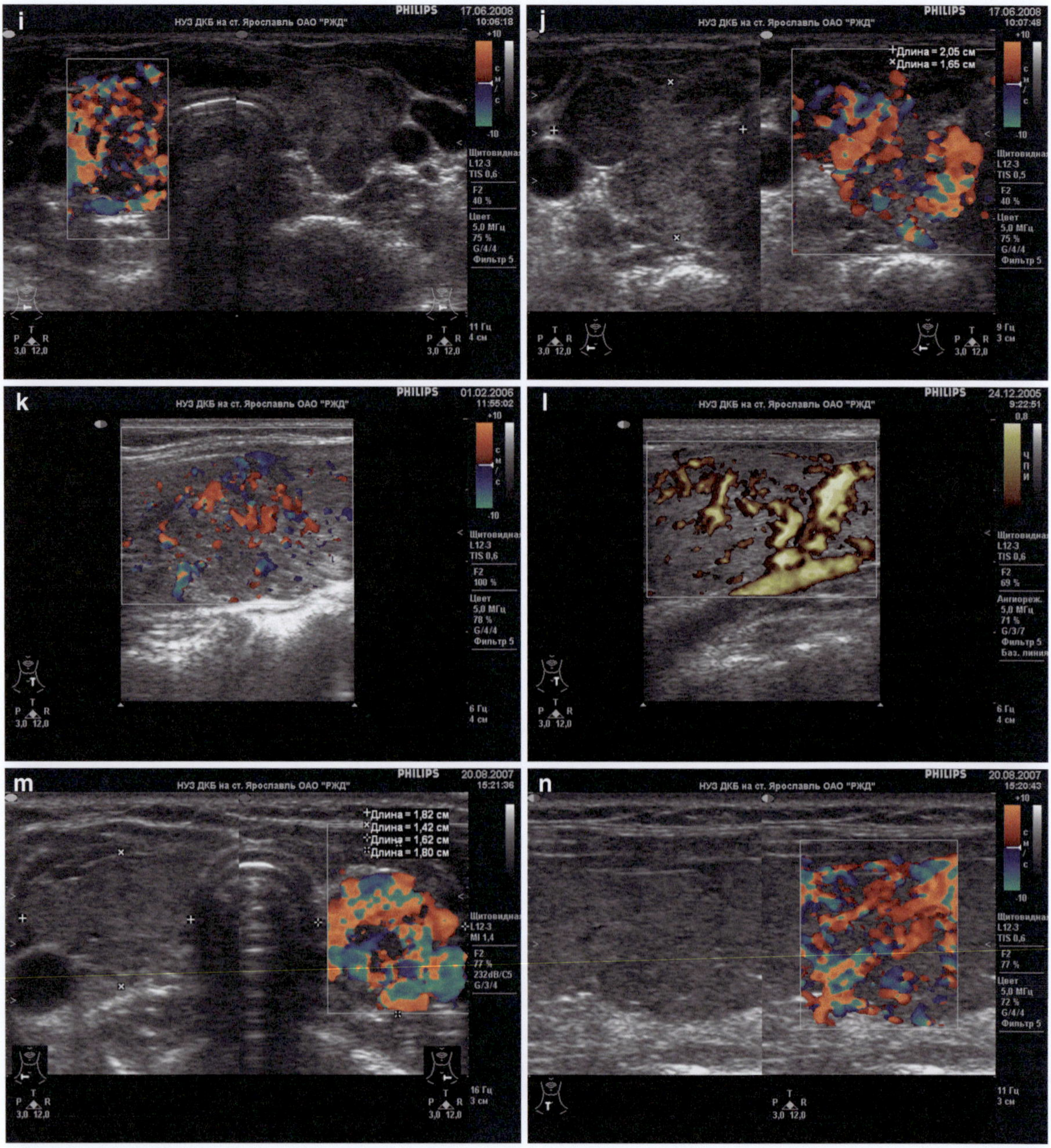

Fig. 5.22 (continued)

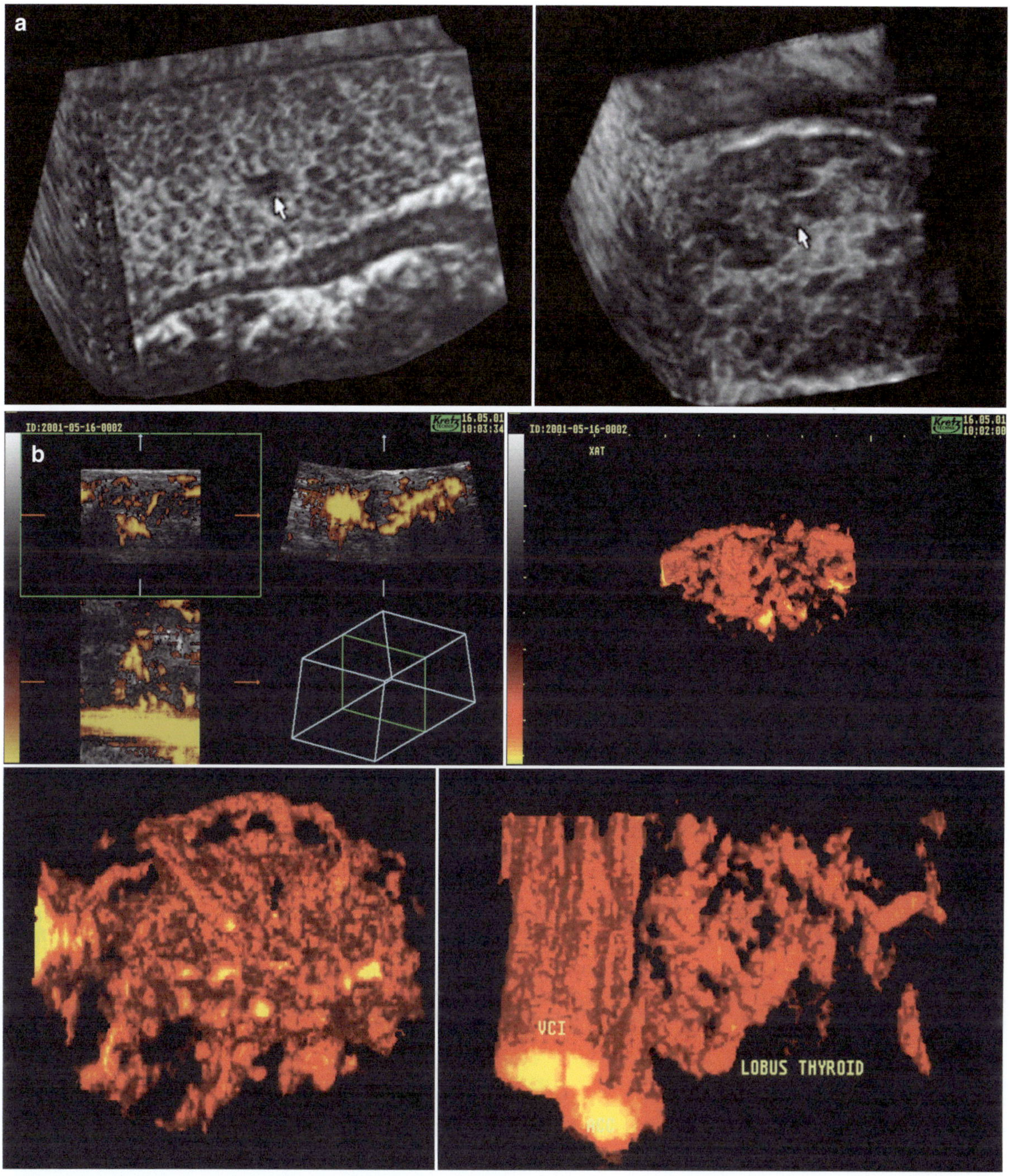

Fig. 5.23 AITD. (**a**) 3D reconstruction. (**b**) 3DPD

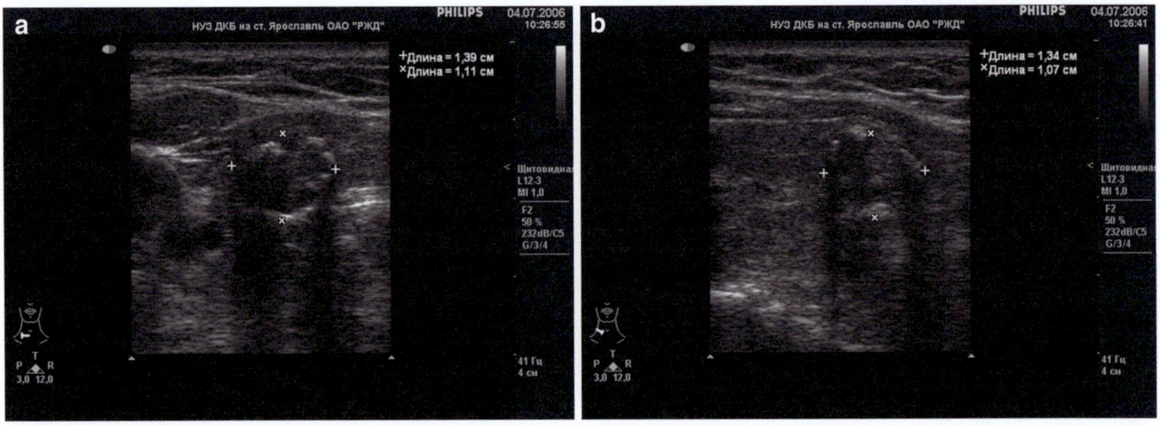

Fig. 5.24 (**a, b**) Thyroid cancer with AITD. Grayscale

The example of US report in AITD

First name, middle initial, last name:
Age:
Date:
The number of case history:
US scanner:
The thyroid gland is typically located with irregular and locally blurred margins.

The depth of the **isthmus** - 13 mm	
Right lobe	**Left lobe**
Depth 27 mm Width 26 mm Length 50 mm	Depth 25 mm Width 24 mm Length 50 mm
Volume 17.5 cm^3	Volume 15.0 cm^3

The total volume 32.5 cm^3 exceeds the upper limit for the endemic region and the WHO recommendations.
The echodensity of the thyroid parenchyma is moderately decreased with heterogeneous echostructure and hypoechoic areas of 0.2-0.7 cm in size with irregular indistinct contours. The stromal component is insignificant. Vascular architectonics of the parenchyma in CDI and PDI is unchanged. Blood flow intensity is significantly increased. CPD is 20-25 %.
The topographic relation of the thyroid gland with the muscles and neck organs is typical.
Several hypoechoic avascular lymph nodes up to 0.5x0.8 cm in size are located close to the inferior poles of both lobes.
The lymph nodes along vascular bundles of the neck are up to 0.8-1.6 cm in size, heterogeneous with regular well-defined margins, unchanged differentiation and vascularity. The lymph nodes in supraclavicular areas are not enlarged.
CONCLUSION: The 3 degree of the increase in thyroid volume. Diffuse changes of the thyroid gland suspicious for autoimmune thyroiditis.
US specialist:

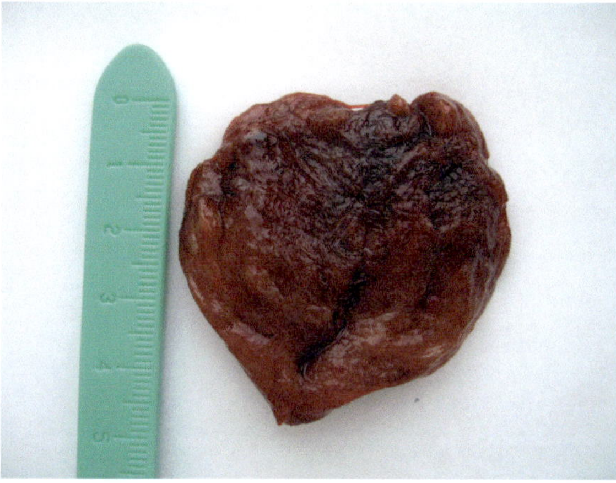

Fig. 5.25 Graves' disease. Macroscopic view

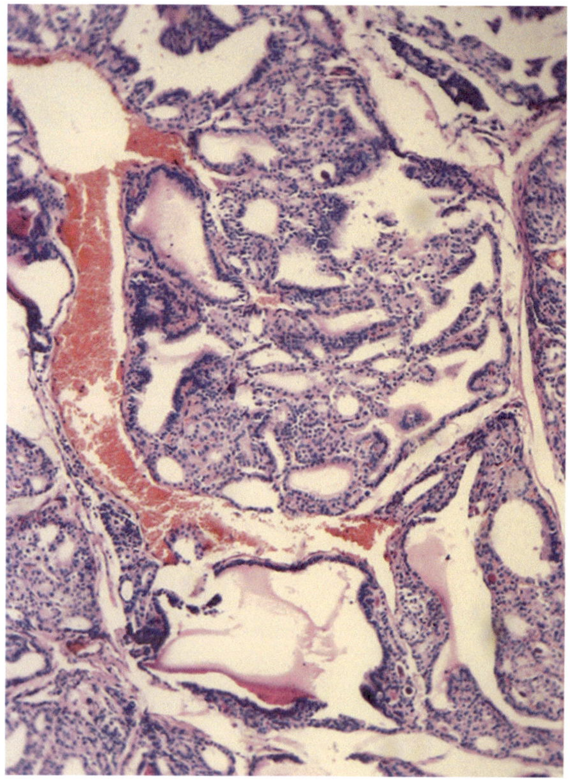

Fig. 5.26 Graves' disease (hematoxylin and eosin stained smears; original magnification, ×200)

and the RI decreases to 0.64 ± 0.11 (Argalia et al. 1997). According to Lelyuk et al. (2007), patients with an active autoimmune process and thyrotoxicosis demonstrate significantly increased blood flow velocity in afferent thyroid arteries (TAMX is 30–180 cm/s), although the resistance index may be increased (RI is 0.7–0.8) or decreased (RI is 0.3–0.5). An increase in blood flow volume velocity in the arteries of parenchyma up to 70–500 mL/min is also characteristic.

The vascularity of the thyroid gland in CDI, PDI, and 3DPD in Graves' disease appears, as a rule, to be significantly increased. According to Ralls et al. (1988), Markova (2001), and Lelyuk et al. (2007), a "thyroid inferno" is often noted due to extreme hypervascularity. The vessels are usually distributed regularly within the parenchyma and show rectilinear character. The number of color cartograms per area unit increases (CPD is 20–50%). The degree of hypervascularization in Graves' disease often depends on the histological type and the clinical development of the disease (Figs. 5.28–5.31) (Castagnone et. al. 1996; Zabolotskaya et al. 2006). Blood flow data from PW Doppler, CDI, PDI, and 3DPD in patients with long-term remission from Graves' disease may remain normal or increased.

Thyroid lesions of various origins may arise in 10–27% of cases of Graves' disease. They are more often observed in patients over 60 years of age with long-term disease (Tsyb et al. 1997). The total frequency of thyroid carcinoma in Graves' disease is about 3.4–12% (Romanchishen et al. 2005; Yano et al. 2007; Erbil et al. 2008).

The specificity of US in grayscale, CDI, PDI, and 3D for the diagnosis of Graves' disease is about 96.3%; its sensitivity is 80.3% and its diagnostic accuracy is 92.9% (Markova 2001).

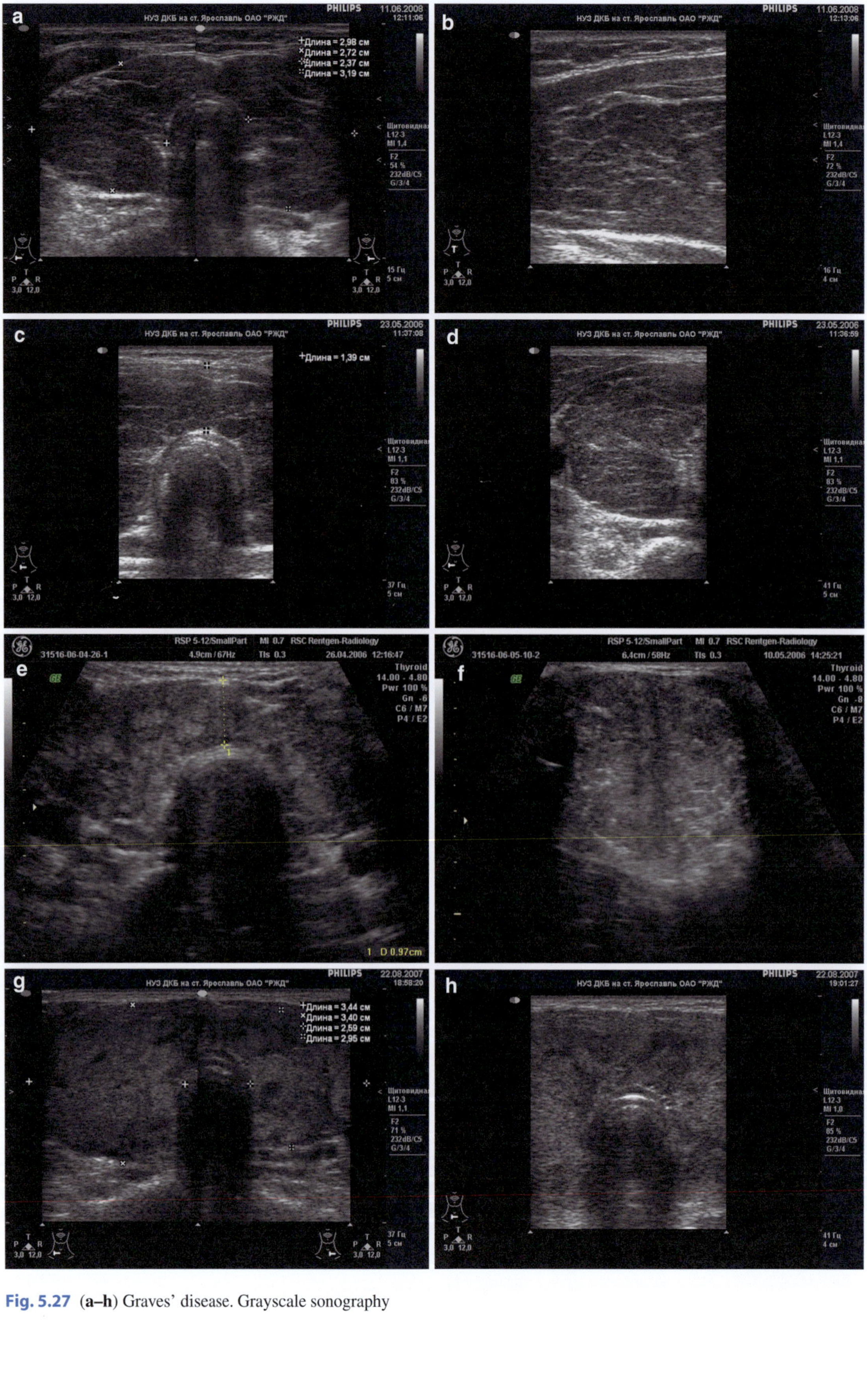

Fig. 5.27 (**a–h**) Graves' disease. Grayscale sonography

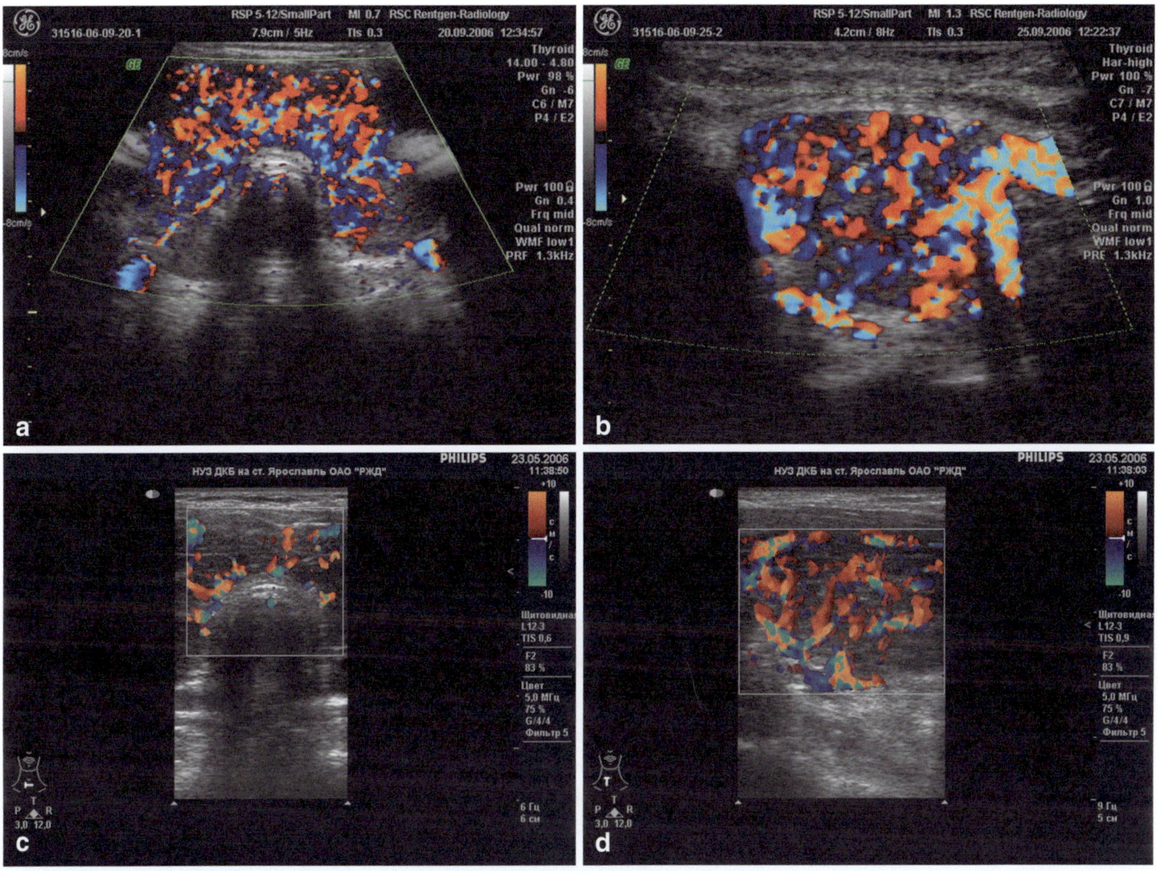

Fig. 5.28 (**a–d**) Graves' disease. Hypervascularity of the parenchyma, the "thyroid inferno" pattern in CDI

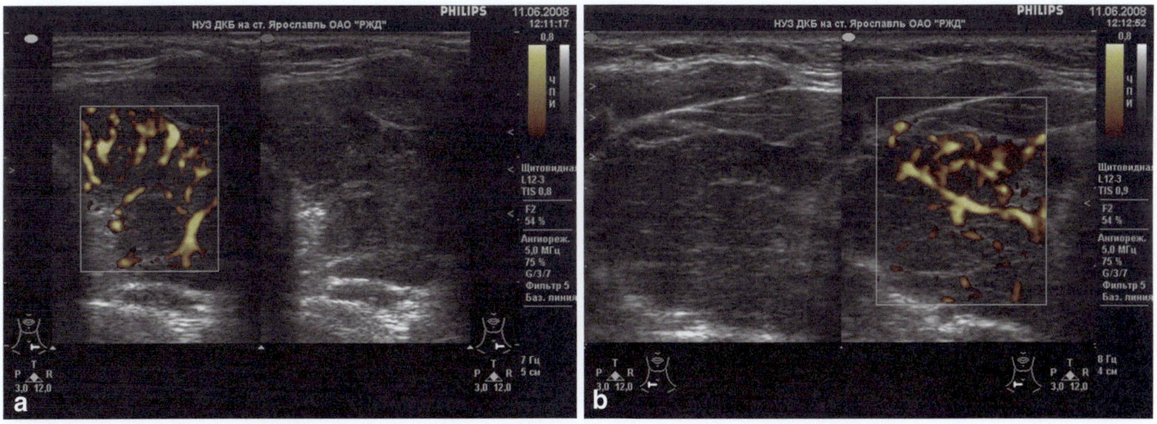

Fig. 5.29 (**a–d**) Graves' disease. PDI

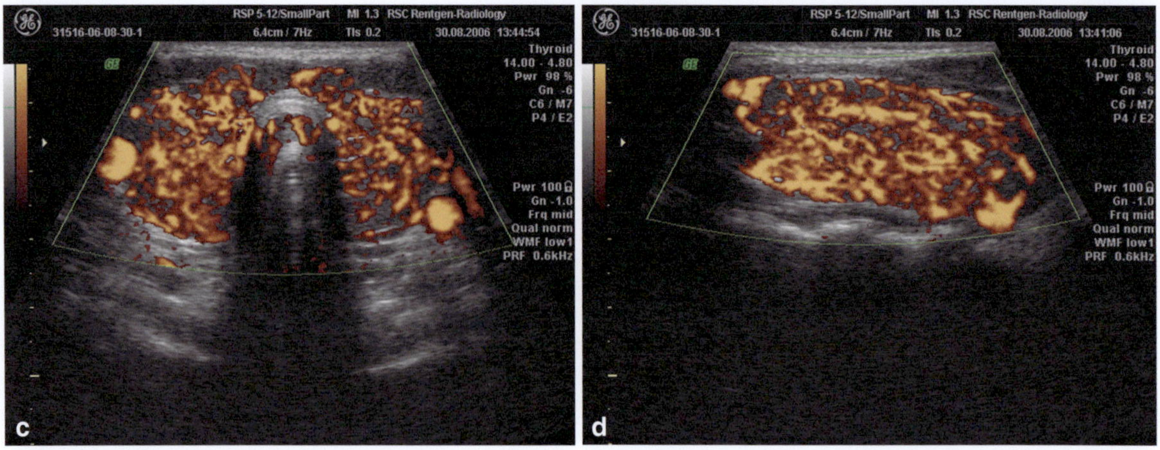

Fig. 5.29 (continued)

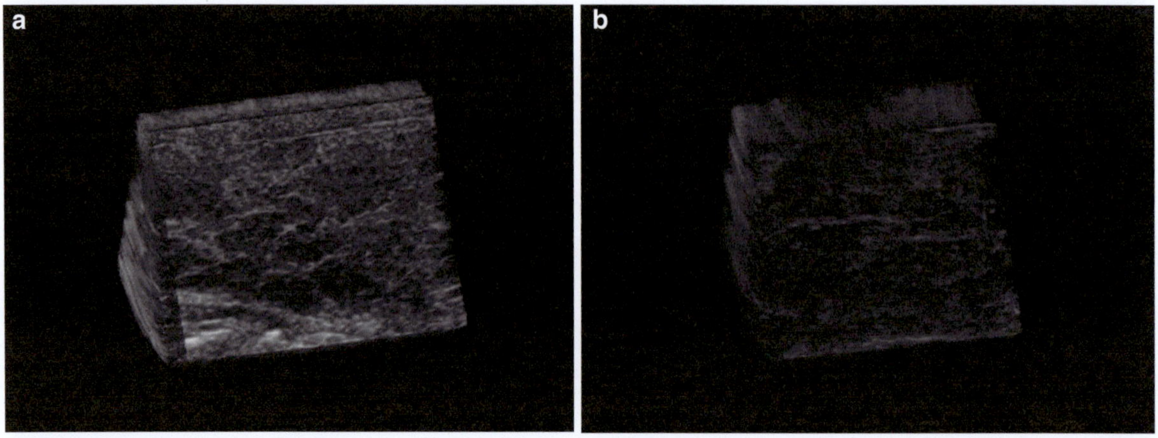

Fig. 5.30 (**a, b**) Graves' disease. 3D reconstruction

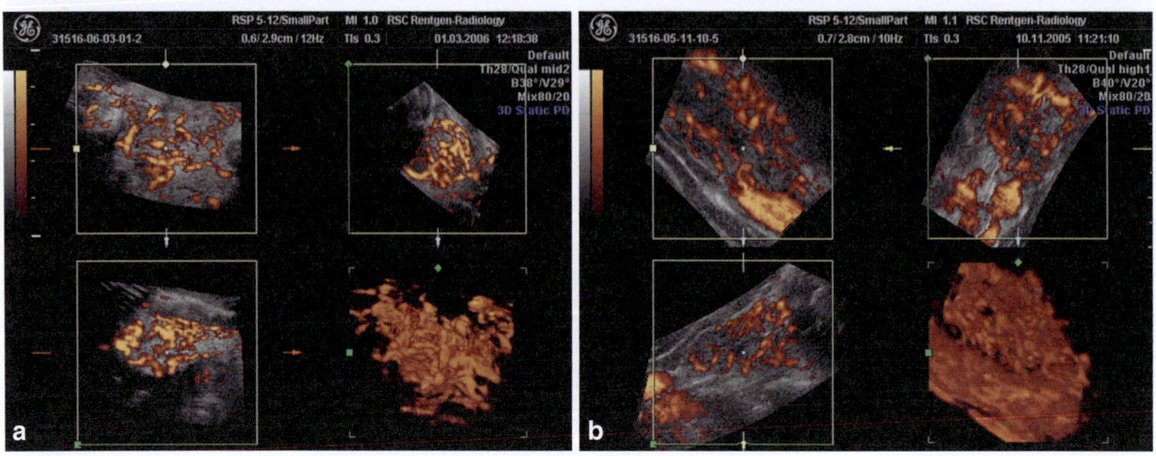

Fig. 5.31 (**a–d**) Graves' disease. 3DPD

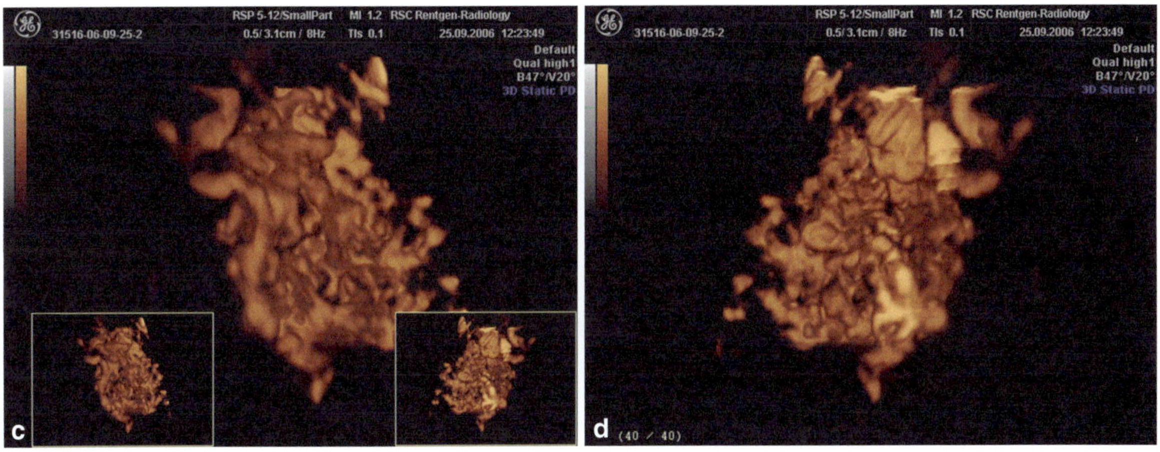

Fig. 5.31 (continued)

The example of US report in Graves' disease

First name, middle initial, last name:
Age:
Date:
The number of case history:
US scanner:
The thyroid gland is typically located with irregular well defined margins and distinct lobular structure.

The depth of the **isthmus** - 14 mm	
Right lobe	**Left lobe**
Depth 27 mm Width 26 mm Length 64 mm	Depth 28 мм Width 24 мм Length 58 мм
Volume 22.5 cm^3	Volume 19.5 см^3

The total volume 42 cm^3 exceeds the upper limit for the endemic region and the WHO recommendations.
The echodensity of the thyroid parenchyma is significantly diffusely decreased and moderately heterogeneous.
The blood flow intensity is significantly increased in CDI, PDI, and 3DPD. CPD is 30-40 %. Vascular pattern is symmetric. Vascular bundles of the neck are moderately displaced laterally.
The lymph nodes along the vascular bundles of the neck are up to 0.4x0.9 cm in size, heterogeneous with regular well-defined margins, unchanged differentiation and vascularity. The lymph nodes in supraclavicular areas are not enlarged.
CONCLUSION: The 3 degree of the increase in thyroid volume. Diffuse changes of the thyroid gland and vascularity suspicious for Graves' disease.
US specialist:

6 Thyroid Lesions

Nodular goiter is a clinical concept that does not always coincide with a morphological definition. In clinical practice it is thought to mean a thyroid lesion of any size having a capsule that may be defined by palpation or by means of any visualization modality (Dedov et al. 2001). According to Gerasimov (1998) and Fadeev (2002), the term "nodular goiter" may be applicable in the case of a thyroid lesion larger than 10 mm in size that is defined by palpation or any diagnostic method. "A multinodular goiter" is characterized by the presence of two or more nodules, which can be located in the isthmus, in one lobe, or in both lobes of the thyroid gland (Kalinin et al. 2004).

Thyroid nodules are detected in 4–15% of the population. The nodules are observed in more than 50% of patients with thyroid pathology; the incidence of nodules can reach 98.9% in endemic regions (Vetshev et al. 2005). Thyroid nodules are identified in more than half of all autopsies (Ashcraft and van Herle 1981; Burch 1995). The incidence of nodular goiter correlates with age.

Thyroid lesions include both colloid nodules and tumors. The latter are divided into the following groups according to the WHO histological classification (1988):

1. Epithelial tumors
   (a) Benign
      - Follicular adenoma
      - Others

   (b) Malignant
      - Follicular carcinoma
      - Papillary carcinoma
      - Medullary carcinoma
      - Undifferentiated (anaplastic) carcinoma
      - Others
2. Nonepithelial tumors
   (a) Benign
   (b) Malignant
3. Malignant lymphomas
4. Miscellaneous tumors
5. Secondary tumors
6. Unclassified tumors
7. Tumor-like lesions

Thyroid lesions are assessed by the following US criteria:

1. Number of nodules
2. Location (in lobes and segments, in relation to the capsule, vascular bundles, or trachea)
3. Dimensions
4. Shape (roundish, oval, irregular)
5. Borders (smooth, rough)
6. Contours (well defined, indistinct)
7. Echodensity
8. Echostructure (the degree heterogeneity)
9. Calcifications (the dimensions, location, and presence of acoustic shadowing)
10. Fluid component (the dimensions and the ratio of fluid to solid components)
11. Peripheral halo
12. Posterior echo change (enhancement or shadowing)
13. Vascularity

Thyroid nodules may be solitary, multiple (two and more), or conglomeratic (when some nodules merge into one lesion).

The dimensions of nodules are measured in three mutually perpendicular planes. Each dimension (length, width, or depth) is the maximum between the opposite margins of the lesion.

V.P. Kharchenko et al., *Ultrasound Diagnostics of Thyroid Diseases*,
DOI: 10.1007/978-3-642-12387-0_6,

Nodule volume is calculated by the standard formula: $V_{nod} = (a \times b \times c) \times 0.52$, where a, b, c are the length, width, and depth of the nodule respectively (Pacella et al. 1995). The calculation of nodule volume in addition to its dimensions is important for precise dynamic follow-up of the thyroid lesions in cases of conservative treatment or minimally invasive modalities.

6.1 Colloid Goiter

Colloid goiter (nontoxic uninodular/multinodular goiter, simple goiter, nodular hyperplasia) accounts for 60–75% of all thyroid lesions (Figs. 6.1 and 6.2).

The basic US features of colloid nodules are as follows (Figs. 6.3, 6.6, and 6.7, Table 6.1):

- Oval (or roundish) shape
- Well-defined, smooth margins
- Intact thyroid capsule
- Decreased or unchanged echodensity in most cases
- Heterogeneous structure, often without large fluid collections
- Possible calcifications within the lesion and peripheral "egg-shell" calcification
- Hypoechoic surrounding ring
- Possible posterior echo enhancement
- A- or hypovascularity in CDI, PDI, and 3DPD (individual color spots)

Obligatory US features of colloid nodule are well-defined margins and intact capsule of both the nodule and thyroid gland. Long-lasting colloid nodules may demonstrate individual calcifications in the periphery of the node, shell-shaped or "egg-shell" impregnations (Evans 1987). A calcium capsule may be observed in 2–4% of cases and can reach 2–3 mm thick (Fig. 6.4). The peripheral calcification significantly differs from microcalcifications and large coarse echogenic inclusions, which are often detected in thyroid cancer.

70–80% of colloid goiters appear to be multinodular (Fig. 6.5). Multiple nodules often show identical echostructure. Combinations of colloid nodules with cysts, adenomas, or thyroid cancer are seen more rarely (Tsyb et al. 1997).

Belashkin et al. (2003) reported that the second harmonic option allowed the quality of visualization of the structure of colloid nodules to be improved in 80% of cases, an absence of additional data was noted in 15%, and a decrease in the quality of visualization in 5% of cases. The improvement in visualization was associated with the increase in sharpness in 33%, clarifying the heterogeneity of the nodules in 13%, detection of

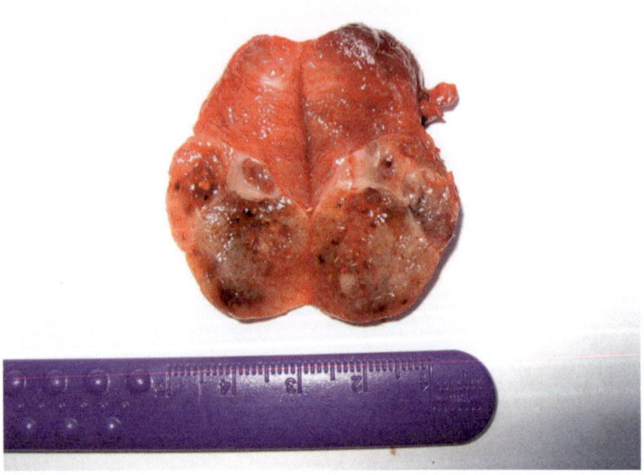

Fig. 6.1 Colloid nodules. Macroscopic view

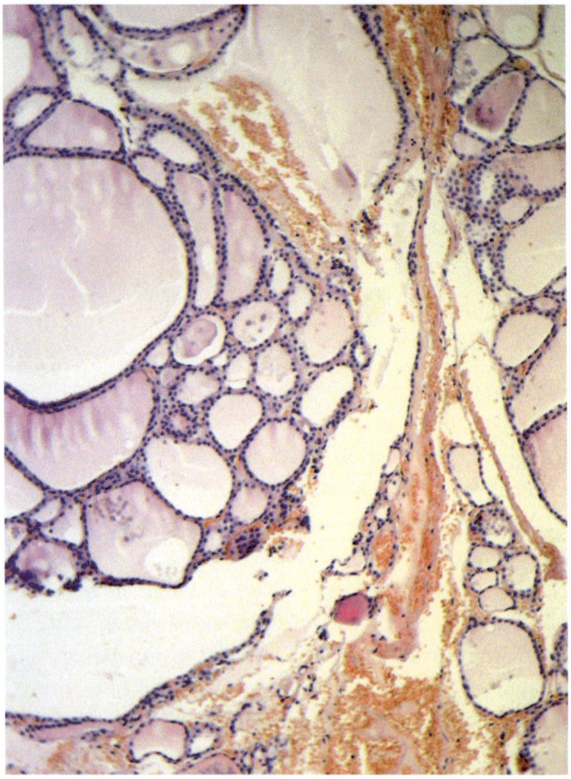

Fig. 6.2 Colloid goiter with fluid component (hematoxylin and eosin stained smears; original magnification, ×200)

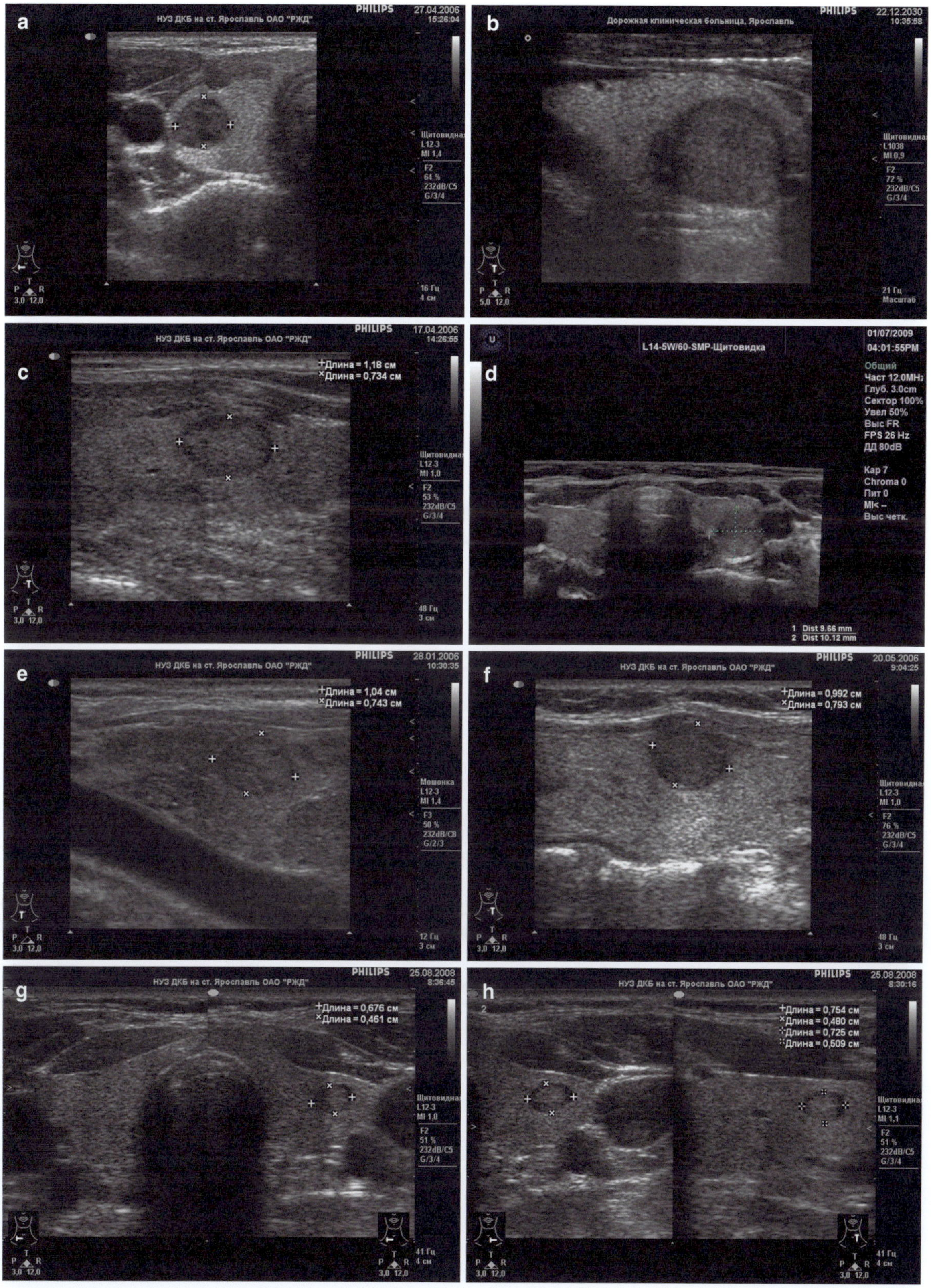

Fig. 6.3 (**a–h**) Colloid nodule. Grayscale sonography

Table 6.1 Sonographic features of colloid goiter

US features	Tsyb et al. (1997) $n=85$	Romanko (1997) $n=85$	Pripachkina (1997) $n=276$	Zubarev et al. (2000) $n=22$	Markova et al. (2001) $n=62$	Pashchevsky (2004) $n=1208$	Own data $n=700$
The shape:							
Oval	84	52–72	43	-	-	98	66.0
Spherical	15	28–31	48				30.3
Irregular	1	0–17	9				3.7
Margins:							
Smooth	98	100	100	82	74.1	96	86.7
Rough	2	–	–	18	25.9	4	13.3
Contours:							
Well defined	100	100	66	–	–	97	89.3
Indistinct	–	–	34			3	10.7
Halo:							
Hypoechoic	62	61	–	–	–	–	58.7
Absent	38	39					41.3
Echodensity:							
Hyper-	–	–	–	5	–	78	3.0
Iso-				59	50		53.3
Hypo-				36	41.9		43.7
An-				–	8.1		–
Echostructure:							
Homogeneous	18	14–23	67	32	–	15	32.3
Heterogeneous	82	67–86	33	68		85	67.7
Calcifications:							
Present	62	3–10	–	14	9.7	–	8.3
Absent	38	90–97		86	90.3		91.7
Posterior enhancement:							
Present	86	41–78	17.8	–	–	–	22.7
Absent	14	22–59	82.2				77.3
Thyroid capsule:							
Unchanged	100	100	–	–	–	99	96.3
Irregular	–	–				1	3.7
Vascularity:							
Avascular	–	–	–	9	27.5		28.7
Hypovascular				27	58		49.0
Hypervascular							22.3

calcifications in 19%, and the fluid component in 10% of cases.

Colloid nodules show a peripheral pattern of blood flow with individual vascular signals in CDI in 40–50% of cases. This pattern is associated with the benign character of the nodules. According to Zubarev et al. (2000) and Markova et al. (2001), the vascular pattern in colloid nodules in CDI and PDI shows rectilinear vascular structures that are normally distributed within the nodule (Figs. 6.6 and 6.7).

The specificities of US in grayscale, CDI, PDI, and 3D at diagnosing colloid nodules are 32.1, 47.6, 69.6, and 84.1%; their sensitivities are 70.7, 61.6, 65.5, and 75.7%, and their diagnostic accuracies are 53.1, 56.5, 70.3, and 79.8%, respectively (Markova 2001). According to Zubarev et al. (1999), Doppler options and 3D reconstruction increase the sensitivity of sonography to colloid nodules by 5% (up to 75.5%), the specificity by 52% (up to 84.1%), and the diagnostic accuracy by 26.7% (up to 79.8%).

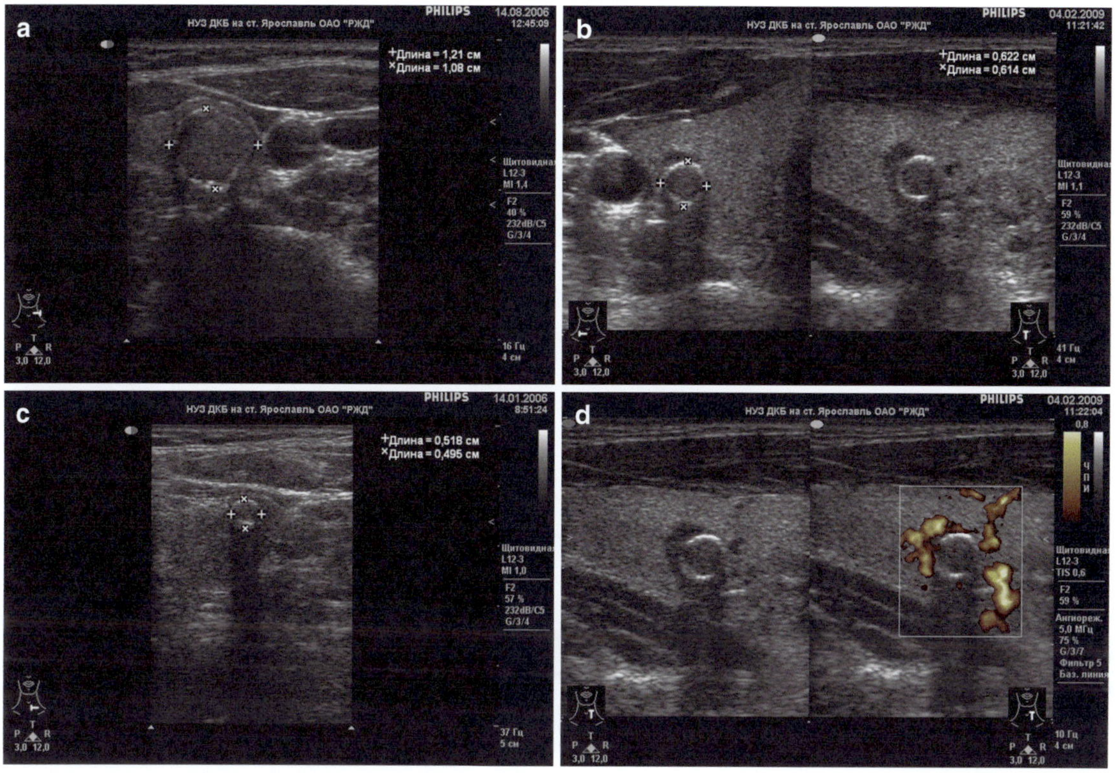

Fig. 6.4 **(a–d)** Colloid nodule. "Egg-shell" calcification. Grayscale and PDI

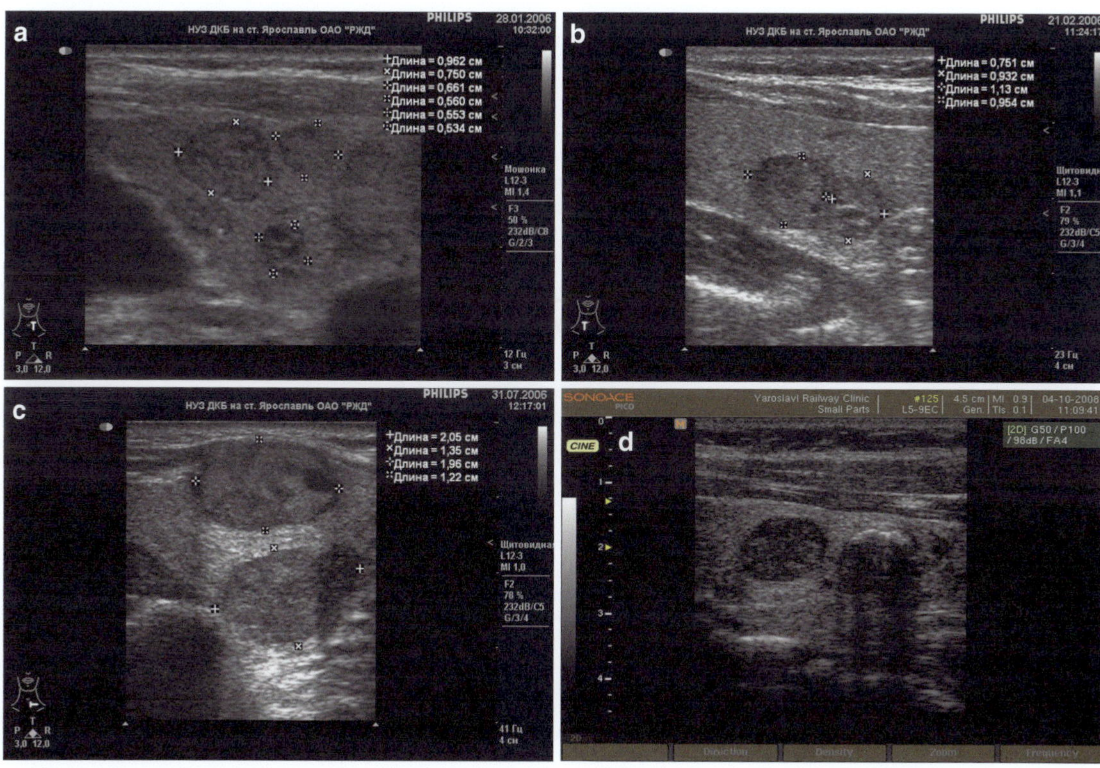

Fig. 6.5 **(a–c)** Multiple colloid nodules. Grayscale sonography

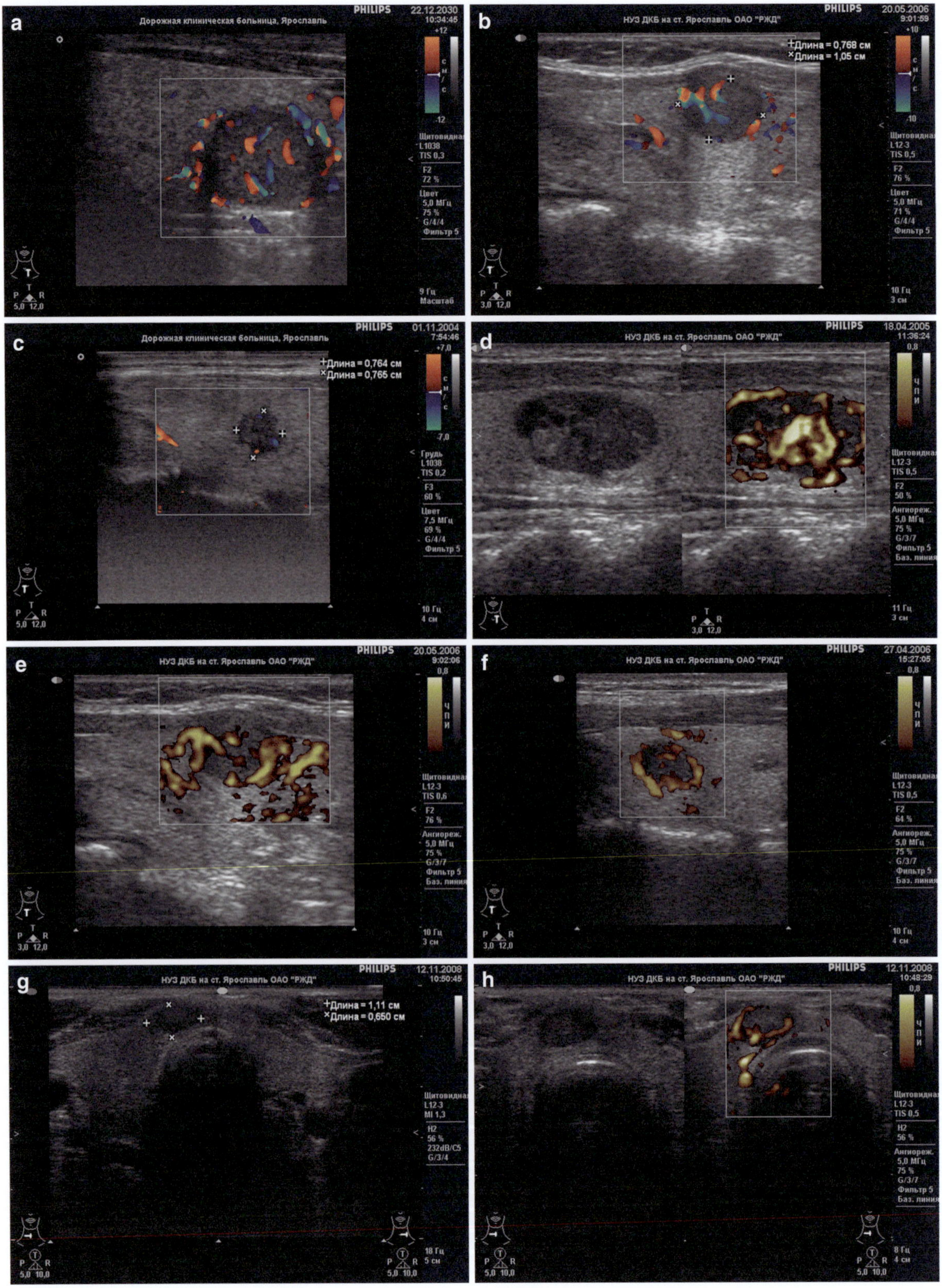

Fig. 6.6 (**a–h**) Colloid nodules. CDI and PDI

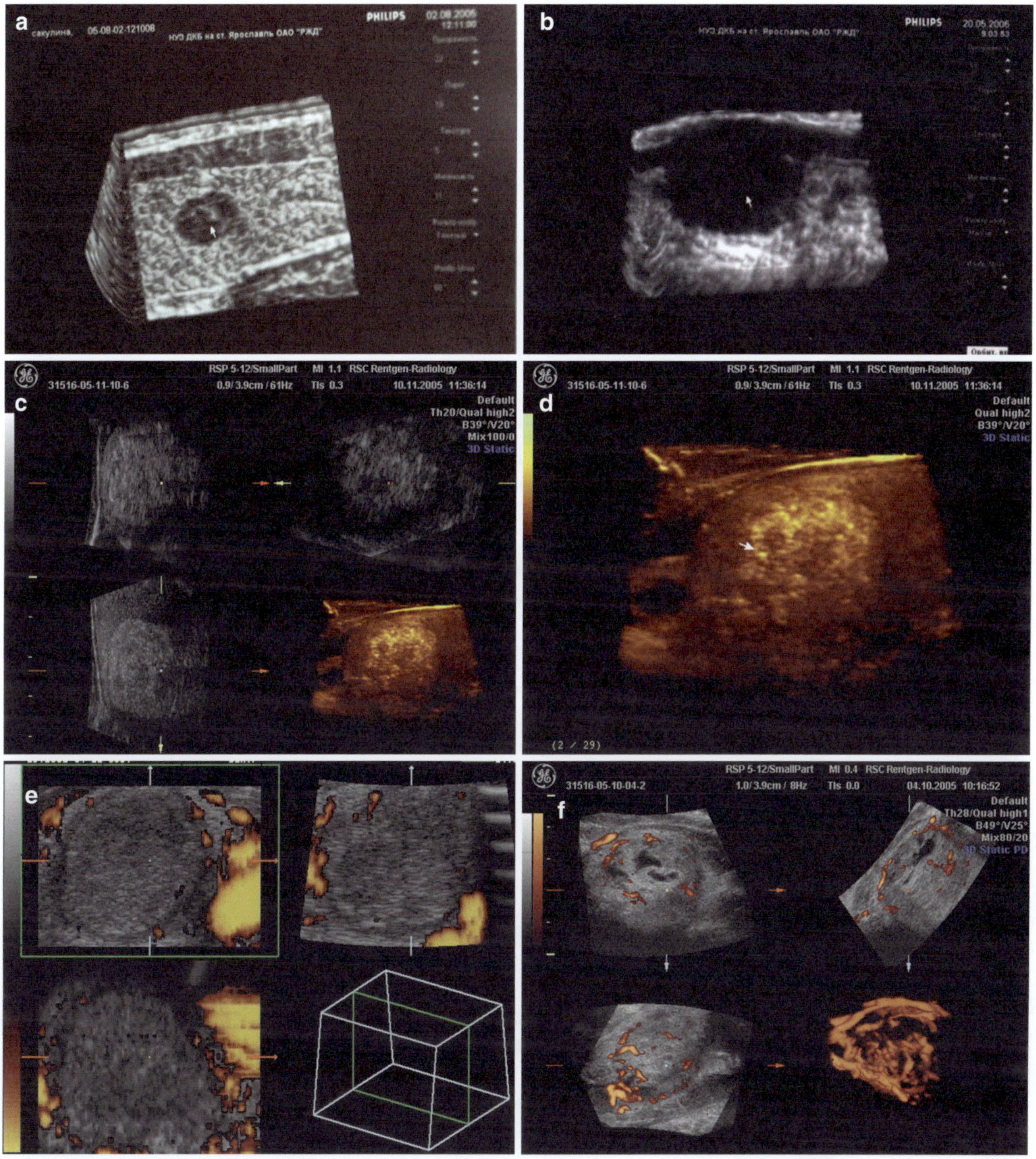

Fig. 6.7 (**a–f**) Colloid nodule. 3D reconstruction and 3DPD

The example of US report in colloid nodules

First name, middle initial, last name:
Age:
Date:
The number of case history:
US scanner:
The thyroid gland is located typically with regular well-defined margins and homogeneous isoechoic structure. The capsule is uniform and continuous on all extent.

<table>
<tr><td colspan="2">The depth of the isthmus - 4 mm</td></tr>
<tr><th>Right lobe</th><th>Left lobe</th></tr>
<tr><td>Depth 12 mm
Width 16 mm
Length 48 mm</td><td>Depth 14 mm
Width 16 mm
Length 50 mm</td></tr>
<tr><td>Volume 4.6 cm^3</td><td>Volume 5.6 cm^3</td></tr>
<tr><td colspan="2">The total volume 10.2 cm^3 does not exceed the upper limit for the endemic region and the WHO recommendations</td></tr>
<tr><td>A hypoechoic heterogeneous hypovascular nodule of 0.5x0.5x0.6 cm in size of roundish shape with well-defined regular margins is located in the middle compartment of the lobe.</td><td>A hypoechoic homogeneous avascular nodule of 0.8x0.7x0.9 cm in size with well-defined regular margins is located in the inferior segment of the lobe.</td></tr>
</table>

The vascular pattern of the parenchyma in CDI and PDI is unchanged.
The topographic relation of the thyroid gland with the muscles and neck organs is typical.
The lymph nodes in the neck and supraclavicular areas are not enlarged.
CONCLUSION: Thyroid nodules, most probably colloid goiter.
US specialist:

6.2 Cysts

Cysts comprise up to 3–5% of all thyroid nodules and account for 4–25% of all lesions removed during thyroid surgery (Tsyb et al. 1997; Zabolotskaya et al. 2006) (Figs. 6.8 and 6.9). True cysts with flat epithelium make up less than 0.5% of all thyroid lesions and, as a rule, are represented by a single cyst (Fig. 6.10). Fluid collections, which are often detected in thyroid nodules, are in most cases a consequence of colloid accumulation or degenerative changes in nodules or adenomas, or more rarely in carcinomas (Fig. 6.11).

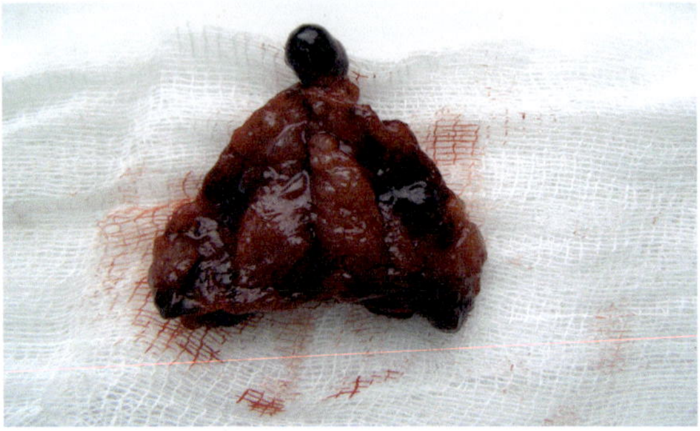

Fig. 6.8 Thyroid cyst with a colloid goiter. Macroscopic view

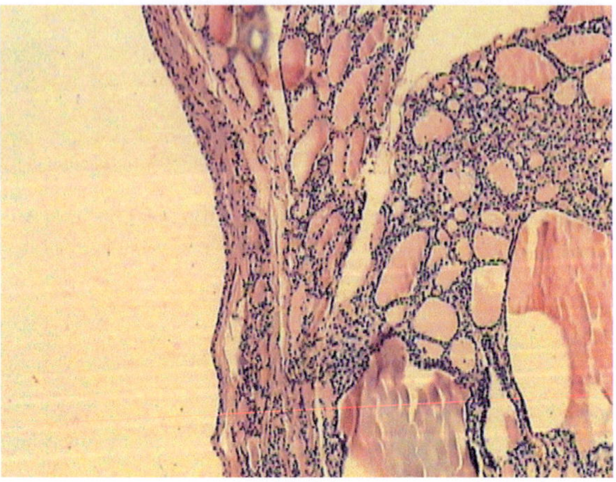

Fig. 6.9 Thyroid cyst (hematoxylin and eosin stained smears; original magnification, ×200)

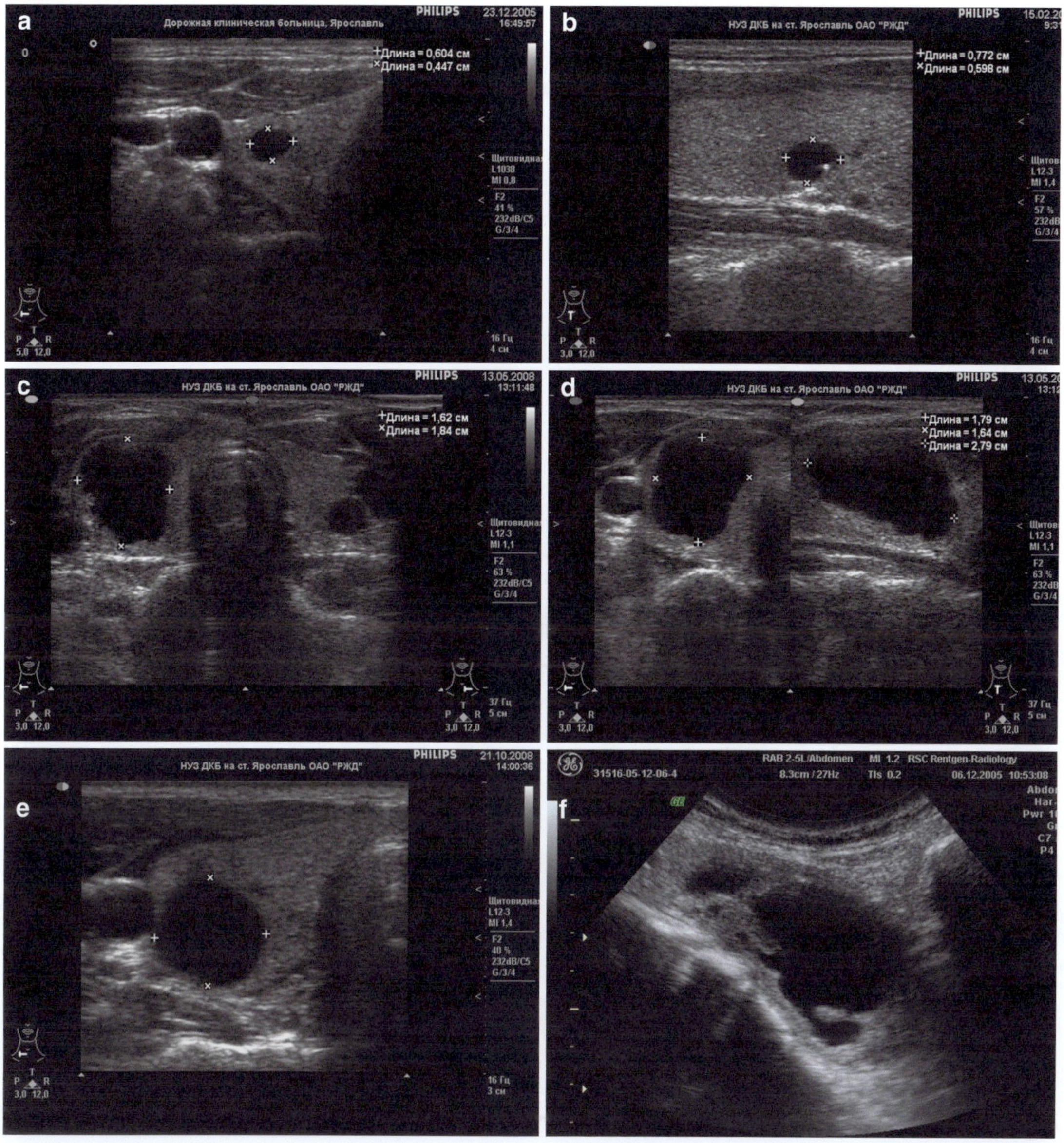

Fig. 6.10 (**a–f**) Thyroid cyst. Grayscale sonography

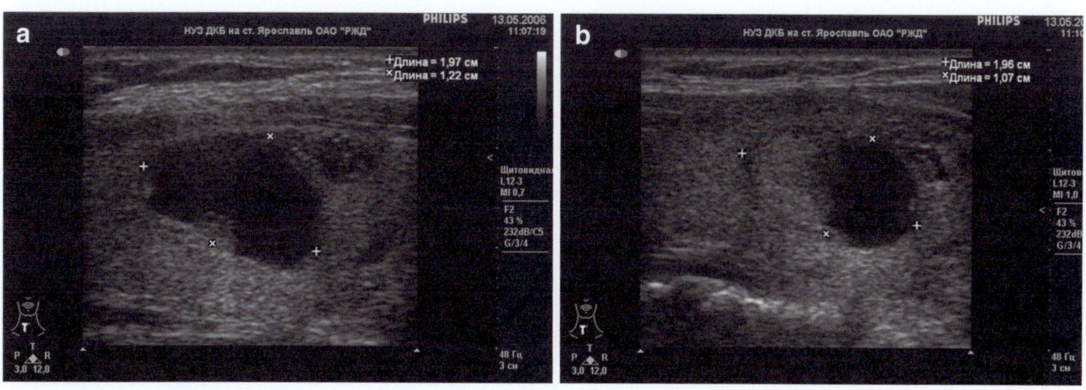

Fig. 6.11 (**a**, **b**) Thyroid nodule with large fluid collection. Grayscale sonography

Thyroid cysts are sonographically characterized by the following typical features (Table 6.2):

- Roundish or oval shape
- Regular, well-defined margins
- Anechoic homogenous inner structure; in rare cases the presence of echogenic inclusions or a solid component is possible
- Dorsal echo enhancement, especially intense in cysts over 5 mm in size
- Lateral acoustic shadows, more often associated with cysts over 10 mm in size
- Avascularity in CDI, PDI, and 3DPD, and in rare cases vascularization of a solid component

Fluid lesions with a minimum diameter of 1 mm can be clearly detected with thyroid sonography.

Thyroid cysts differ in their origins and morphological structures. The following types can be defined (Barsukov et al. 2000) (Figs. 6.12–6.16):

1. Simple colloid cysts
2. Complex cysts
    - Result from previous inflammatory processes in thyroid parenchyma
    - Filled with transudate
    - Contain the products of hemorrhages
    - The connective tissue component merges into the lumen
    - Have an epithelial component

Thyroid nodules that contain dense colloid may be observed as anechoic lesions with regular (or

Table 6.2 Sonographic features of thyroid cysts, based on data from different authors

US features	Markova et al. (2001) $n=34$	Pashchevsky (2004) $n=202$	Own data $n=300$
Shape:			
Oval	–	–	33.7
Spherical	–	–	62.3
Regular	–	99	–
Irregular	–	–	4
Margins:			
Smooth	100	96	96
Contours:			
Well defined	–	99	97.3
Halo:			
Hypoechoic	–	–	–
Absent	–	–	100
Echodensity:			
Hyper-	–	–	–
Iso-	–	–	–
Hypo-	–	–	–
An-	100	100	100
Echostructure:			
Homogeneous	–	60	34.7
Heterogeneous	–	–	65.3
Calcifications:			
Present	–	–	–
Absent	–	–	100
Posterior enhancement:			
Present	–	–	–
Absent		99	76.7
Thyroid capsule:			
Unchanged	–	99	100
Irregular	–	1	–
Vascularity:			
Avascular	85.3	–	73.7
Hypovascular solid component	14.7	–	16
Hypervascular solid component	–	–	10.3

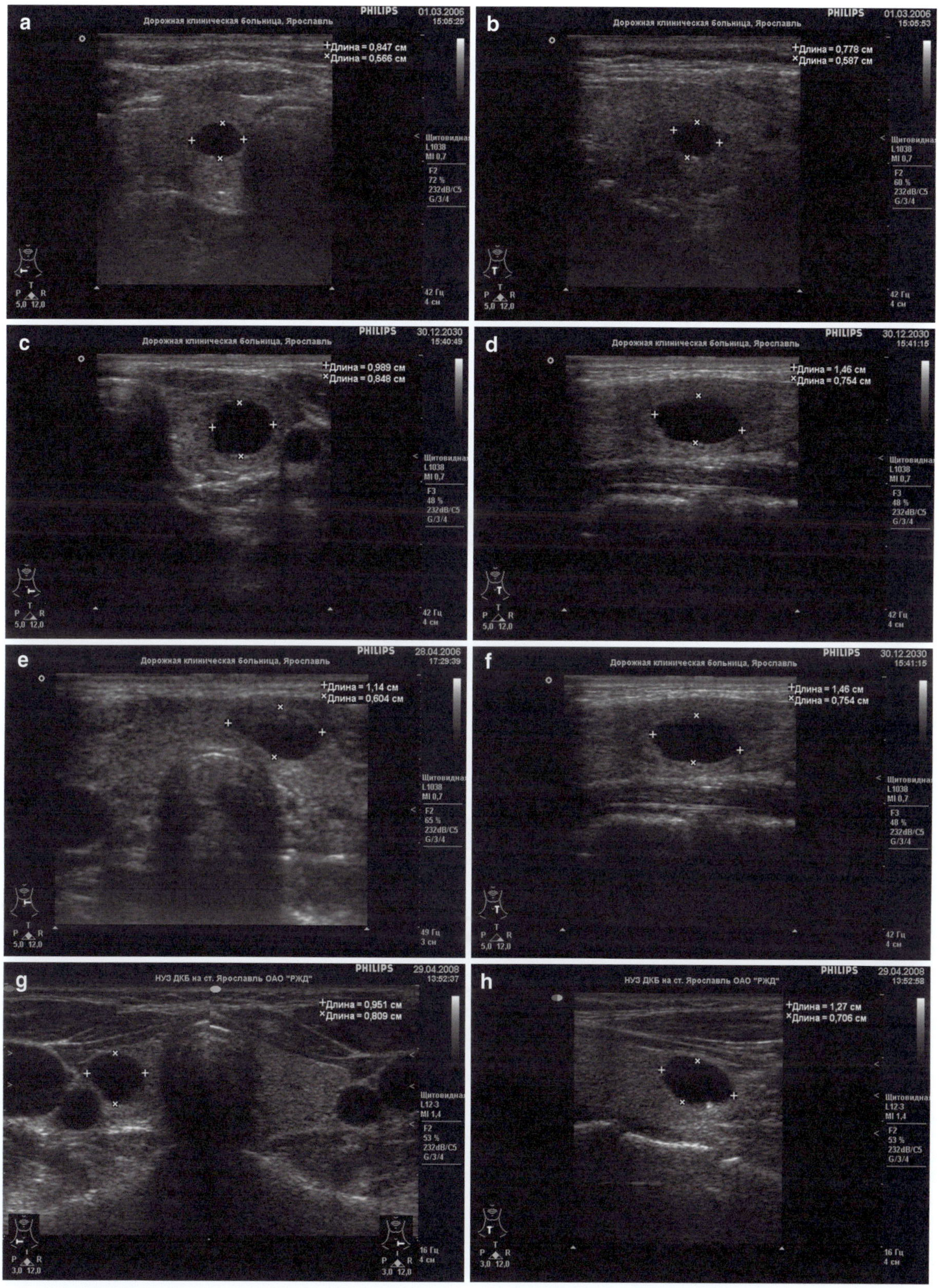

Fig. 6.12 (**a–h**) Simple thyroid cyst. Grayscale sonography

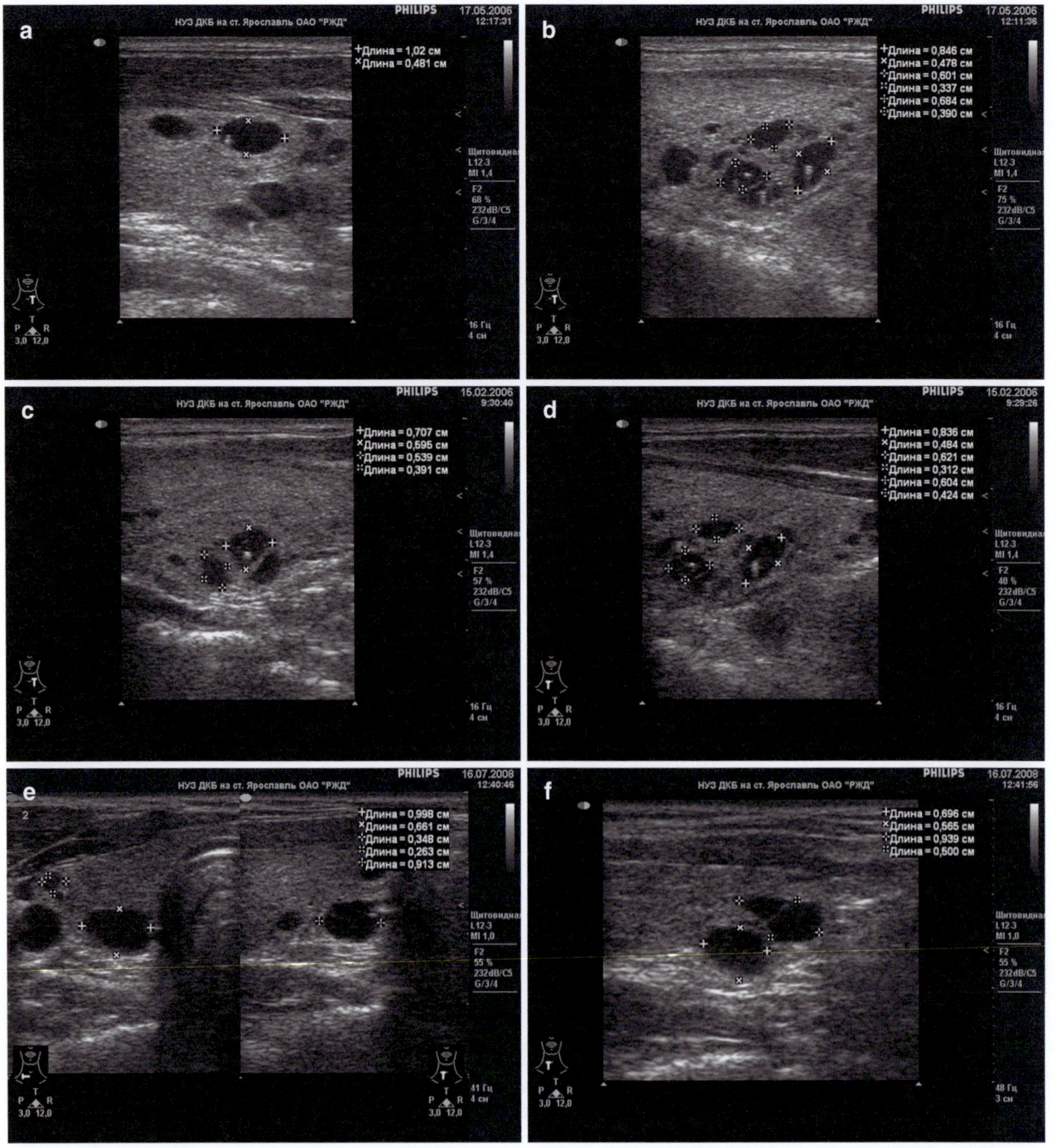

Fig. 6.13 (**a–f**) Multiple colloid cysts of the thyroid. Grayscale sonography

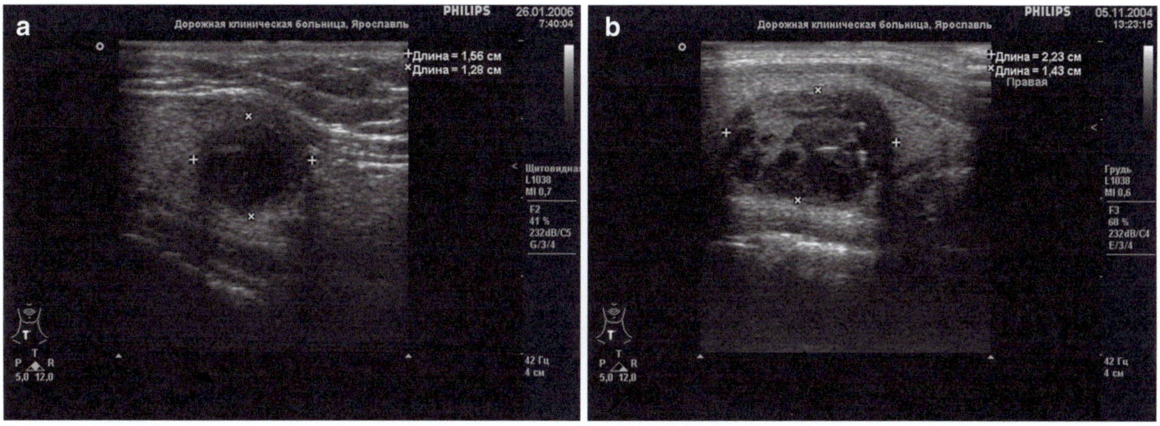

Fig. 6.14 (**a, b**) Complex thyroid cyst containing products of hemorrhage. Grayscale sonography

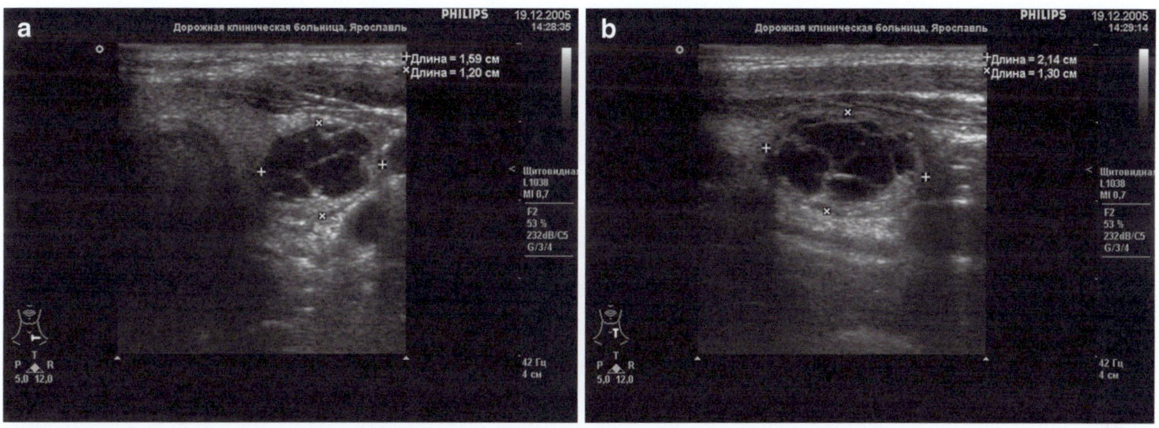

Fig. 6.15 (**a, b**) Complex thyroid cyst with connective tissue component. Grayscale sonography

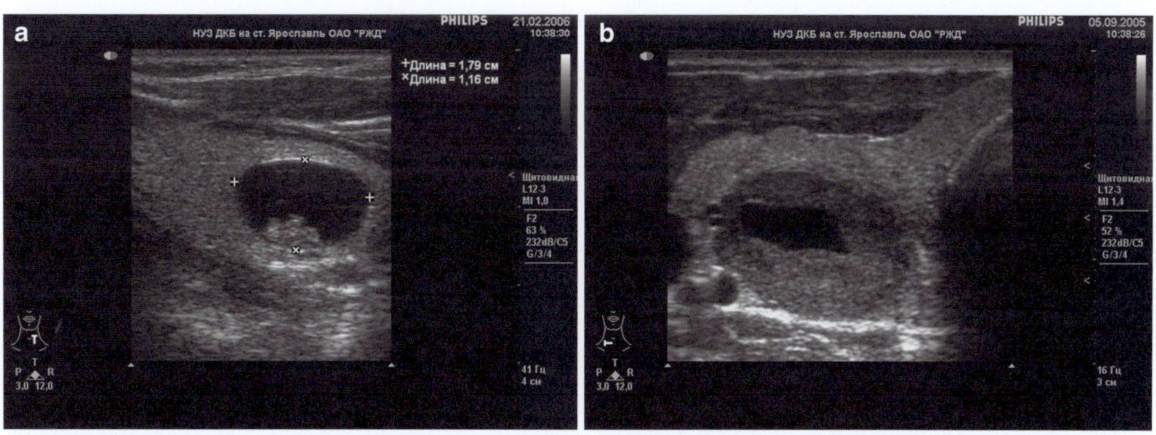

Fig. 6.16 (**a, b**) Complex thyroid cyst with epithelial component. Grayscale sonography

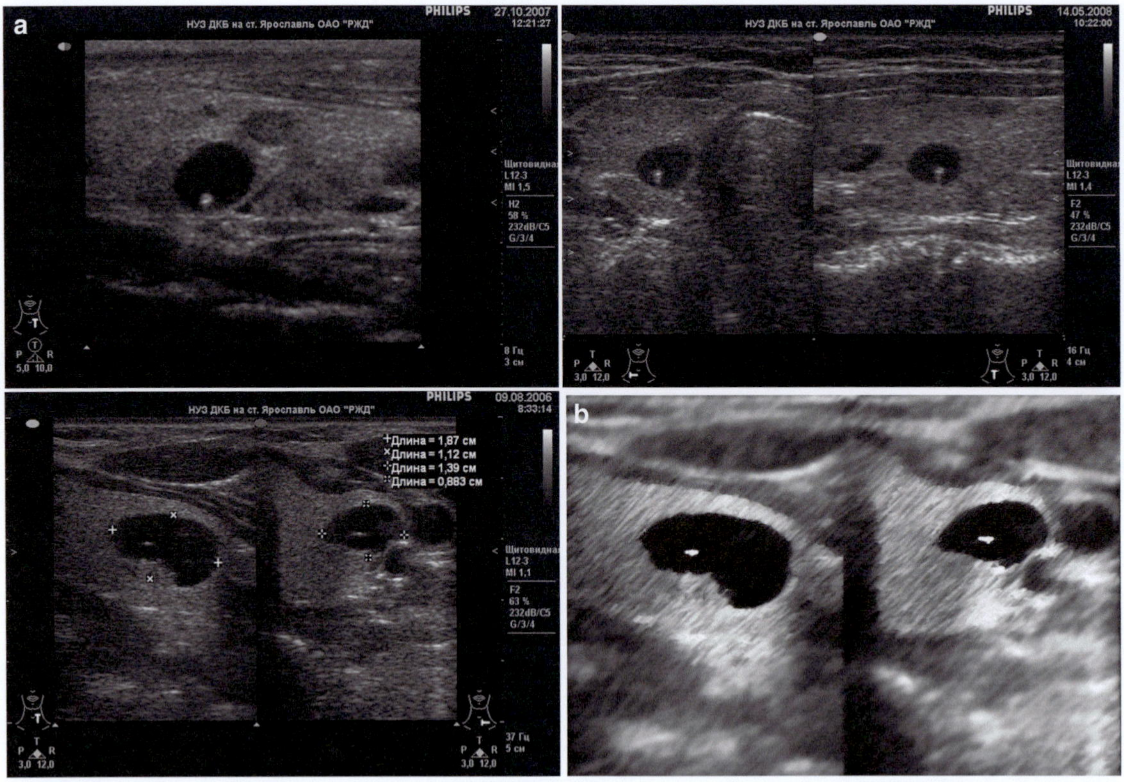

Fig. 6.17 Colloid cyst with "comet tail." (**a1–3**) Sonogram. (**b**) Scheme

irregular) shapes and smooth, well-defined margins. They usually measure up to 1 cm in size and often show distinct point-like echogenic signals with a "comet tail," which characterize dense colloid contents (Ahuja et al. 1996). The "comet tail" is an acoustic phenomenon that results from ultrasound reverberation. It is observed when the US wave is caught between two or multiple reflecting surfaces. Reverberations occurring in grayscale sonography are detected as a short hyperechoic trace ("tail") behind the source of the artifact (Fig. 6.17). Thus, nonexistent surfaces on the screen arise behind the second reflection shield at a distance equal to that between the first and second reflectors. The artifact usually appears when the US beam passes through fluid containers. The above mentioned colloid lesions are normally multiple and correspond morphologically to enlarged follicles (macrofollicles).

As a rule, cysts appear avascular in CDI, PDI, and 3DPD (Figs. 6.18 and 6.19).

The incidence of malignancy in a cyst is about 7–19% (Bellantone et al. 2004). In cases with a solid component within the cyst, CDI and PDI are required to exclude carcinoma (Fig. 6.20). Up to 20–30% of papillary thyroid cancers demonstrate fluid collections (Ahuja 2000). According to Solbiati et al. (1995), connective tissue septa and a solid component with increased vascularity may be observed in the cystic type of papillary thyroid cancer (Fig. 6.21). In a benign process, these septa are normally observed to be avascular. This is an important feature that permits differentiation from cystadenocarcinoma.

The specificities of US in grayscale, CDI, PDI, and 3D for thyroid cysts are 26, 63, 63, and 63%, with sensitivities of 95.6, 90.4, 90.4, and 90.4% and diagnostic accuracies of 64.3, 80.5, 80.5, and 80.5%, respectively (Markova 2001).

Sonography permits not only cyst detection but also preliminary assessment of the nature of these lesions. However, it is often impossible to determine the morphological nature of the solid part of a complex cyst with a single US examination. Therefore, any suspicion of thyroid malignancy should be followed by US-guided FNAB.

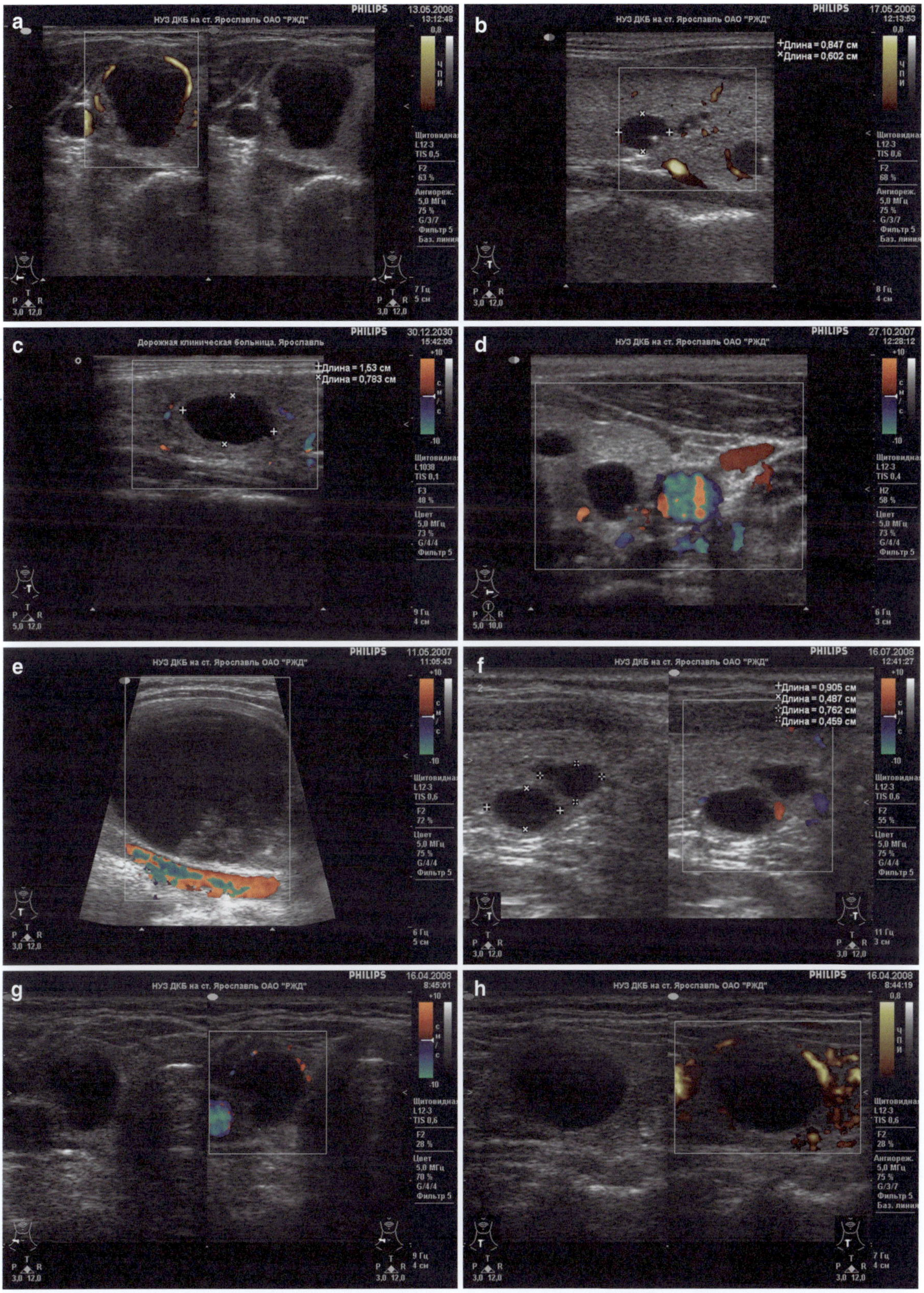

Fig. 6.18 (**a–h**) Thyroid cysts. Avascularity in CDI and PDI

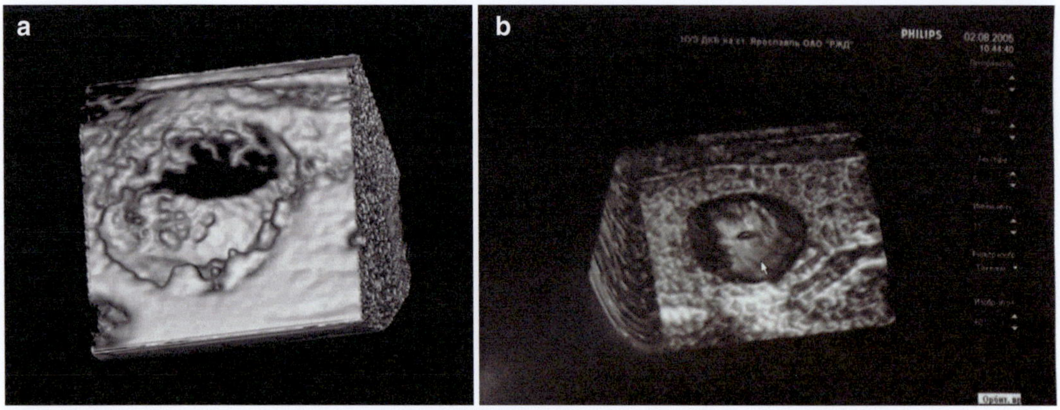

Fig. 6.19 Thyroid cyst. Solid component. 3D reconstruction

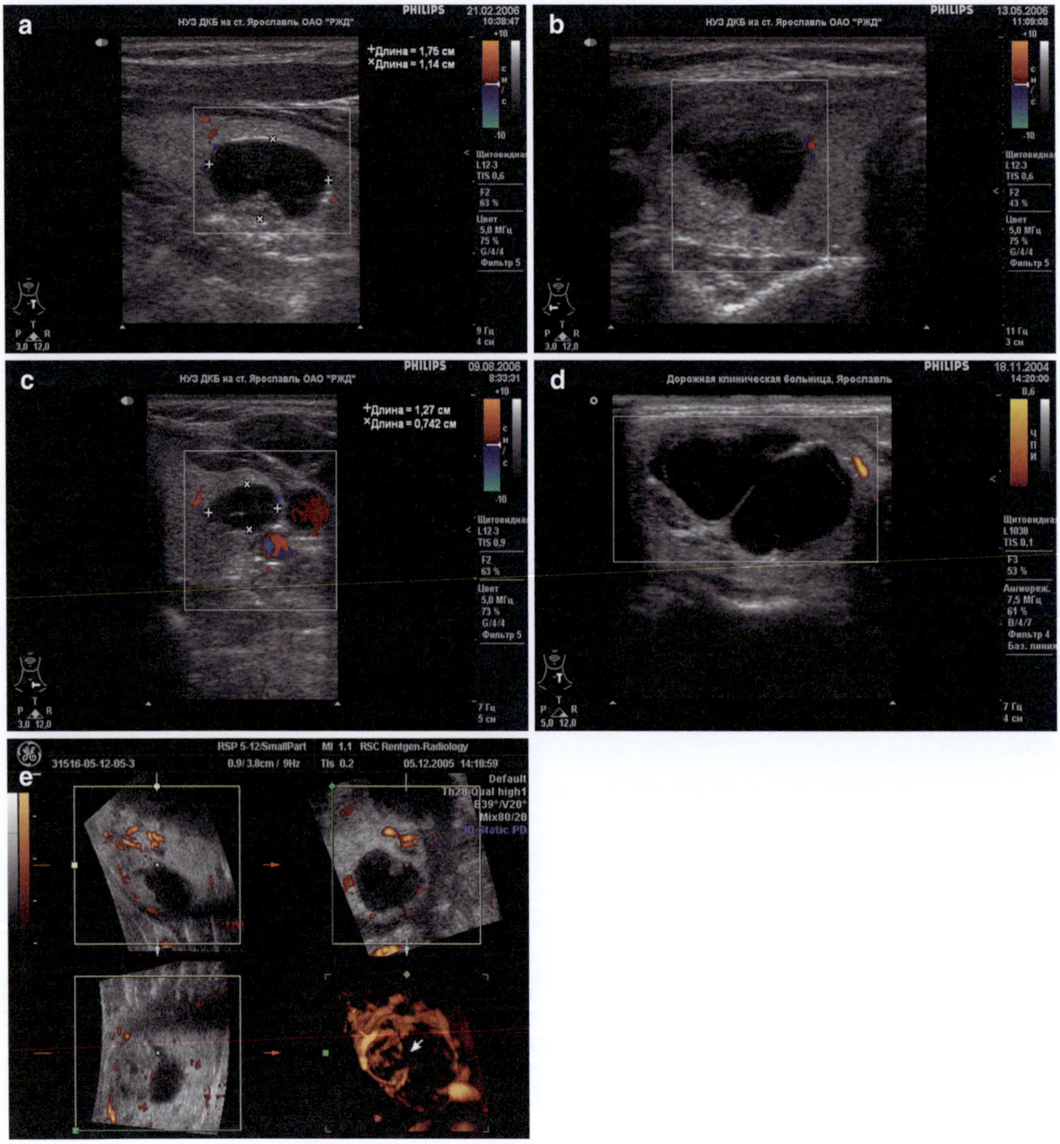

Fig. 6.20 (a–e) Complex thyroid cyst. Avascularity of the solid component. CDI, PDI, and 3DPD

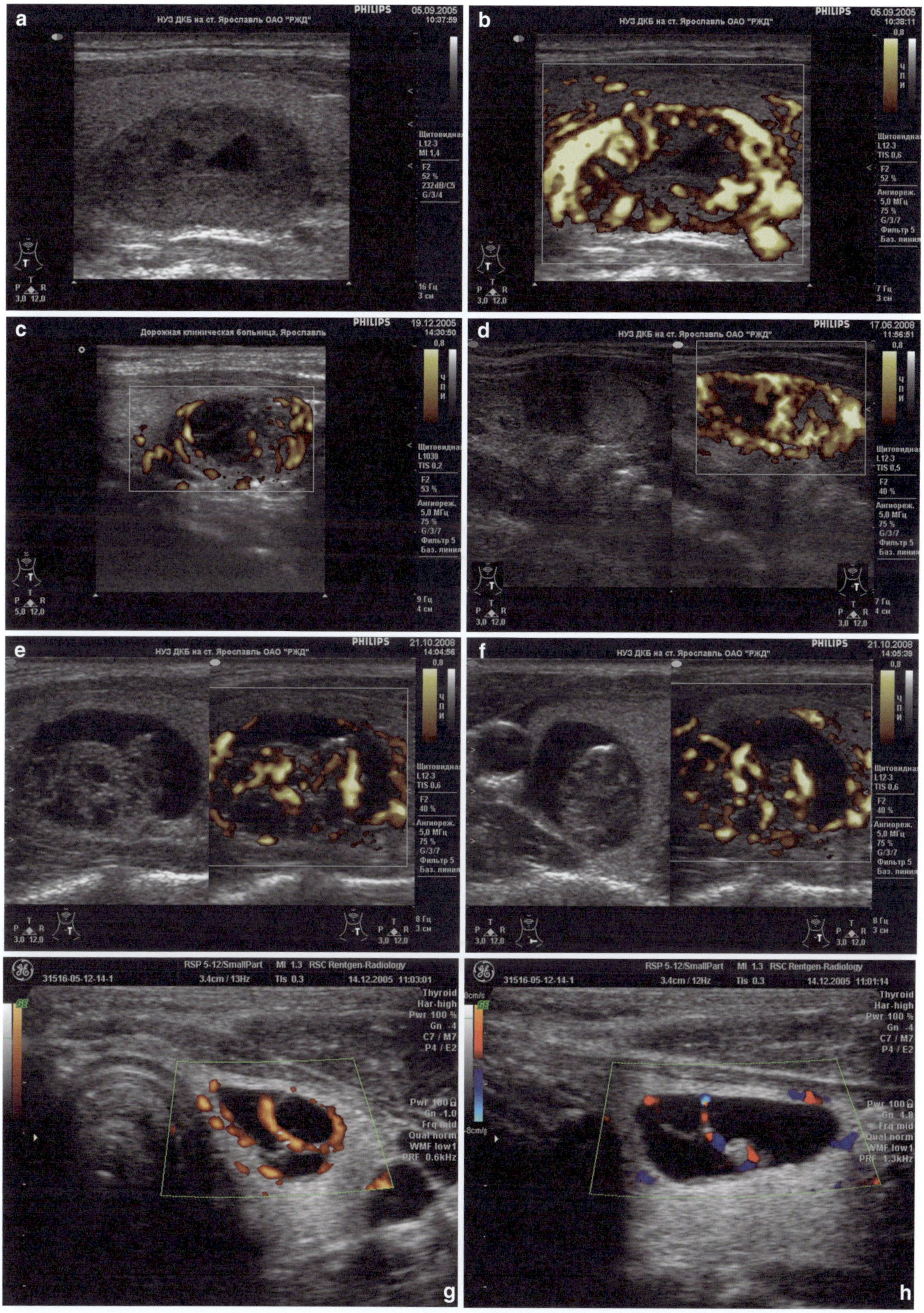

Fig. 6.21 (**a–h**) Papillary cancer of the thyroid gland with fluid collection. Hypervascularity of the solid component. Grayscale, PDI, and CDI

The example of US report in thyroid cysts

First name, middle initial, last name:
Age:
Date:
The number of case history:
US scanner:
The thyroid gland is typically located with regular well-defined margins and homogeneous isoechoic structure. The capsule is uniform and continuous on all extent.

The depth of the **isthmus** - 3 mm	
Right lobe	**Left lobe**
Depth 20 mm Width 21 mm Length 50 mm	Depth 17 MM Width 21 MM Length 52 MM
Volume 10.5 cm^3	Volume 9.3 CM^3
The total volume 19.8 cm^3 exceeds the upper limit for the endemic region and the WHO recommendations.	
A homogenous anechoic avascular lesion of 0.9x0.8x0.5 cm in size of roundish shape with well-defined regular margins is located in the inferior segment of the lobe.	A homogenous anechoic avascular lesion of 0.9x1.0x0.8 cm in size with well-defined regular margins and a single echogenic signal within its central compartment is located in the middle segment of the lobe. Similar lesion of 0.7x0.4x0.7 cm is located in the inferior segment.

The vascular pattern of the parenchyma in CDI and PDI is unchanged.
The topographic relation of the thyroid gland with the muscles and neck organs is typical.
The lymph nodes in the neck and supraclavicular areas are not enlarged.
CONCLUSION: Diffuse thyroid enlargement of 1 stage. Thyroid lesions, most probably colloid cysts.
US specialist:

6.3 Adenomas

Thyroid adenomas are benign tumors that appear as a result of local thyrocyte hyperplasia and proliferation due to genetic mutation (or some other genetic abnormality) in a single precursor cell. Adenomas occupy 16–25% of all thyroid lesions (Vetshev et al. 2005). They are typically represented by a solitary nodule (Figs. 6.22 and 6.23). Multiple lesions are rare.

Thyroid adenomas are histologically typed according to the following classification (Yamasita and Ito 1996):

(a) Follicular adenoma
- Simple adenoma (colloid macrofollicular adenoma)
- Microfollicular adenoma
- Fetal adenoma
- Embryonal (trabecular) adenoma

(b) Papillary adenoma
(c) Variants
- Oxyphilic (Hürthle cell) adenoma
- Clear cell adenoma
- Functioning adenoma (Plummer's disease, toxic multinodular goiter)
- Others

Various morphological types of adenomas cannot be sonographically differentiated. Follicular adenoma is the predominant benign thyroid tumor, accounting

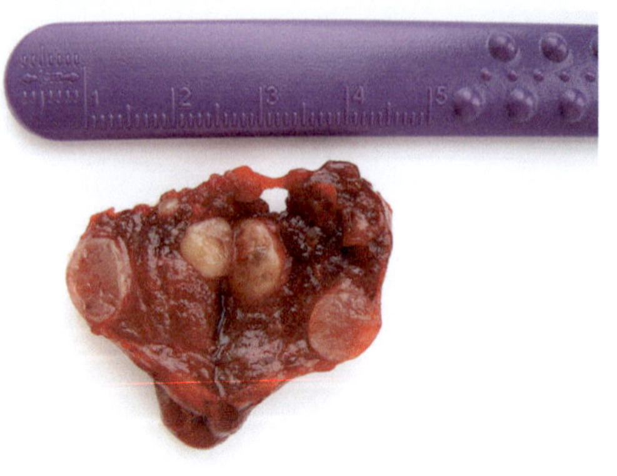

Fig. 6.22 Follicular adenoma of the thyroid gland

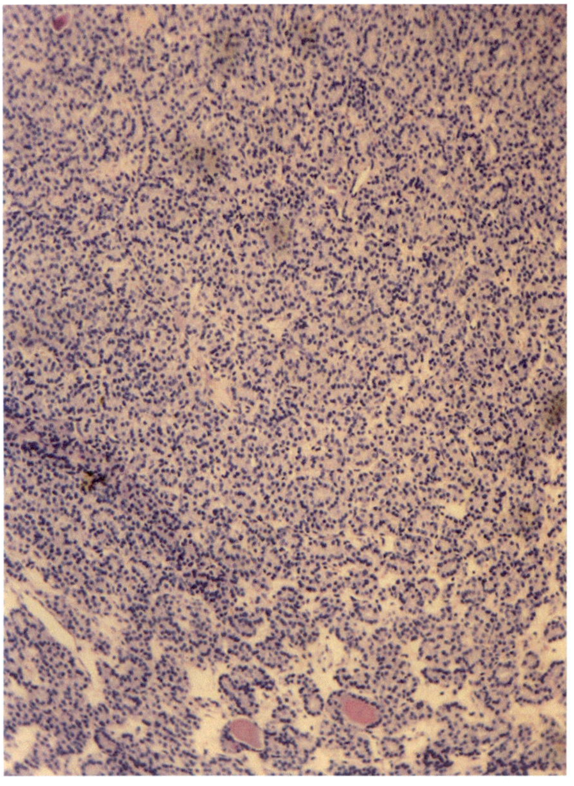

Fig. 6.23 Follicular adenoma of the thyroid gland (hematoxylin and eosin stained smears; original magnification, ×200)

for over 85% of all benign neoplasms of the gland (Bronstein 1997).

Typical US features of thyroid adenoma are as follows (Fig. 6.24, Table 6.3):

- Oval or spherical shape.
- Low echodensity.
- Homogeneous or moderately heterogeneous echostructure.
- Regular, well-defined margins.
- Hypoechoic halo 1–3 mm in width.
- Intact thyroid capsule.
- Absence of calcifications.
- Hypervascularity with a mixed (central and peripheral) pattern and a regular distribution of vessels within the nodule in CDI, PDI, and 3DPD is usually seen. A perinodular vascular ring corresponding to a halo is characteristic. Radial vessels connected with the peripheral ring (a "basketball basket" sign) are often detected.

Thyroid adenomas tend to grow, so they are normally large (over 2–3 cm in size) by the time they are diagnosed.

The majority of adenomas show a peripheral hypoechoic ring (halo) in grayscale sonography. A halo is present in 87.7% of thyroid adenomas. It corresponds to histological capsule, edema of the surrounding normal parenchyma (especially in fast-growing lesions), or to nodule vessels (Fig. 6.25). Becker et al. (1997) showed that the hypoechoic peripheral ring is associated with parenchyma vessels that are displaced by the nodule.

Adenomas can undergo degeneration with cystic or hemorrhagic changes or calcination. Leisner et al. (1987) consider that adenomas with increased echodensity consist of macrofollicular tissue, and those that are hypoechoic consist of microfollicular tissue. Cystic degeneration in adenomas was observed more often (62%) than in thyroid cancer (38%), while calcifications were detected at almost the same rate as in thyroid cancer (11% vs. 17%, respectively). Adenomas with a significantly decreased echodensity are often difficult to differentiate from colloid nodules and malignant tumors. Hypoechoic areas in adenomas are a consequence of hemorrhages into the nodule. The anechoic component in central or peripheral compartments of the lesion with typical fluid echostructure is thought to be associated with cystic degeneration (Fig. 6.26).

According to Struchkova et al. (2003), blood flow velocities in the main thyroid arteries and peripheral vessels of micro- and macrofollicullar adenomas, as measured with PW Doppler, are increased compared to micro- and macrofollicular goiters (PSV = 19.3–40.1 cm/s vs. 10.9–30.6 cm/s, EDV = 5.6–13 cm/s vs. 3.3–10.8 cm/s, RI = 0.45–0.6 vs. 0.6–0.8, and PI = 0.8–1.2 vs. 0.7–1.1, respectively). Kotlyarov et al. (2001) did not find any significant change in blood flow parameters in the vessels of adenomas with PW Doppler (Fig. 6.27).

According to Zubarev et al. (2000), most adenomas show the mixed type of of vascularity with perinodular and intranodular hypervascularization (88.9–100% of cases). The vessels within adenomas appear visually dilated and wavy, with a centripetal direction. According to Kotlyarov et al. (2001), the assessment of blood flow in adenomas with 3DPD suggests a regular pattern without disorganization, as opposed to thyroid cancer (Fig. 6.28).

Thyroid adenomas show a typical vascular pattern in CDI, PDI, and 3DPD: a perinodular vascular ring (corresponding to a halo, which is not always evident in grayscale) with centripetal radial vessels. This

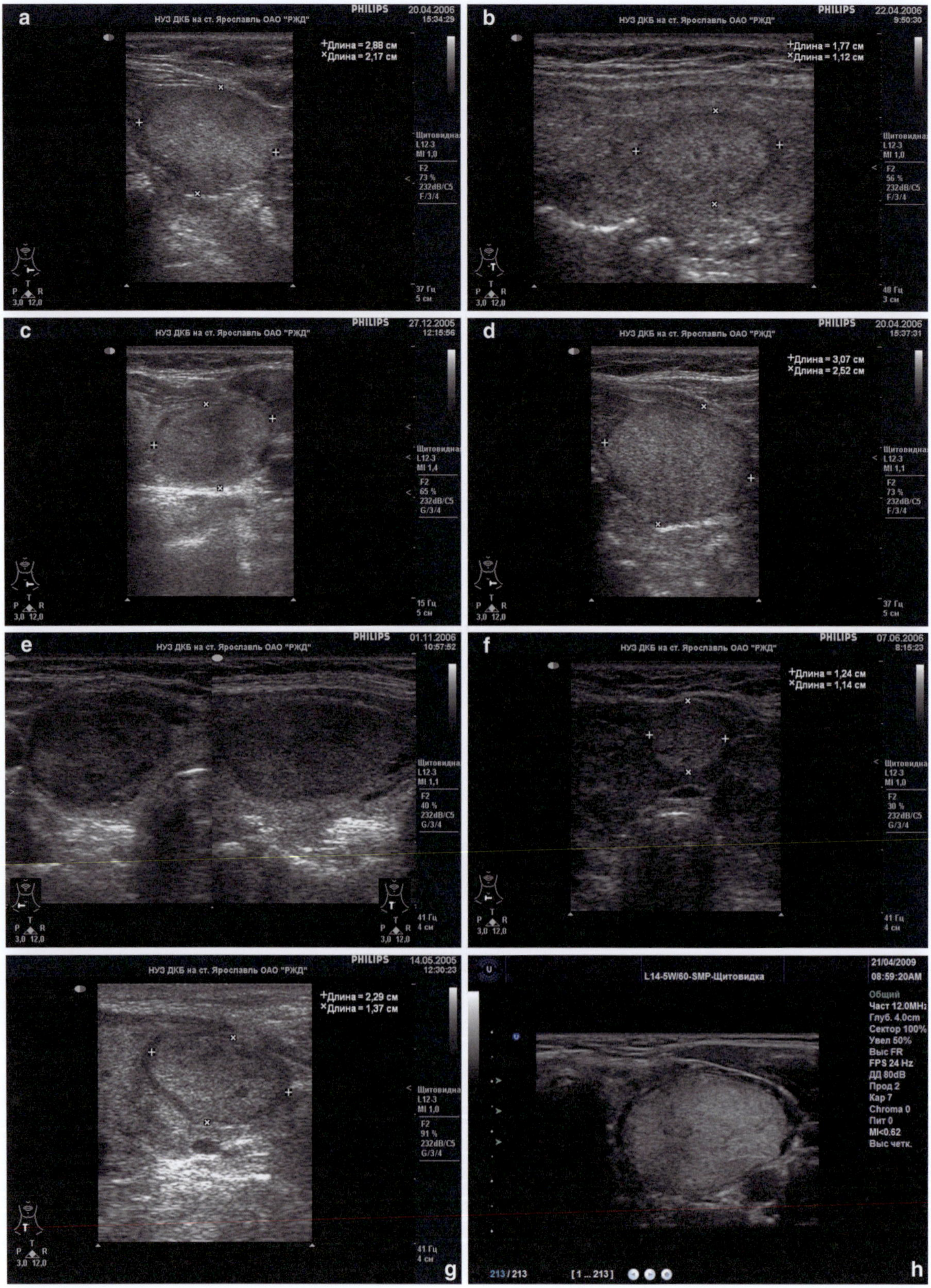

Fig. 6.24 (**a–h**) Thyroid adenoma. Grayscale sonography

Table 6.3 Important sonographic features associated with thyroid adenoma

US features	Tsyb et al. (1997) $n=51$	Pripachkina (1997) $n=134$	Abdulhalimova et al. (1999) $n=65$	Markova et al. (2001) $n=18$	Abalmasov and Ionova (2007) $n=45$	Own data $n=138$
Shape:						
Oval	70	100	–	–	–	60.1
Spherical	20	–	–	–	–	28.3
Irregular	10	–	–	–	–	11.6
Margins:						
Smooth	100	90.3	–	77.8	93.3	89.9
Rough	–	9.7	–	22.2	6.7	10.1
Contours:						
Well defined	91	84.3	81.5	–	95.6	91.3
Indistinct	9	15.7	18.5	–	4.4	8.7
Halo:						
Present	100	81.6	90.8	–	31.1	87.7
Hypo-, anechoic	14	23.9	90.8	–	68.9	87.7
Hyperechoic	86	56.7	–	–		–
Absent	–	19.4	9.2	–		12.3
Echodensity:						
Hyper-	–	56.7	16.9	11.1	4.4	11.6
Iso-	–	19.4	38.5	55.6	42.2	25.4
Hypo-	–	23.9	32.3	22.2	40.0	63.0
Mixed	–	–	12.3	–	13.3	–
Echostructure:						
Homogeneous	–	17.2	–	–	22.2	55.0
Heterogeneous	–	82.8	–	–	77.8	45.0
Calcifications:						
Present	10	–	–	–	31.1	12.3
Absent	90	–	–	100	68.9	87.7
Posterior enhancement:						
Present	37	–	–	–	–	68.1
Absent	63	–	–	–	–	31.9
Thyroid capsule:						
Unchanged	100	–	–	–	100	95.65
Irregular	–	–	–	–	–	4.35
Vascularity:						
Avascular	–	–	–	–	–	10
Hypovascular	–	–	–	–	53.3	25
Hypervascular:	–	–	–	–	46.7	65
Perinodular	–	–	55.4	–	–	–
Mixed	–	–	44.6	100	–	–

pattern was named a "basketball basket" (Figs. 6.29 and 6.30). According to Sencha (2008), this sign is observed in 24.6% of all thyroid adenomas.

The specificities of sonography in grayscale, CDI, PDI, and 3D in the diagnosis of thyroid adenomas are about 30, 56.6, 68.7, and 79.2%, with sensitivities of 79.9, 84, 89.5, and 93.4% and diagnostic accuracies of 38.2, 61.5, 72, and 82%, respectively (Markova 2001). According to Zubarev et al. (2001), combining Doppler options with 3D increases the sensitivity of US to adenomas by 13.5% (up to 93.4%), its specificity by 49.2% (up to 79.2%), and its diagnostic accuracy by 43.8% (up to 82%). According to Pinsky et al. (1999), a sonographic conclusion of thyroid adenoma appears to be correct in 23.9% of cases. Sonoelastography can obviously help to diagnose thyroid adenoma, but its efficacy is still to be investigated (Fig. 6.31).

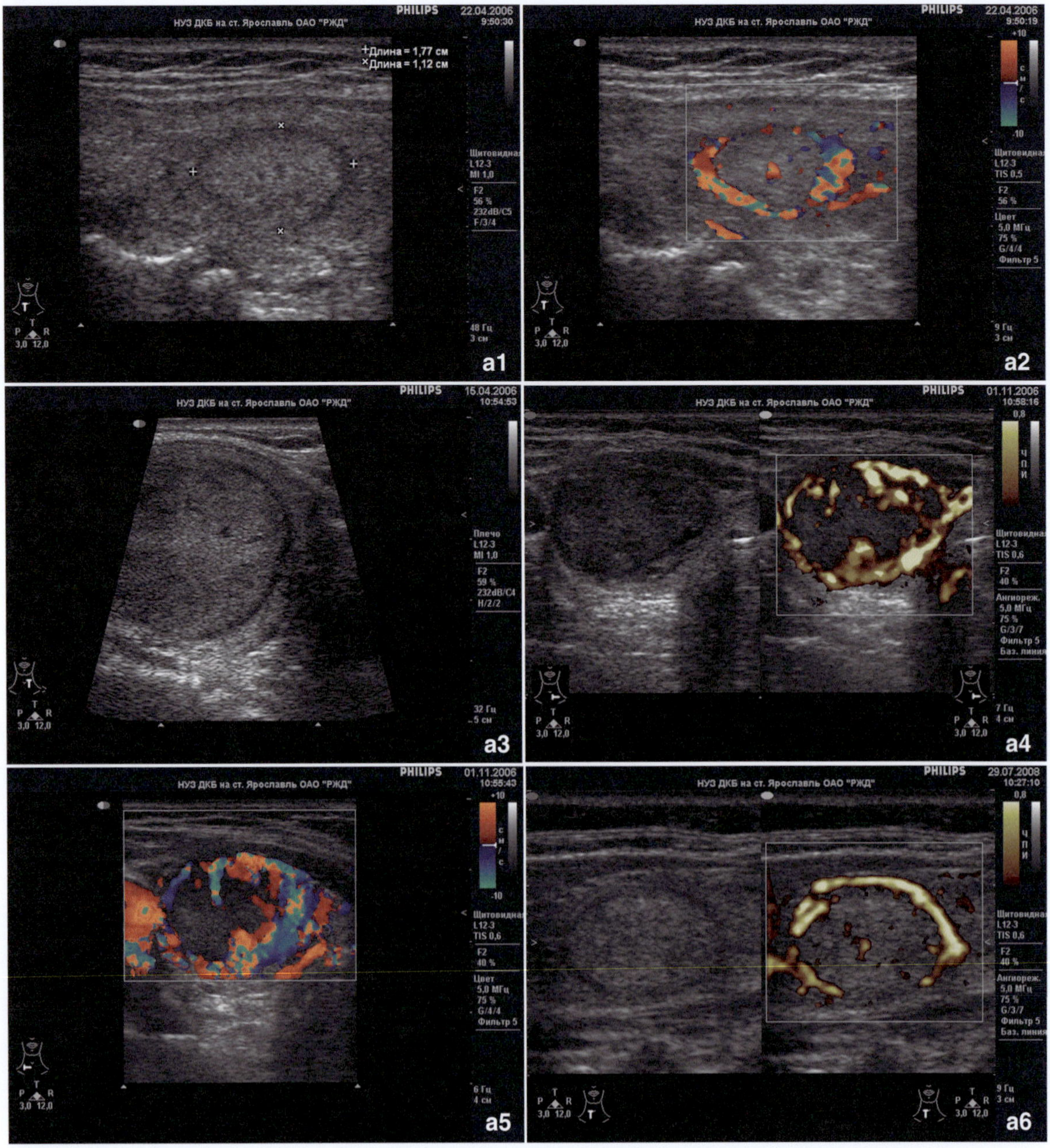

Fig. 6.25 Thyroid adenoma. Peripheral halo. (**a1–a8**) Sonograms. Grayscale, CDI, PDI, and sonoelastogram. (**b**) Scheme

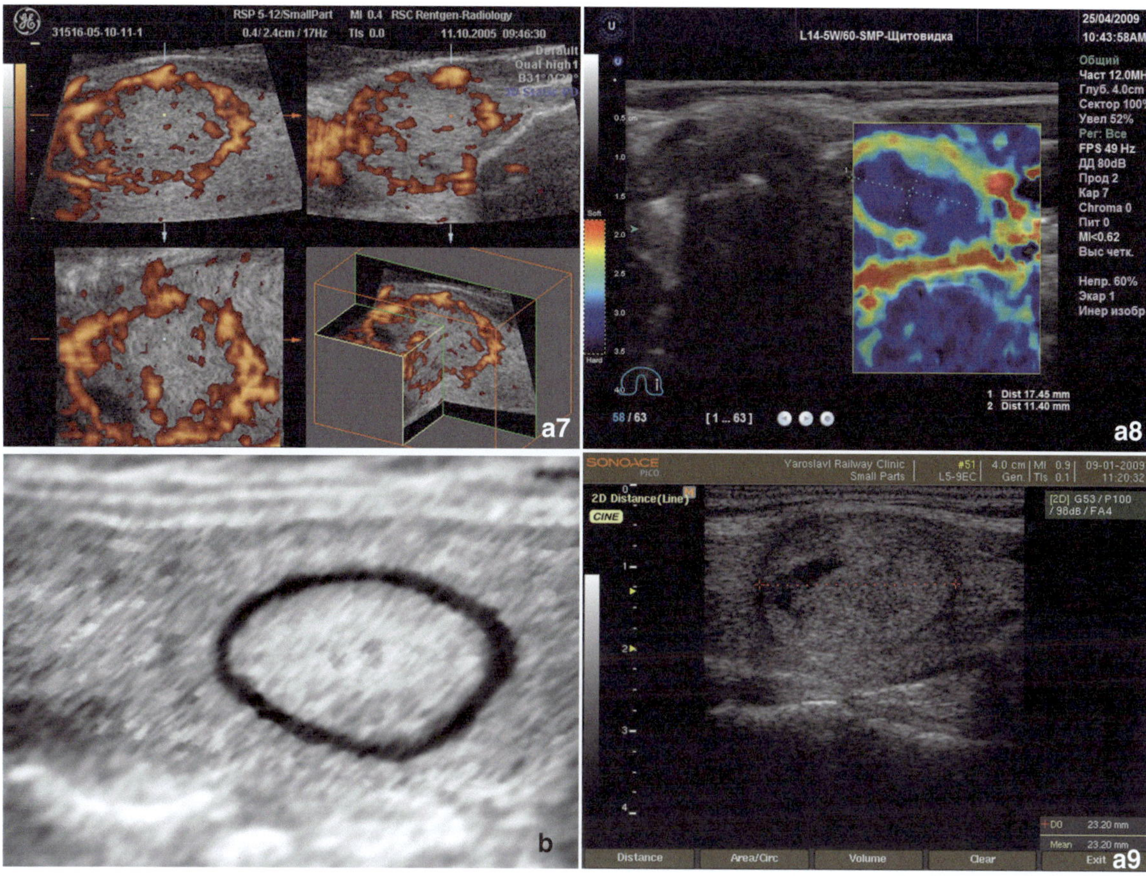

Fig. 6.25 (continued)

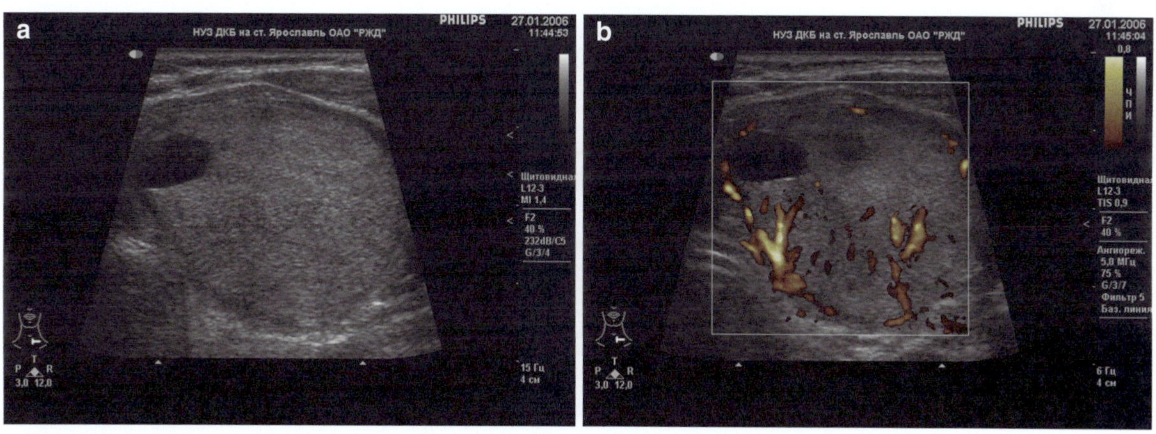

Fig. 6.26 (a–f) Thyroid adenoma. Cystic degeneration. Grayscale, PDI, and CDI

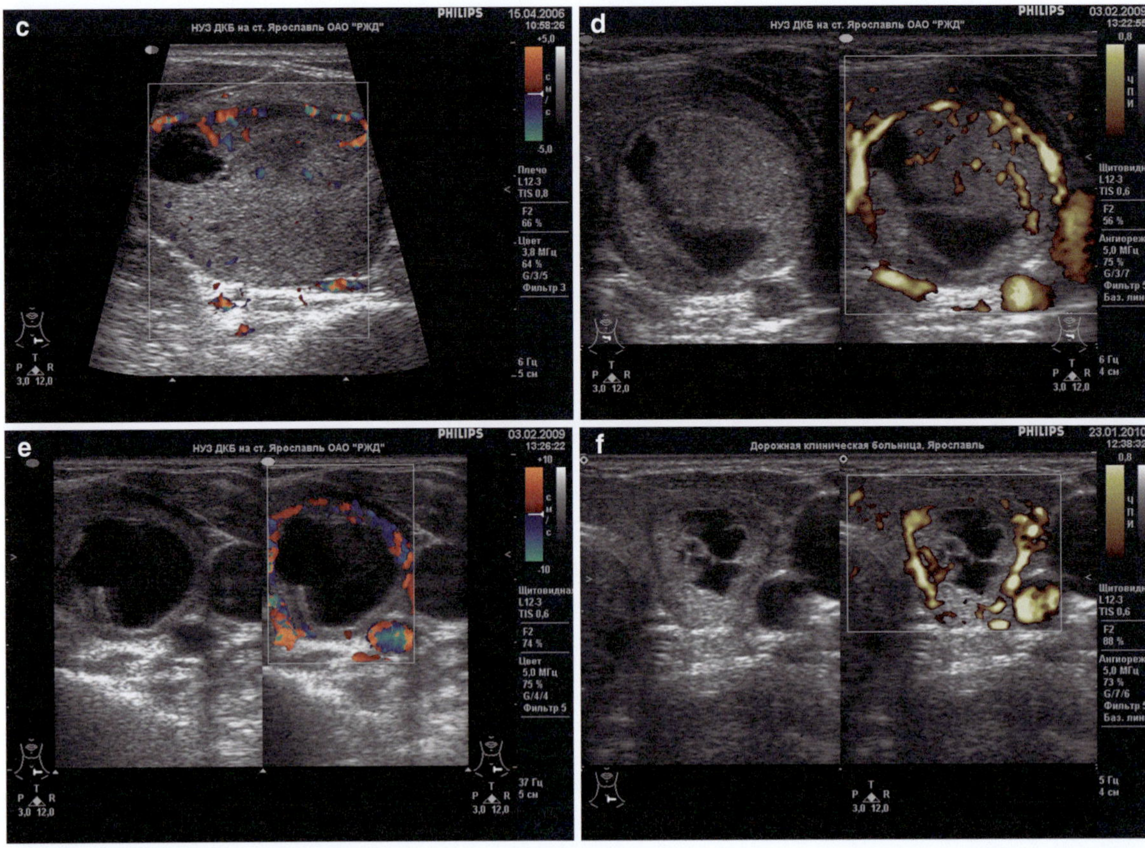

Fig. 6.26 (continued)

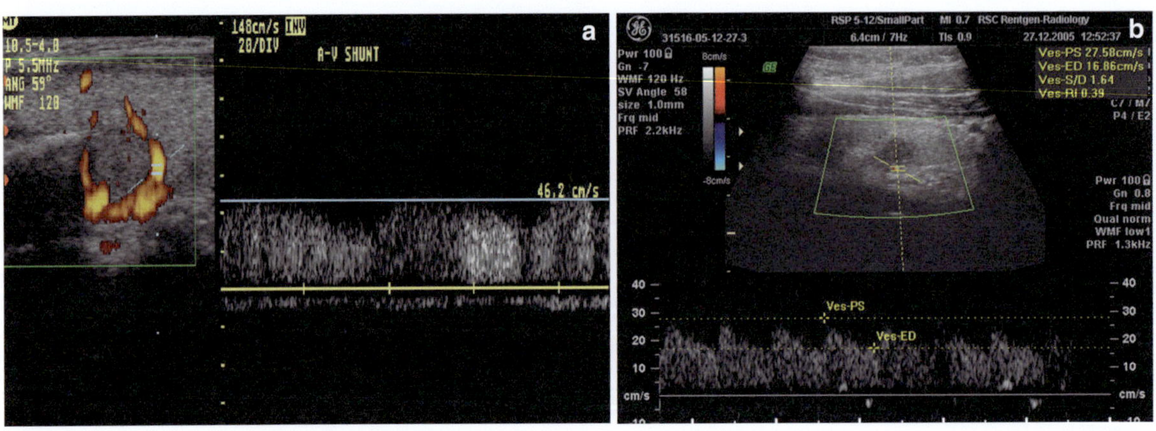

Fig. 6.27 (a, b) Thyroid adenoma. PW Doppler

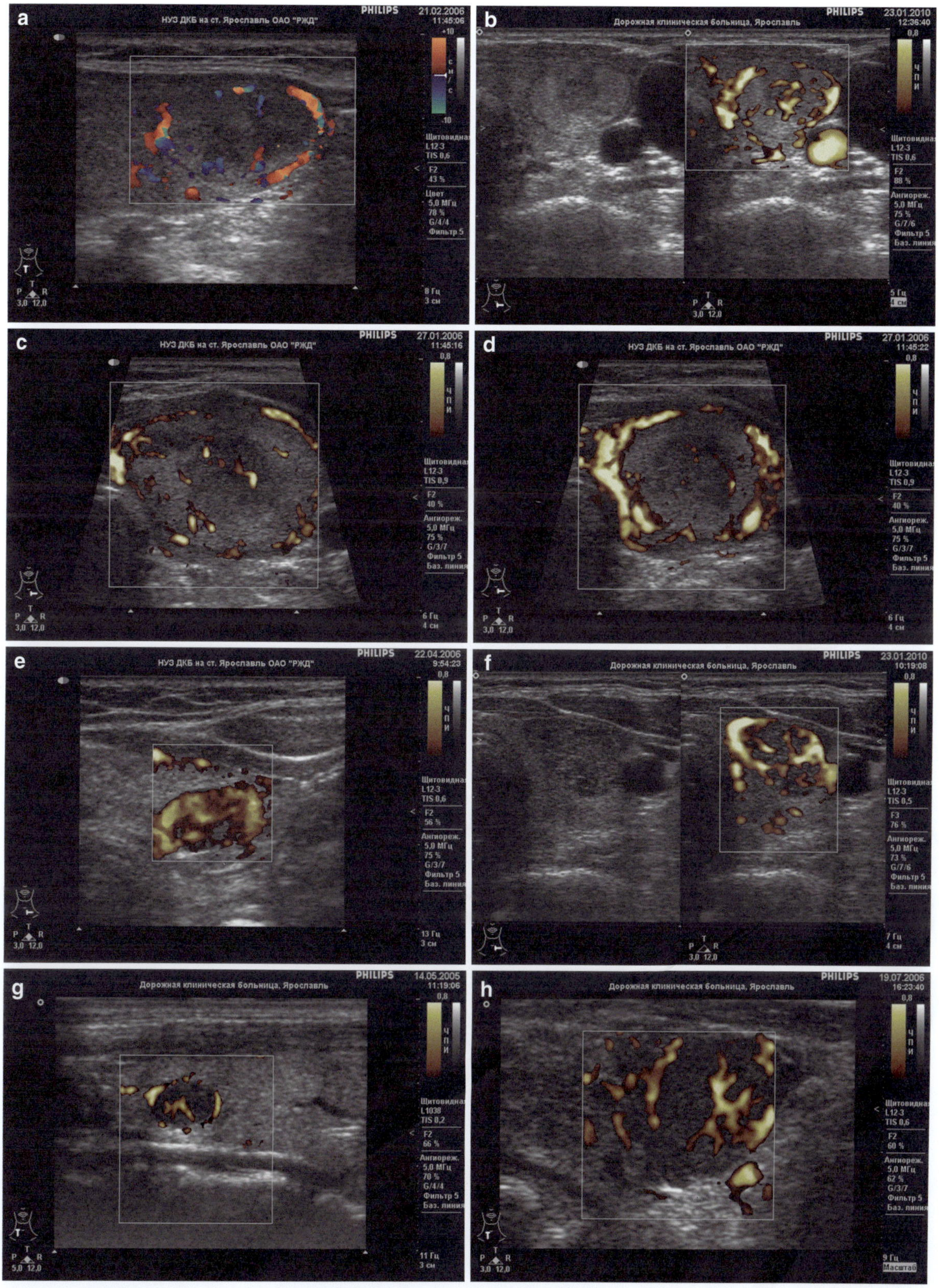

Fig. 6.28 (**a–j**) Thyroid adenoma. Nodule hypervascularity. CDI and PDI

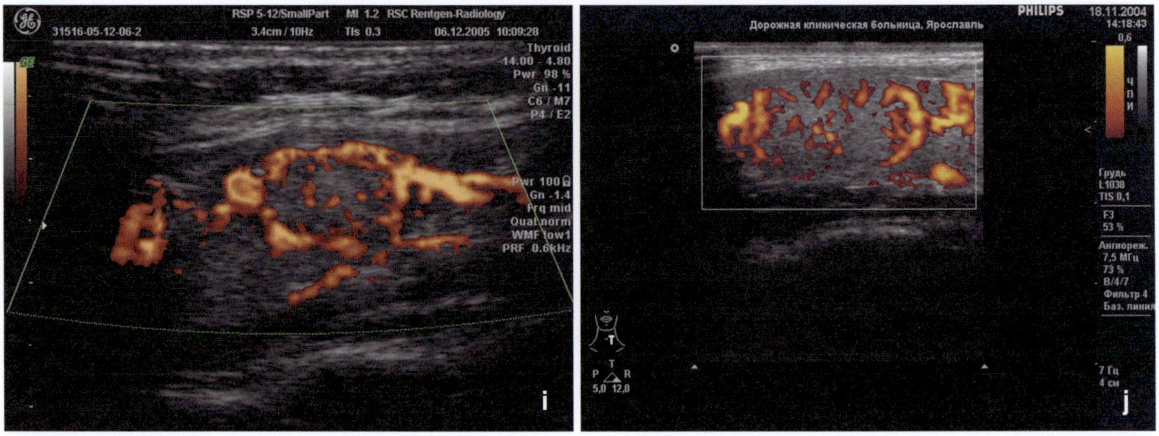

Fig. 6.28 (continued)

The literature and our own experience prove that none of the features listed above can serve as an absolute criterion of the benign character of a thyroid nodule. The cytology often permits the benign nature of the obtained cells to be specified, but this is quite a problem in several cases, such as for follicular tumors and others. Thus, the role of US is often limited to the selection of the patients with nodules that are suspicious for a tumor and subsequent US-guided FNAB.

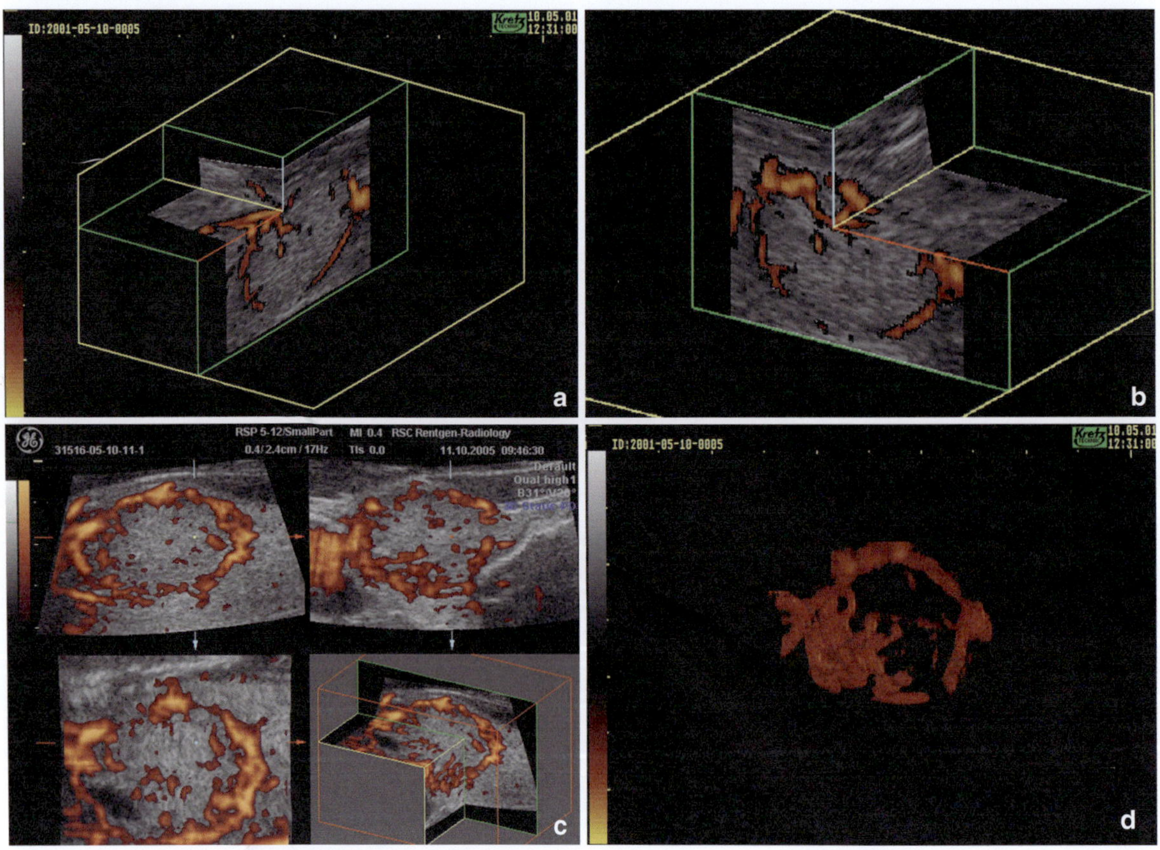

Fig. 6.29 **(a–f)** Thyroid adenoma. The "basketball basket" sign. 3DPD

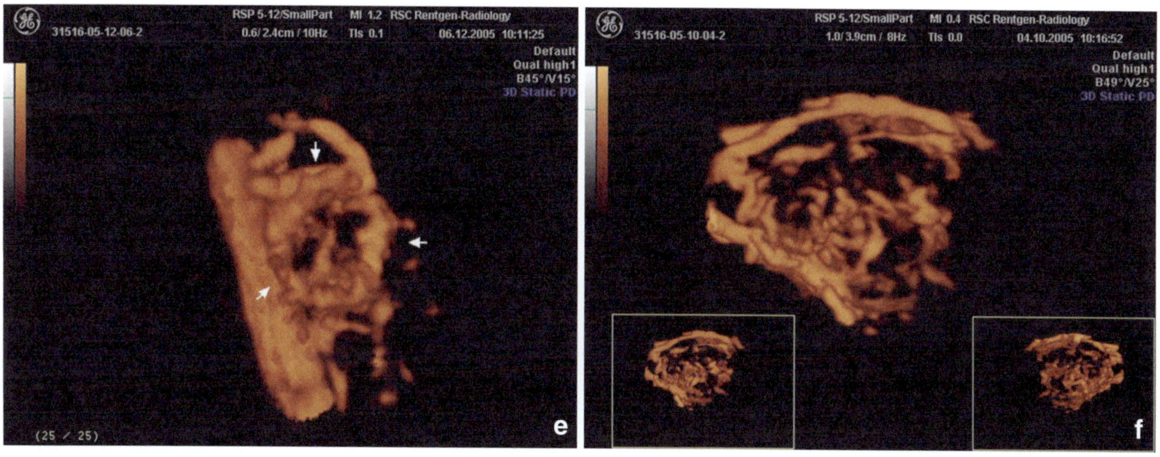

Fig. 6.29 (continued)

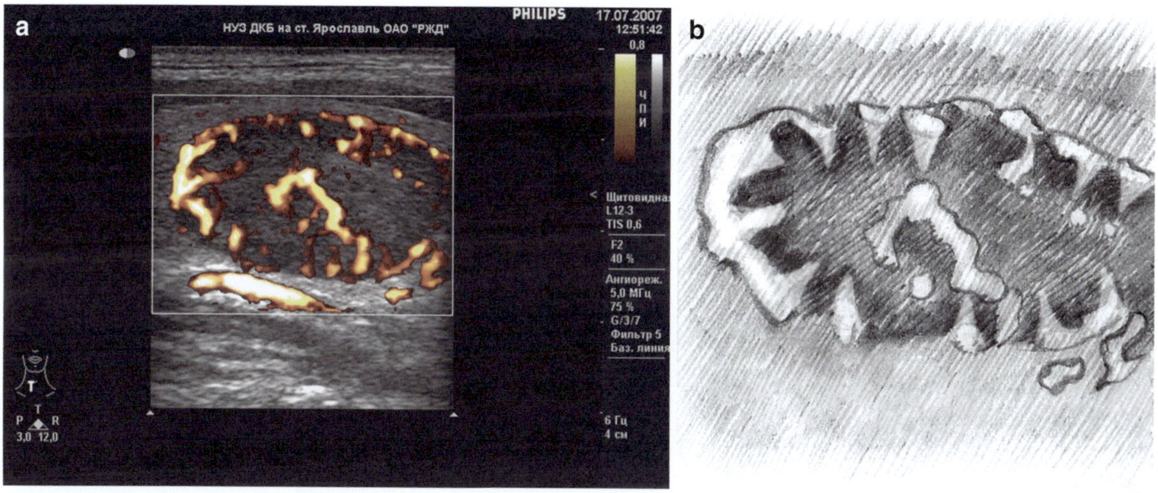

Fig. 6.30 The "basketball basket" sign. (**a**) PDI. (**b**) Scheme

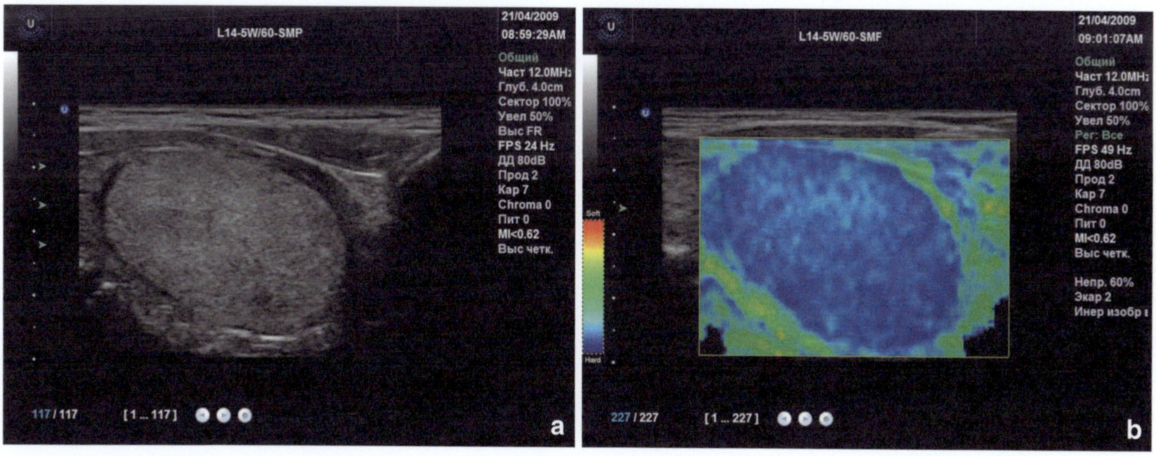

Fig. 6.31 (**a, b**) One type of thyroid adenoma with sonoelastography

The example of US report in thyroid adenoma

First name, middle initial, last name:
Age:
Date:
The number of case history:
US scanner:
The thyroid gland is typically located with regular well-defined margins and homogeneous isoechoic structure. The capsule is uniform and continuous on all extent.

The depth of the **isthmus** - 2 mm	
Right lobe	**Left lobe**
Depth 18 mm Width 18 mm Length 51 mm	Depth 14 mm Width 14 mm Length 50 mm
Volume 8.3 cm^3	Volume 4.9 cm^3
The total volume 13.2 cm^3 does not exceed the upper limit for the endemic region and the WHO recommendations.	
A moderately heterogeneous isoechoic lesion of 1.5x1.5x1.7 cm in size of roundish shape with well-defined regular margins and hypoechoic peripheral ring (halo) is located in the inferior segment of the lobe. The vascularization of the lesion is increased in CDI and PDI with predominantly perinodular pattern and a "basketball basket" sign. 3DPD reveals regular distribution of the vessels within the nodule.	No lesion is observed.

The vascular pattern of the parenchyma in CDI and PDI is unchanged.
The topographic relation of the thyroid gland with the muscles and neck organs is typical.
The lymph nodes in the neck and supraclavicular areas are not enlarged.
CONCLUSION: The nodule in the right thyroid lobe. The image may correspond to thyroid adenoma.
US specialist:

6.4 Thyroid Cancer

Thyroid cancer is the most widespread tumor of the endocrine system. It accounts for about 1.5–2% of all head and neck malignancies and 1–4% of all malignant tumors. Thyroid cancer is detected in 7.3–23.4% of thyroid surgeries (Hundahl et al. 2000) (Figs. 6.32 and 6.33). Nevertheless, thyroid cancer appears to be the cause of death in only 0.3–1% of all cases of malignancy (Mazzaferri 1993; Bronstein 1997; Dymov 2007; Morozova 2007). Importantly, up to 10% of patients with thyroid cancer are younger than 21 years of age (Gorlin and Sallan 1990).

Twenty-five to 55 new cases of differentiated thyroid cancer per million are recorded annually. According to the WHO, the incidence of thyroid cancer doubled during the last decade due to the increased detection of "obscure" variants.

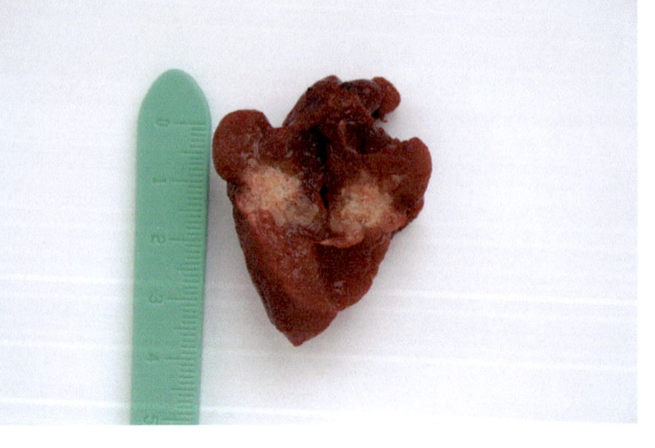

Fig. 6.32 Papillary thyroid carcinoma. Macroscopic view

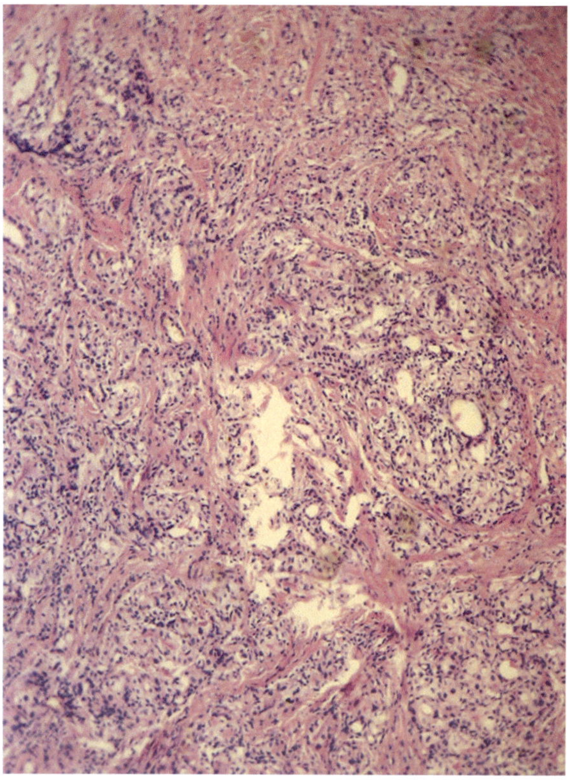

Fig. 6.33 Papillary thyroid carcinoma, the sclerosing variant (hematoxylin and eosin stained smears; original magnification, ×200)

Thyroid cancer is more common in women, with a ratio of 6:1 (Moon et al. 2008). Follicular cancer is particularly rare in men (with a ratio of 1:17), although medullary and diffuse sclerosing types of papillary cancer can be observed more often in men. Among children, thyroid cancer is also more common in girls, with an incidence ratio of 1:1.6–2.

According to Sherman (1990), thyroid cancer exhibits two peaks in all countries: a smaller peak between the ages of seven and 20, and a larger peak between the ages of 40 and 65. The incidence of thyroid cancer increases again between the ages of 41 and 50 years (Moon et al. 2008).

As a rule, the neoplasm is located in the lateral lobes of the thyroid. The inferior compartments of the lobes tend to be affected more often. Follicular and medullary carcinomas arise twice and 2.5 times as often in the right lobe as they do in the left lobe, respectively. Papillary cancer is more often detected in the isthmus. Solitary lesions in cases of thyroid cancer are often 1–3 cm in size.

The following US features are suspicious for thyroid malignancy (Fig. 6.34, Table 6.4):

1. Single lesion
2. Irregular shape of the lesion
3. Tuberous borders
4. Indistinct contours
5. Decreased echodensity
6. Heterogeneity of echostructure
7. Echogenic inclusions and microcalcifications that are smaller than 2 mm in size, without acoustic shadowing
8. Posterior shadowing behind the lesion
9. Absence of the peripheral halo
10. Hypervascularity of large lesions and hypo- or avascularity of small lesions in CDI, PDI, and 3DPD
11. Irregular distribution of vessels within the lesion, disorganization of the vascular pattern, nonlinear wavy course with a nonuniform gauge and pathological transformation of the vessels in CDI, PDI, and especially 3DPD
12. Enlargement of the regional lymph nodes

According to Romanko (1997), a subcapsular nodule location is observed in 55% of all thyroid cancers. Ilyin et al. (1997) state that the following additional sonographic features should lead to a suspicion of carcinoma merging into the thyroid capsule:

1. Adhesion
2. Thyroid deformation
3. Blurred margins of the lesion and the thyroid gland

According to Abdulhalimova et al. (1999), and Zabolotskaya et al. (2006), the echostructure of thyroid cancer can vary: it can be solid hypoechoic, solid isoechoic, solid hyperechoic, mixed, or cystic. Messina et al. (1996) consider that 60–70% of thyroid cancers are characterized by hypoechoic solid structure, 15–25% of neoplasms are isoechoic, 2–4% are hyperechoic, and 5–10% show mixed echostructure.

The tumor margins in thyroid carcinoma are often uniformly or locally indistinct. Microcalcifications and anechoic fields corresponding to necrotic cavities may be observed. The presence of fine echogenic inclusions can be a sign of malignancy, although calcifications of different sizes, shapes, and heterogeneities may be

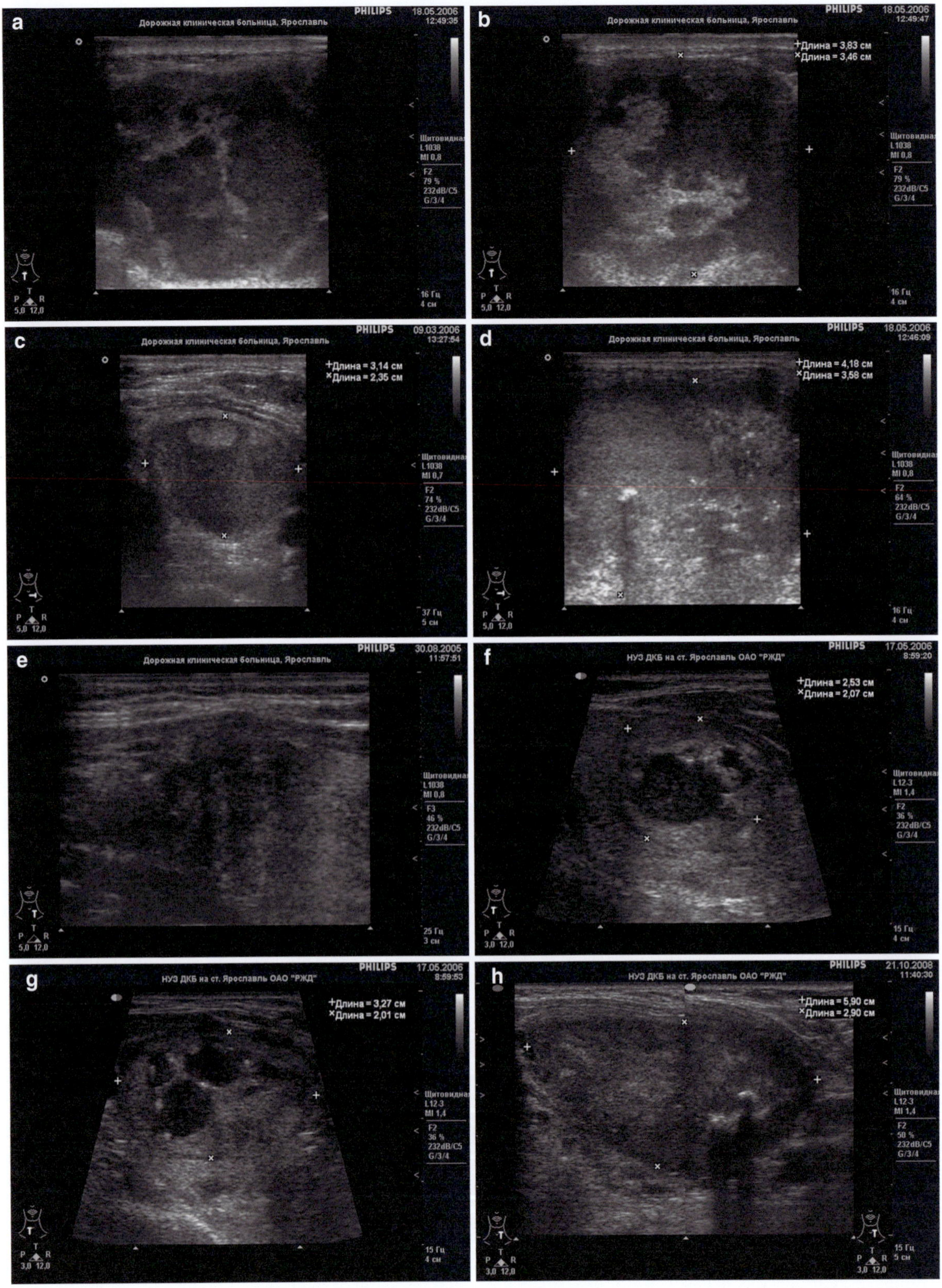

Fig. 6.34 (**a–h**) Thyroid carcinoma. Grayscale sonography. Decreased echodensity, irregular blurred margins, posterior shadowing, multiple microcalcifications, and deformation of the capsule of the thyroid gland

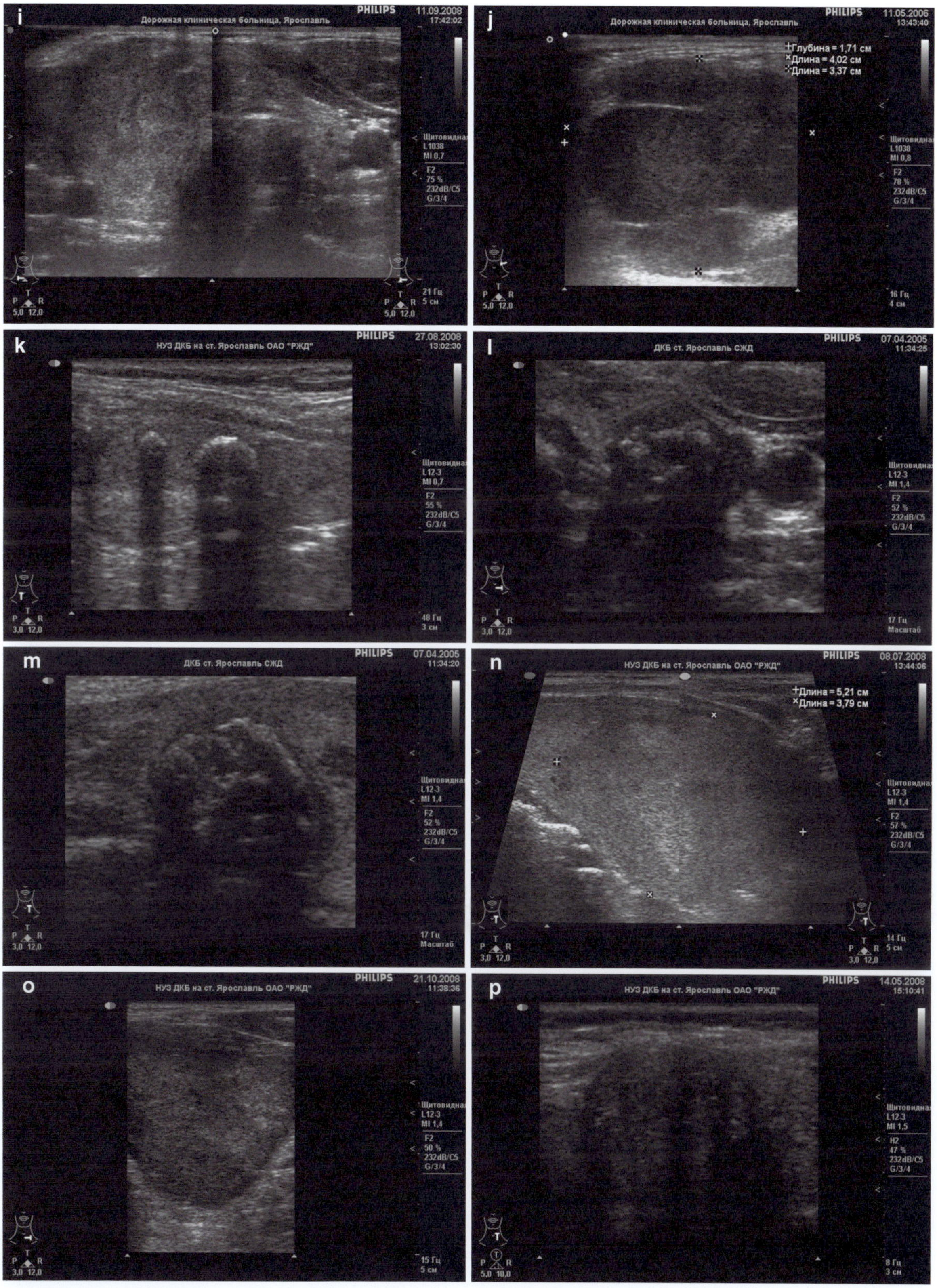

Fig. 6.34 (**i–p**) (continued)

Table 6.4 Sonographic features (frequency, %) of thyroid cancer according to different authors

US features	Romanko (1997) Tsyb et al. (1997) $n=74$	Pripachkina (1997) $n=130$	Markova et al. (2001) $n=34$	Pashchevsky (2004) $n=86$	Ershova (2004) $n=120$	Korenev et al. (2005) $n=148$	Abalmasov and Ionova (2007) $n=56$	Own data $n=300$
Shape:								
Oval	8	17.7	–	14	–	–	–	15.33
Spherical	14	66.9	–	21	–	–	–	9.33
Irregular	78	15.4	–	65	–	–	–	75.34
Margins:								
Smooth	19	34.6	20.6	24	–	–	64.3	18.7
Rough	81	65.4	79.4	76	–	46.2	35.7	81.3
Contours:								
Well defined	31	56.9	–	37	–	19.8	75	28.3
Indistinct	69	43.1	–	63	72	46.2	25	71.7
Halo:								
Present	–	–	–	–	–	–	–	–
Hypo-,	4	39.2	–	52	–	34	10.7	28.3
anechoic	–	–	–	6	–	–	–	–
Hyperechoic	96	–	–	42	–	–	89.3	71.7
Absent								
Echodensity:								
Hyper-	–	6.2	–	10	–	6.1	3.6	11.7
Iso-	–	2.3	20.6	22	–	21.6	23.2	5.0
Hypo-	–	83.8	73.5	68	86	60.85	71.4	83.3
An-	–		5.9	–	–	11.5	–	–
Mixed-	–		–	–	–	–	1.8	–
Echostructure:								
Homogeneous	4	–	–	8	–	–	25	13
Heterogeneous	96	100	–	92	86	52	75	87
Calcifications:								
Present	46	76.2	79.4	43	58	26.4	41.1	25.3
Absent	54	–	–	57	–	–	58.9	74.7
Posterior enhancement:								
Present	23	6.2	–	29	–	–	–	29.0
Absent	77	–	–	71	48	–	–	71.0
Thyroid capsule:								
Unchanged	45	–	–	–	–	–	8.9	61.7
Irregular	55	–	–	–	22	–	91.1	38.3
Vascularity:								
Avascular	–	–	–	–	–	–	3.6	3.0
Hypovascular	–	–	–	–	–	–	21.4	11.3
Hypervascular	–	–	–	–	72	–	75.0	85.7
Lymph nodes:								
Homolateral	–	–	–	–	–	–	–	36
On both sides	–	–	–	–	–	–	–	12

sometimes detected in the normal thyroid gland (Fig. 6.35).

Hyperechoic inclusions within thyroid carcinoma are often microcalcifications (up to 2 mm without acoustic shadowing). Coarse amorphous echogenic calcium (larger than 2 mm with acoustic shadowing) may be sometimes identified. Severskaya (2002) reports that calcifications are equally often observed in thyroid cancer and nodular goiter. According to Burch (1995), peripheral "egg-shell" calcification suggests that the nodule is benign. Alternatively, microcalcifications in the central part of the lesion should increase the investigator's suspicion of malignancy. Takashima et al. (1995) report that microcalcifications showed the greatest

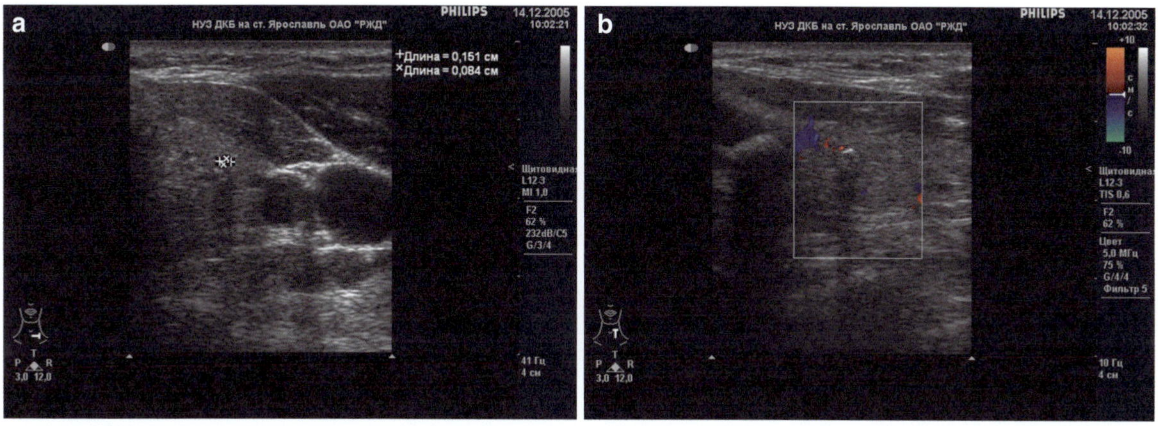

Fig. 6.35 (**a**, **b**) Calcifications in the normal thyroid. Grayscale and CDI

accuracy (76%) and specificity (93%) for diagnosing a malignancy among all US features, but the sensitivity of this approach appeared low, at 36%. According to Moon et al. (2008), macro- and microcalcifications are statistically significant features of thyroid cancer and demonstrate sensitivities of 44.2% and 9.7% along with specificities of 90.8% and 96.1%, respectively.

A sonographic study alerts to a suspected thyroid cancer in 65% of cases. The greatest probability (77%) is achieved with the combination of the following four sonographic features: decreased echodensity, irregular shape, indistinct borders, and irregular contours (Severskaya 2002). However, Bazhenova et al. (2002) report that the main US features of thyroid cancer (hypoechodensity, heterogeneity, and irregular margins) were detected in only 37% of patients with T1N0M0-stage thyroid cancer.

Indistinct contours and disorganization of the US architectonics of the affected muscles in cases of invasion of thyroid cancer may serve as accessory signs (Tsyb et al. 1997). The suspicion of a tumor merging into the trachea may arise in cases where more than 10 mm of a malignant lesion appears adjacent to the trachea.

The tissue harmonic option permits the improved visualization of the lesions in 28–30% of cases, the detection and localization of calcifications, and the differentiation of fluid collections in lesions with solid hypoechoic structure. However, its value for the differential diagnosis of thyroid cancer is insignificant. This option is especially effective when assessing the echostructures of large and small lesions (larger than 30 mm and smaller than 5 mm in size, respectively).

Over 90% of all malignant lesions demonstrate an intranodular blood flow pattern, while Zubarev et al. (2000) state that the majority of neoplasms (82.4%) show perinodular hypervascularization and intranodular hypovascularization with a chaotic disorganized pattern. According to Kotlyarov et al. (2001), lesions smaller than 0.8 cm in size appear avascular in CDI and PDI in 98%, and lesions of size 0.8–3 cm are hypovascular in 92% of cases. Tumors larger than 3 cm in size corresponded to hypervascular lesions in 99% of cases (Figs. 6.36–6.38).

According to Kotlyarov et al. (2001), no regularity in blood flow velocity, indices, and other data from PW Doppler was recorded for thyroid cancers of any size (Fig. 6.39).

3D reconstruction increases the diagnostic value of US (Fig. 6.40). It permits an assessment of the number and structure of malignant lesions, allows their location to be specified in relation to the thyroid capsule, vascular bundles, trachea, enables an analysis of the vascularity, growth and invasiveness, and can be used to calculate the volume of the affected and intact thyroid tissue. It clearly shows blurred, irregular, and tuberous margins, calcifications, and interruptions of the thyroid capsule along with merging into adjacent structures. 3D and panoramic scans also allow for a more precise follow-up of a lesion of any origin (Fig. 6.41). In several cases it may assist in reducing the follow-up period and the early diagnosis of thyroid malignancies (Zubarev et al. 2000; Drozd et al. 2000). 3DPD permits accurate assessment of pathological transformations and the density of vessels irregularly distributed within the neoplasm, the definition of the character of and the disturbance to the vascular pattern, and the detection of vessels with corkscrew courses (Fig. 6.42). Sonoelastography specifies the dense structure of the lesion (Fig. 6.43).

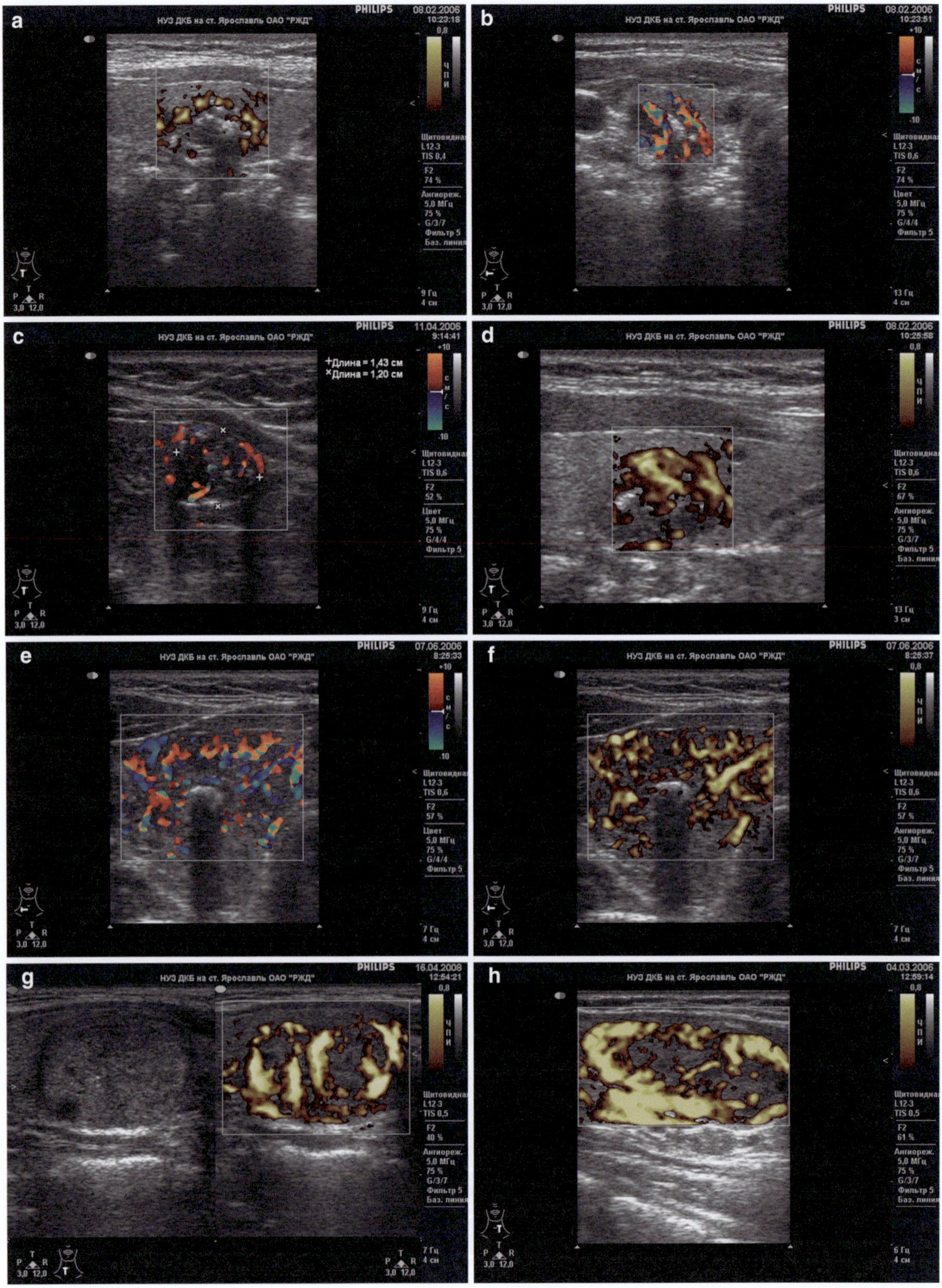

Fig. 6.36 (**a–h**) Thyroid cancer. Hypervascularity in CDI and PDI

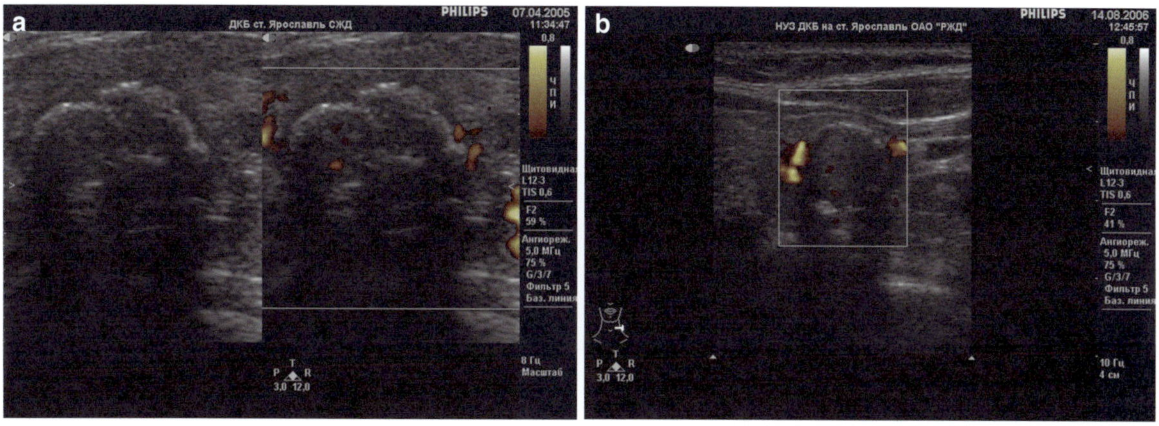

Fig. 6.37 (**a**, **b**) Thyroid cancer. Hypovascularity in CDI and PDI

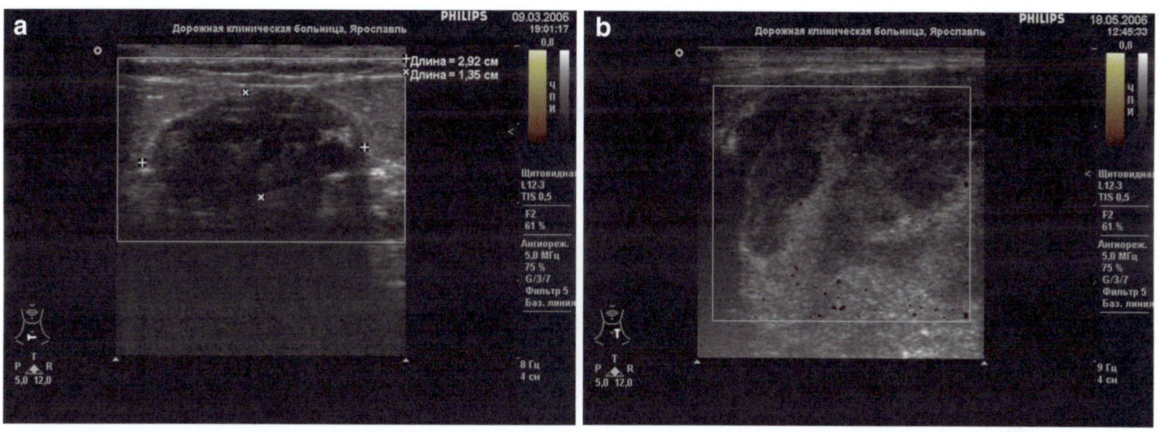

Fig. 6.38 (**a**, **b**) Thyroid cancer. Avascularity in CDI and PDI

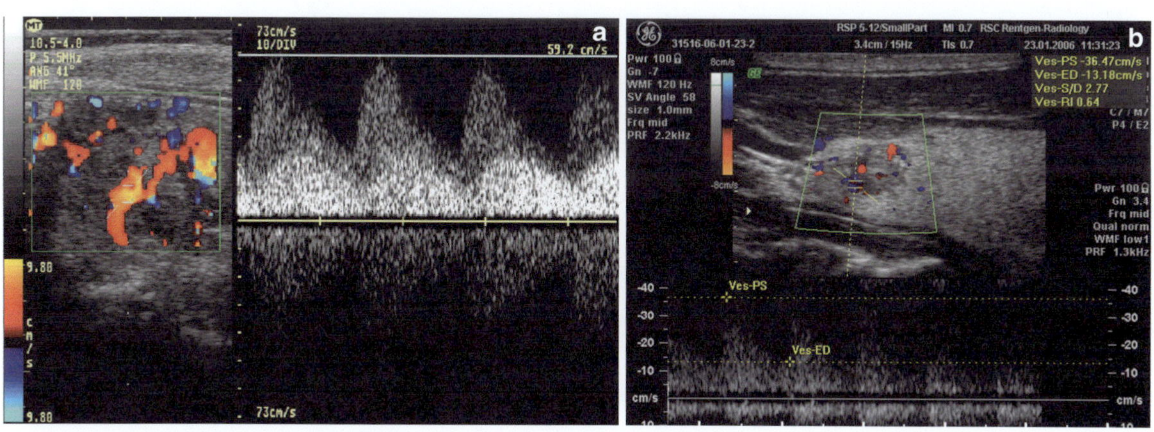

Fig. 6.39 (**a**, **b**) Thyroid cancer. PW Doppler

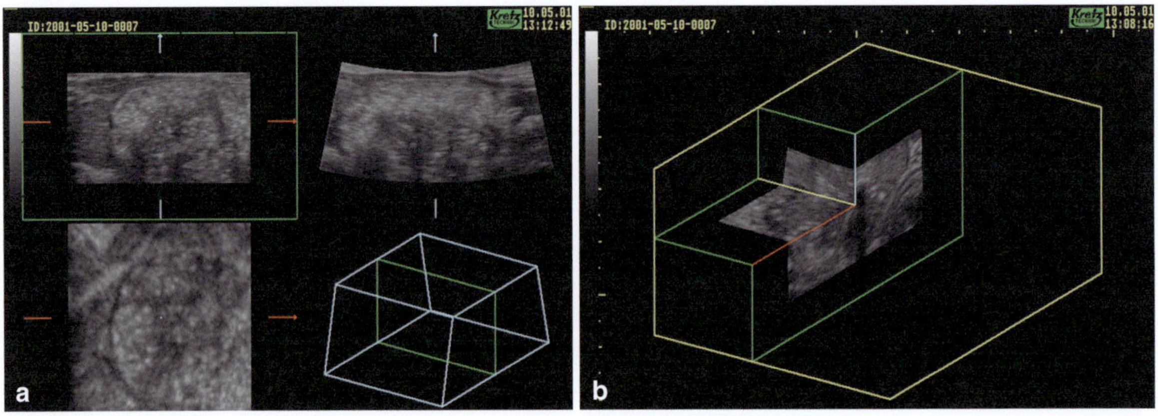

Fig. 6.40 (**a**, **b**) Thyroid cancer. 3D reconstruction

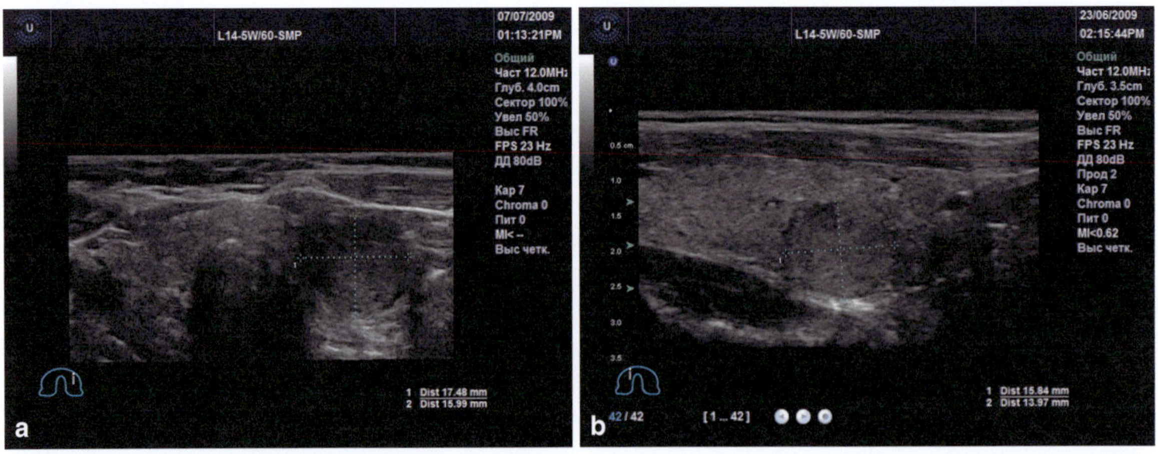

Fig. 6.41 (**a**, **b**) Thyroid cancer. Panoramic scan

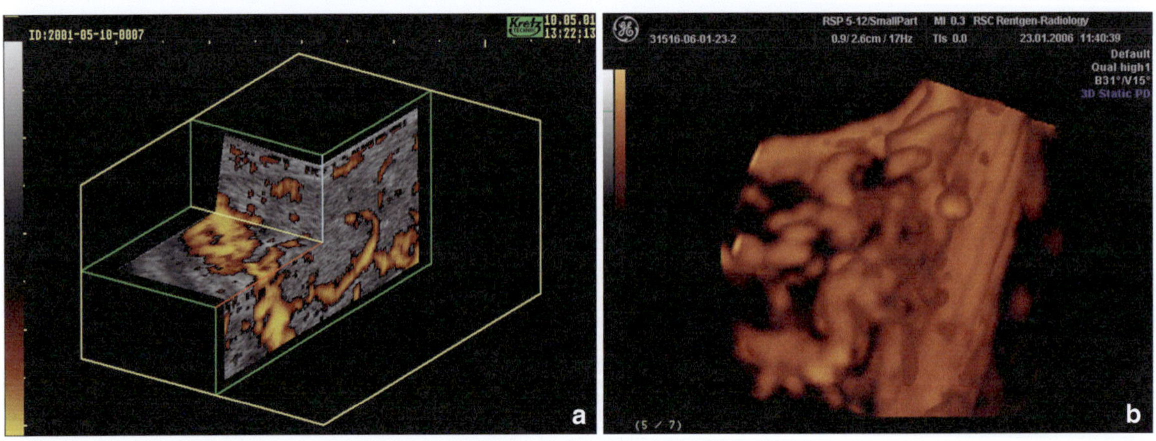

Fig. 6.42 (**a–h**) Thyroid cancer. Disorganized and asymmetric vascular pattern in 3DPD

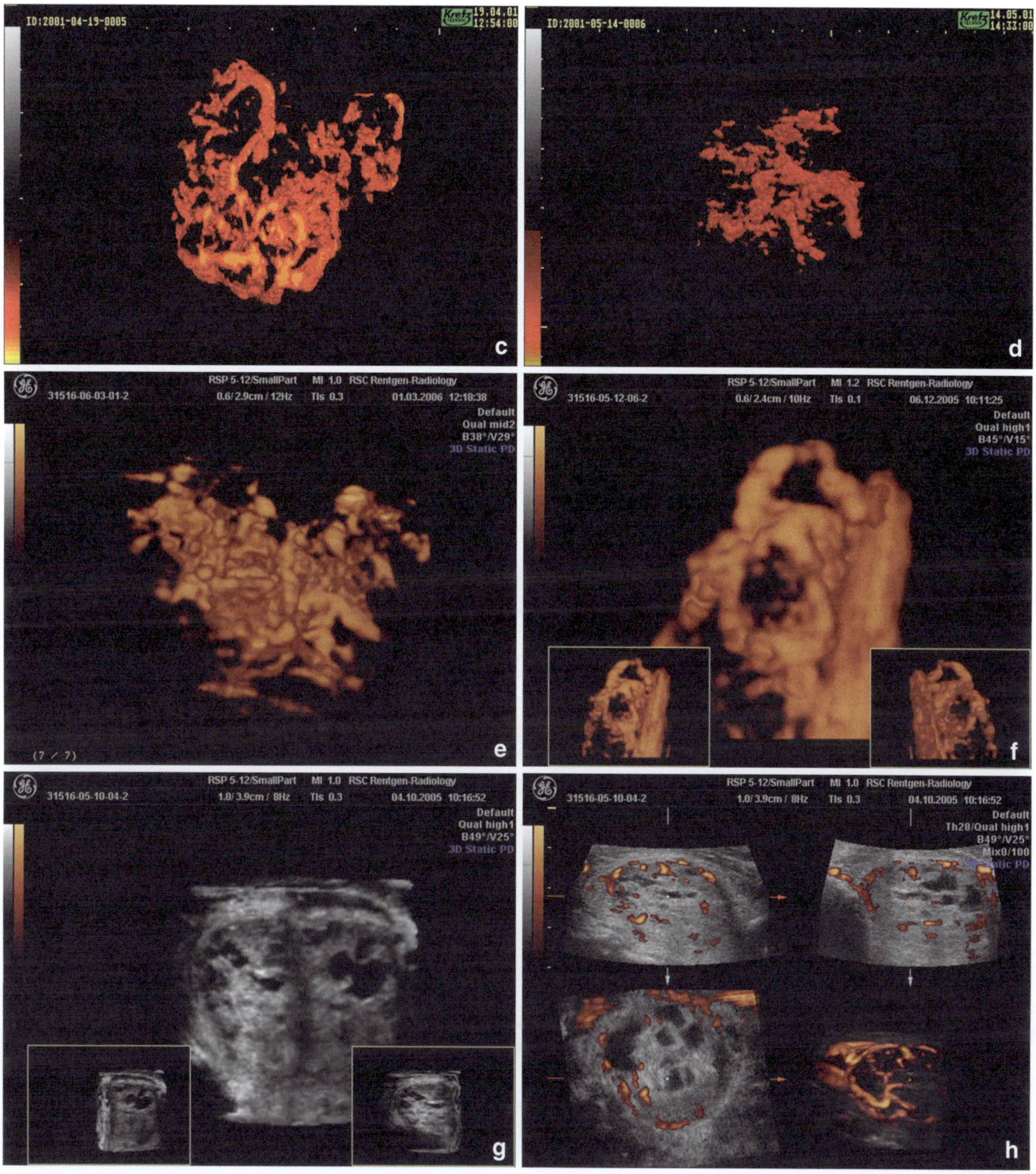

Fig. 6.42 (continued)

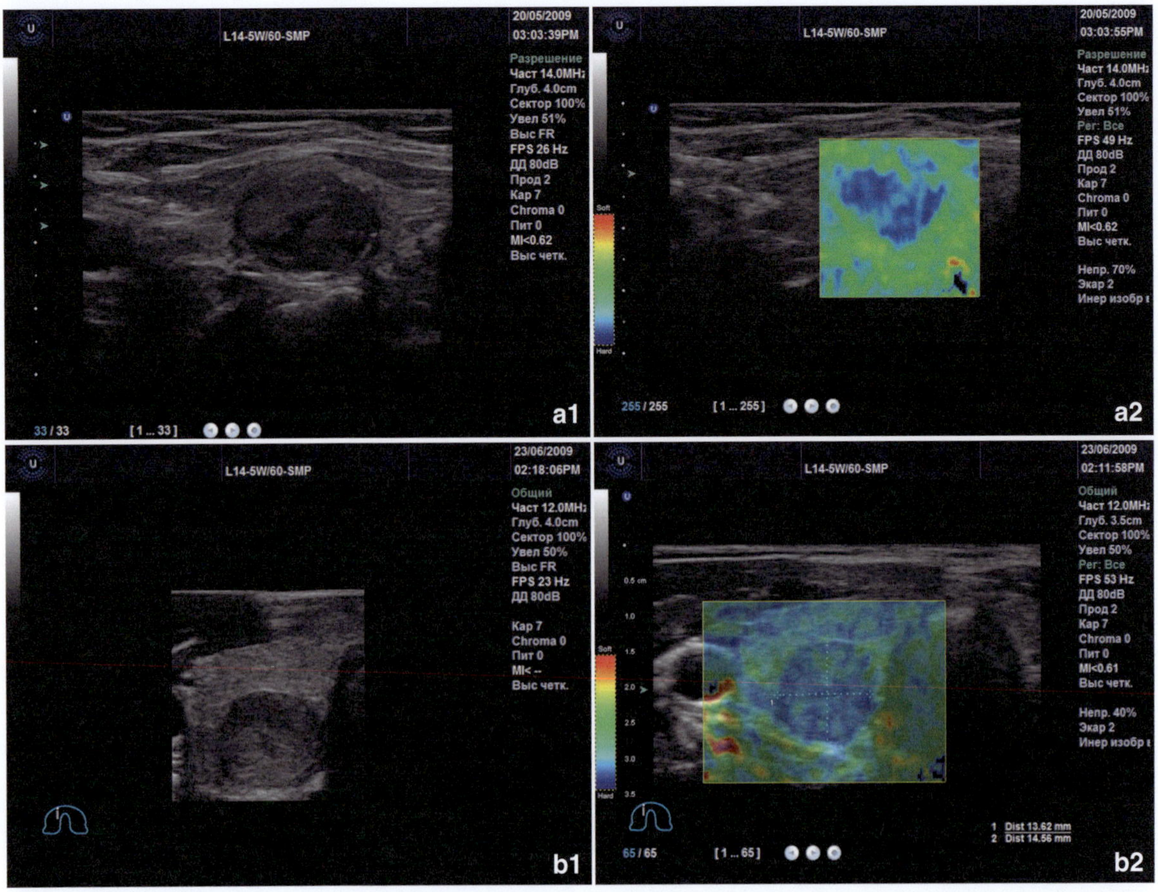

Fig. 6.43 (**a1,2–b1,2**) Thyroid cancer. Sonoelastography

The advantages of 4D US in thyroid cancer are linked to fast accurate spatial visualization of blood flow in the lesion with better differentiation of artifacts in real time. This permits the detailed differential diagnosis of mixed or incomplete types of vascularity of the lesion (Drozd et al. 2000).

Thyroid cancer is classified based on cell type as follows:

1. Follicular epithelial cell
   (a) Well-differentiated carcinomas
   - Papillary thyroid carcinoma (PTC)
     – Pure papillary
     – Follicular variant
     – Diffuse sclerosing variant
     – Tall-cell, columnar-cell variants
   - Follicular thyroid carcinoma (FTC)
     – Minimally invasive
     – Widely invasive
     – Hürthle-cell carcinoma (oncocytic)
     – Insular thyroid carcinoma

   (b) Anaplastic thyroid carcinoma (ATC)
2. C-cell (calcitonin-producing)
   (a) Medullary thyroid carcinoma (MTC)
   - Sporadic
   - Familial
   - MEN-2
3. Other cancers
   (a) Lymphoma
   (b) Sarcoma
   (c) Metastases
   (d) Others

Attempts to elucidate the morphological structure of a neoplasm based on its US image were undertaken. The sonographic features that were found for different morphological types of thyroid cancer are listed below (Zabolotskaya et al. 2006).

1. Papillary carcinoma is the most common type of thyroid malignancy. It accounts for 60–80% of all thyroid cancers and most often affects women of childbearing age. It appears extremely aggressive in children and adults over 50 years (McDougall 2006). It is well differentiated and frequently exhibits multicentricity and lymph node involvement. Papillary carcinoma is characterized by the following US features (Lu et al. 1994; Zabolotskaya et al. 2006):
   - Multicentricity
   - Hypoechoic echostructure (up to 90%)
   - Irregular indistinct margins in cases of invasive cancer or microcarcinoma
   - Microcalcifications up to 1 mm in size (85–90%)
   - Fluid collections with papillary vegetations and microcalcifications
   - Metastases in lymph nodes, which demonstrate microcalcifications in 80–90% of cases
   - Hypervascularity of peripheral and central patterns in CDI and PDI (up to 90%)
2. Follicular carcinoma accounts for about 10–30% of all thyroid cancers. Two subtypes are described: minimally invasive (indolent) and widely invasive (aggressive) carcinoma. Follicular carcinoma is characterized by capsular invasion and high risk of hematological spread and distant metastases (lungs, bones, and other sites). Metastases in neck lymph nodes are uncommon. Follicular thyroid cancer is characterized by the following US features (Zabolotskaya et al. 2006):
   - Frequently arises in adenomas.
   - Solid structure (up to 70%).
   - Isoechodensity (60%) or hypoechodensity (40%).
   - Homogeneous echostructure (up to 80%).
   - Irregular, tuberous borders.
   - Wide peripheral halo with irregular width.
   - Signs of invasion into the surrounding muscles.
   - Absence of microcalcifications within the lesion.
   - Rare metastases in lymph nodes (8–10%).
   - A mixed blood flow pattern (intranodular and perinodular) in CDI, PDI, and 3DPD is usually characteristic. Intranodular blood flow is mainly represented by wavy arterial vessels of irregular gauge, which are randomly distributed within the lesion.
3. Medullary carcinoma originates from thyroid parafollicular C-cells and accounts for 2–10% of all thyroid neoplasms (McDougall 2006). It shows a more aggressive character than other well-differentiated cancers. It can be both sporadic (3.5–80%) and familial (4.5–38%). According to Ilyin et al. (2000), the average ratio is 1:1.4 in men and women respectively in both types of MTC. Sporadic cancer usually occurs in patients over 40–50 years of age, and presents with a monofocal (unilateral) thyroid lesion. The familial type is autosomal dominant, and usually initiates below 35 years of age. It predominantly affects the thyroid bilaterally and shows multiple lesions, which are usually located in the upper parts of the lobes. It may occur as part of a multiple endocrine neoplasia (MEN) syndrome. MTC is characterized by early regional metastases (40–55%). The sonographic features of medullary thyroid cancer are as follows (Zabolotskaya et al. 2006):
   - Frequent multicentricity or diffuse affection of both lobes
   - Hypoechoic solid structure
   - Irregular contours
   - A peripheral hypoechoic halo with irregular width is often noted
   - Presence of microcalcifications with acoustic shadowing (80–90%)
   - Frequent postoperative recurrence
   - Intranodular blood flow pattern in CDI, PDI, and 3DPD
4. Anaplastic thyroid carcinoma accounts for 1.6–12% of all malignant tumors of the thyroid gland. It occurs most often in people over 60 years of age, and mainly in women. It is a very aggressive neoplasm.
5. Malignant lymphoma accounts for about 5% of all thyroid cancers, and more often occurs in the elderly (McDougall 2006). It is a fast-growing tumor that often (in 70–80%) arises in women with pre-existing Hashimoto's thyroiditis (Privalov et al. 1995). Thyroid lymphomas are associated with the following sonographic features:
   - Large size
   - Pressure effects on trachea and esophagus
   - Decreased echodensity
   - Tuberous contours
   - Heterogeneous echostructure with large anechoic areas
6. Metastatic tumors of the thyroid gland may be detected in patients with breast cancer (21%), renal

cancer (10%), melanoma (39%), and other tumors (Zabolotskaya et al. 2006). Such tumors are most often characterized by the following sonographic features:

- Hypoechoic heterogeneous solid lesion more than 4 cm in size (up to 80%)
- More often with a hypoechoic halo
- Changes in regional neck lymph nodes are seen

7. Rare types of thyroid cancer include squamous carcinoma, reticulosarcoma, fibrosarcoma, angiosarcoma, teratoma, etc.

The sensitivity of US in the diagnosis of thyroid cancer is 69–98%, and it has a specificity of 50–92% and a diagnostic accuracy of 80–99% (Pripachkina 1997; Erdem et al. 1997; Zubarev et al. 2000; Kotlyarov et al. 2001; Pashchevsky 2004; Moon et al. 2008). According to Agamov et al. (2003), the popularization of sonography resulted in an increase in the proportion of patients with stage T1–2N0M0 thyroid cancer from 57.4% (in 1991) to 70.6% (in 2000). According to Kotlyarov et al. (2001), grayscale sonography shows positive predictive value for thyroid cancer in 85.5% of cases. CDI, PDI, and 3D reconstruction increase the efficacy of US up to 95%. Markova (2001) reported that the specificities of sonography in grayscale, CDI, PDI, and 3DPD for the diagnosis of thyroid cancer are 73, 78.8, 81.1, and 86.1%, with sensitivities of 76.6, 85.4, 89.8, and 92.9%, and diagnostic accuracies of 72.4, 78.6, 81.7, and 86.9%, respectively.

According to Kumar et al. (1992), Pripachkina (1997), and Abdulhalimova et al. (1999), US imaging does not reveal any specific features for thyroid cancer, but it does allow the detection of nonpalpable nodules of malignant tumors in 20.6% of patients. Common US features in malignant and benign thyroid nodules are observed in 8–45% of cases (Romanko 1997).

Mistakes in the differential diagnosis of thyroid malignancies are reported in 25–75% of cases. Thyroid carcinomas demonstrate atypical US features

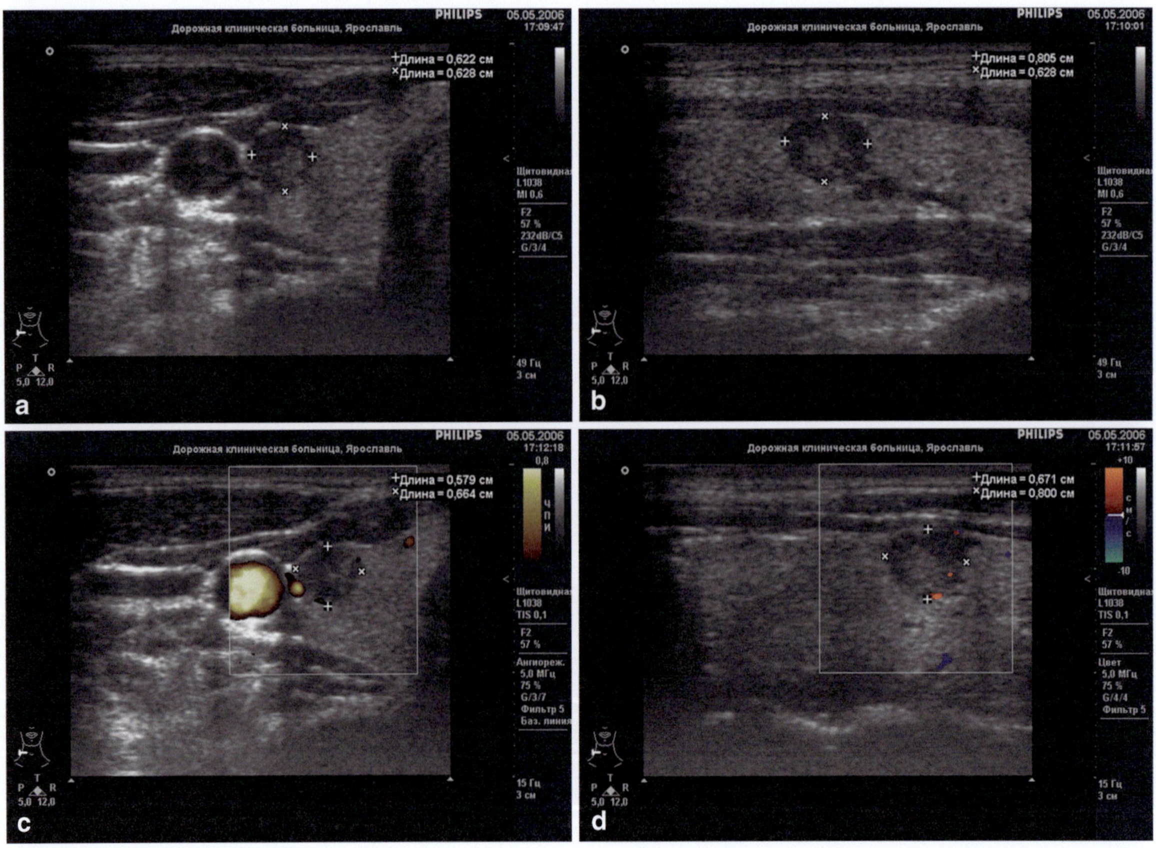

Fig. 6.44 (**a–d**) Papillary thyroid cancer. Grayscale, CDI, and PDI. US image not characteristic of thyroid cancer. Roundish shape; accurate, well-defined margins; homogeneity; absence of posterior acoustic change; and avascularity

in 4.7% of patients (Fig. 6.42). Most authors agree that the lack of absolute pathognomonic features of thyroid cancer makes it impossible to reliably differentiate malignant and benign lesions by US examination only. Therefore, US reports are regarded as suggestive.

The experience and skills of sonographers and radiologists along with those of other specialists, as well as the advantages of new US options and modalities, permit the early diagnosis and rational management of thyroid neoplasms.

The example of US report in thyroid cancer

First name, middle initial, last name:
Age:
Date:
The number of case history:
US scanner:
The thyroid gland is substernally located (the left lobe), asymmetric with irregular margins. The contours are locally indistinct, the capsule is not detected in the upper and middle segments of the left lobe. The margin between the lobe and trachea is blurred, the structure of the adjacent muscles is disorganized, heterogeneous, and hypoechoic.

The depth of the **isthmus** - 5 mm	
Right lobe	**Left lobe**
Depth 19 mm Width 11 mm Length 42 mm	Depth 52 mm Width 72 mm Length 80 mm
Volume 4.4 cm^3	Volume 149.8 cm^3
The total volume 154.2 cm^3 exceeds the upper limit for the endemic region and the WHO recommendations.	
No lesions detected.	The lobe is substituted by a hypoechoic lesion of 8.0x7.2x5.2cm in size with irregular margins and substernal inferior part. The lesion is extremely heterogeneous with hyperechoic inclusions up to 0.9cm in size with posterior shadowing, isoechoic irregular areas up to 3.0cm in size. The vascularity of the lesion is disorganized, asymmetric with locally hypervascular areas and irregularly distributed vessels. 3DPD reveals the pathological transformation of the vessels within the lesion.

The trachea and esophagus are dislocated to the right with compression. The esophagus follows along the right side of the trachea. The blood flow in the left CCA is not detected. The left internal jugular vein is partially compressed with the lesion, demonstrates significant spontaneous echo contrast without thrombus. The right vascular bundle is unchanged.
The lymph nodes of the central neck (pretracheal) and lateral neck (left internal jugular chain) are enlarged up to 0.9x2.0cm, hypoechoic, heterogeneous, hypovascular with moderate chaotic vascularization throughout the cortex, of irregular shape with the tendency to merging at the left side. The lymph nodes in supra- and infraclavicular areas are not enlarged.
CONCLUSION: The image suggests the carcinoma of the left thyroid lobe with the thyroid enlargement of the 3 stage with invasion into trachea, left CCA, and neck muscles, compression of the left IJV and the esophagus. Bilateral metastases into the lymph nodes of the neck.
US specialist:

7 Ultrasound Examination After Thyroid Surgery

US of the postoperative neck requires a certain degree of experience on behalf of the sonographer. It is important to take the type of operation and the time that has elapsed since the surgery into account. The examination may benefit from reviewing the history of the disease, the results of preoperative US, and the data from the histological assessment of the removed specimen.

Below is a guide to interpreting the US changes in the region of the operation:

1. Detection of thyroid tissue in the thyroid bed (residue or fragments)
   - Number of thyroid fragments
   - Location of each fragment and relations to surrounding structures
   - Size
   - Margins
   - Echodensity and echostructure
   - Vascularity of the thyroid residue and fragments
2. Detection of pathological lesions in the remaining thyroid tissue (location, size, shape, borders, contours, echodensity, echostructure, vascularization, and relations to surrounding organs and tissues)
3. Mutual relations of neck organs and structures
4. Status of cervical, supra- and subclavicular lymph nodes

The immediate postsurgical period is characterized by the infiltration of the thyroid bed and subcutaneous fat, with visualization of hematomas and suture material. Granulomas, calcifications, and fluid structures may appear later. This may lead to US hyperdiagnosis of disease recurrence within the first two months. Sonography normally reveals thickening and heterogeneity of fat with a decrease in echodensity due to edema and infiltration. These changes may be misinterpreted as preserved thyroid tissue, or they can also mask the thyroid residue (its margins are poorly differentiated against the changes in the structure of the surrounding tissue). Hemorrhages can be seen as hypoechoic lesions in the thyroid bed. They are most often observed as heterogeneous structures with hypo- and hyperechoic areas, often with anechoic fluid collections of different shapes and sizes (Fig. 7.1). They show fast changes in US appearance, which are also typical of hematomas with other localizations. Suture material is often visualized as dot-shaped

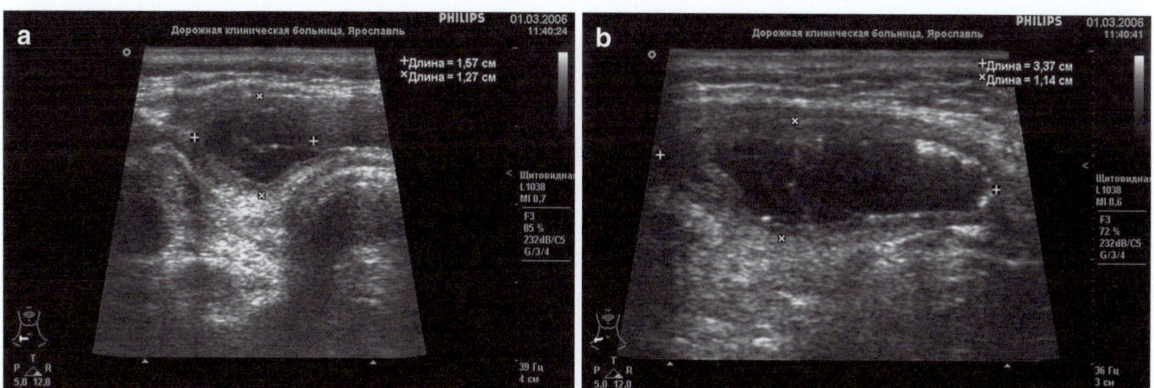

Fig. 7.1 (**a**, **b**) Status one month after thyroid surgery. Postoperative hematomas. Grayscale, CDI, and PDI

V. P. Kharchenko et al., *Ultrasound Diagnostics of Thyroid Diseases*,
DOI: 10.1007/978-3-642-12387-0_7, © Springer-Verlag Berlin Heidelberg 2010

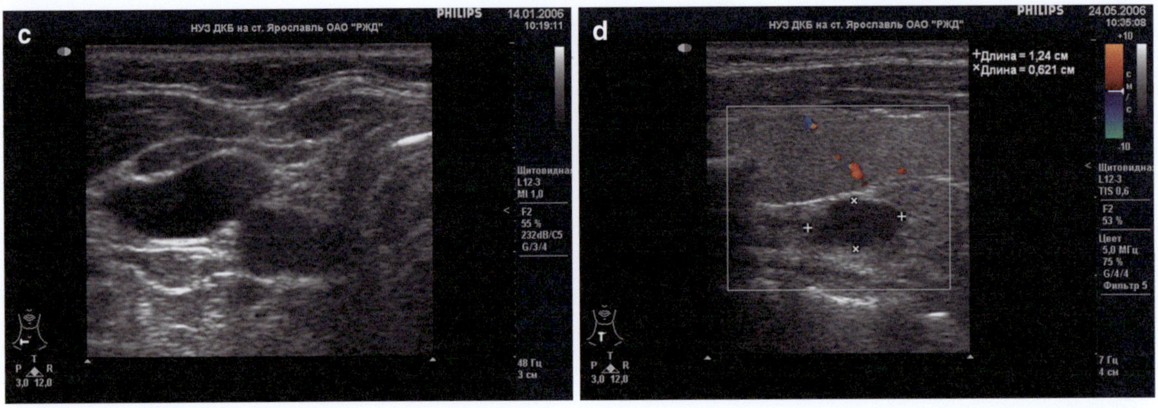

Fig. 7.1 (continued)

echogenic inclusions with indistinct or absent acoustic shadows located in the bed of the thyroid lobe or attached to the capsule of the thyroid residue.

Sonography of the thyroid bed more than three months after surgery reveals full or partial absence of thyroid tissue. The site shows diffuse fibrous changes with vascular bundles displaced medially (Fig. 7.2). The fields of hemorrhage, as a rule, are no longer defined. Organizational features can be detected at the locations of former hematomas, and these show an increase in echodensity, heterogeneous structure, and indistinct and irregular contours. Three months after surgery, sutures and ligatures can only be defined in a few cases. Fine, roundish fields of increased echodensity up to 5 mm in

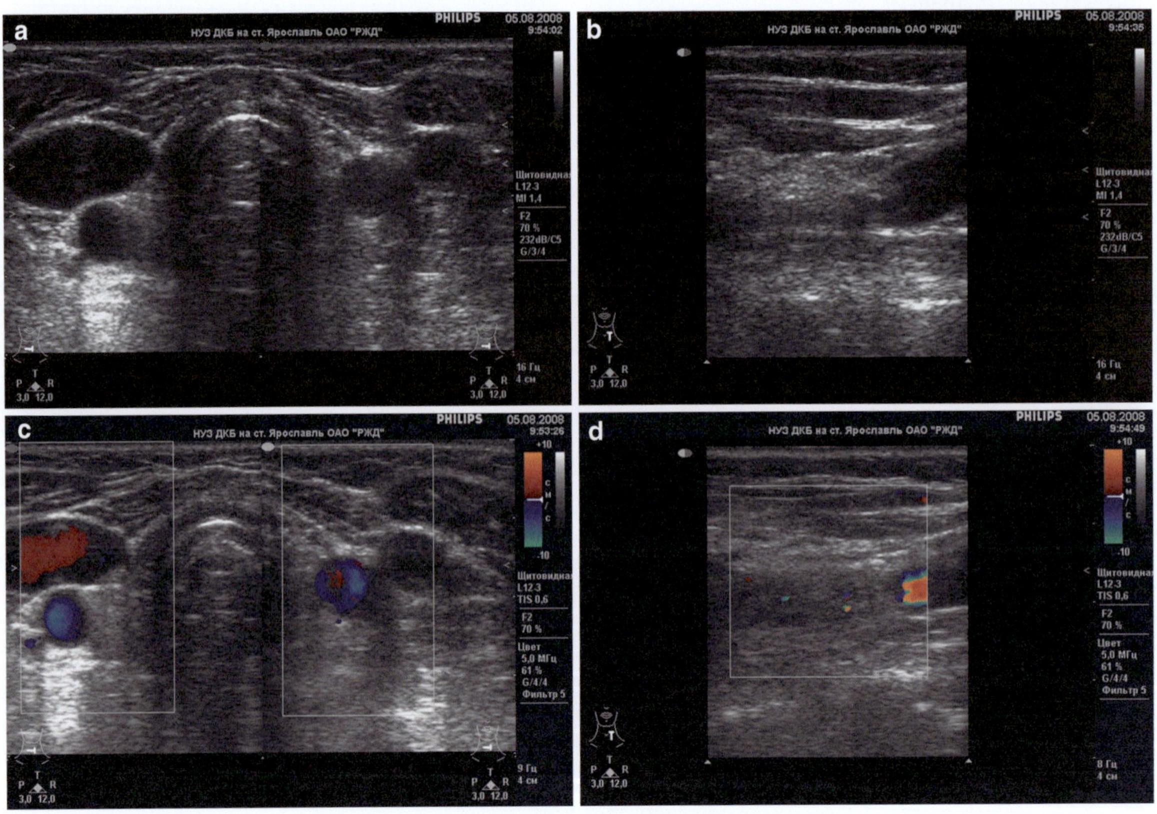

Fig. 7.2 (**a–d**) Status three months after thyroid resection. Grayscale, CDI, and PDI

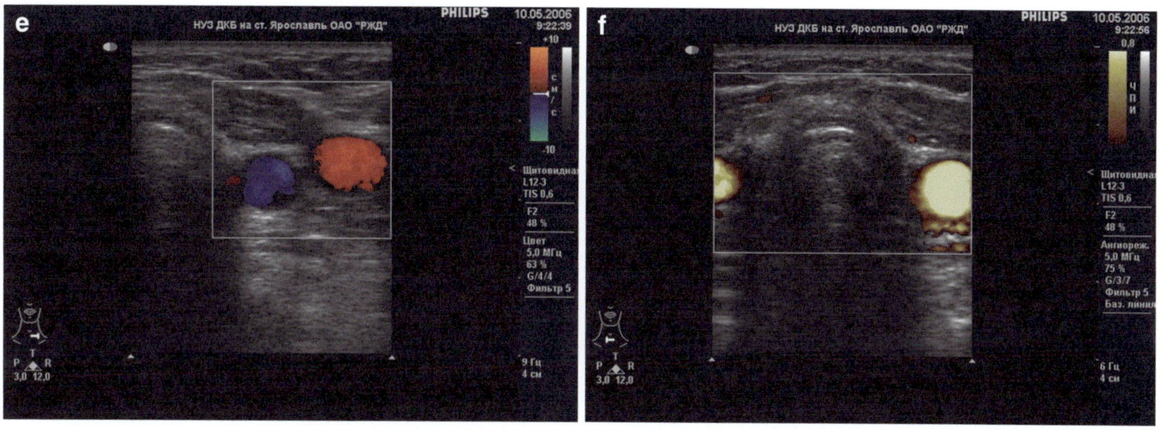

Fig. 7.2 (continued) (**e, f**) Status three months after thyroid resection. Grayscale, CDI, and PDI

size with regular distinct margins may be noted in some patients at the locations of former sutures. These may be regarded as suture granulomas. Anechoic lesions, such as fine cysts and organized fluid collections, may be seen in rare cases (Altunina 1996; Kotlyarov et al. 2001).

The US image of the thyroid bed three months after organ-saving operations (subtotal resection, hemithyroidectomy) depicts the thyroid residue with regular margins, homogeneous structure, and unchanged or slightly decreased/increased echodensity (Fig. 7.3).

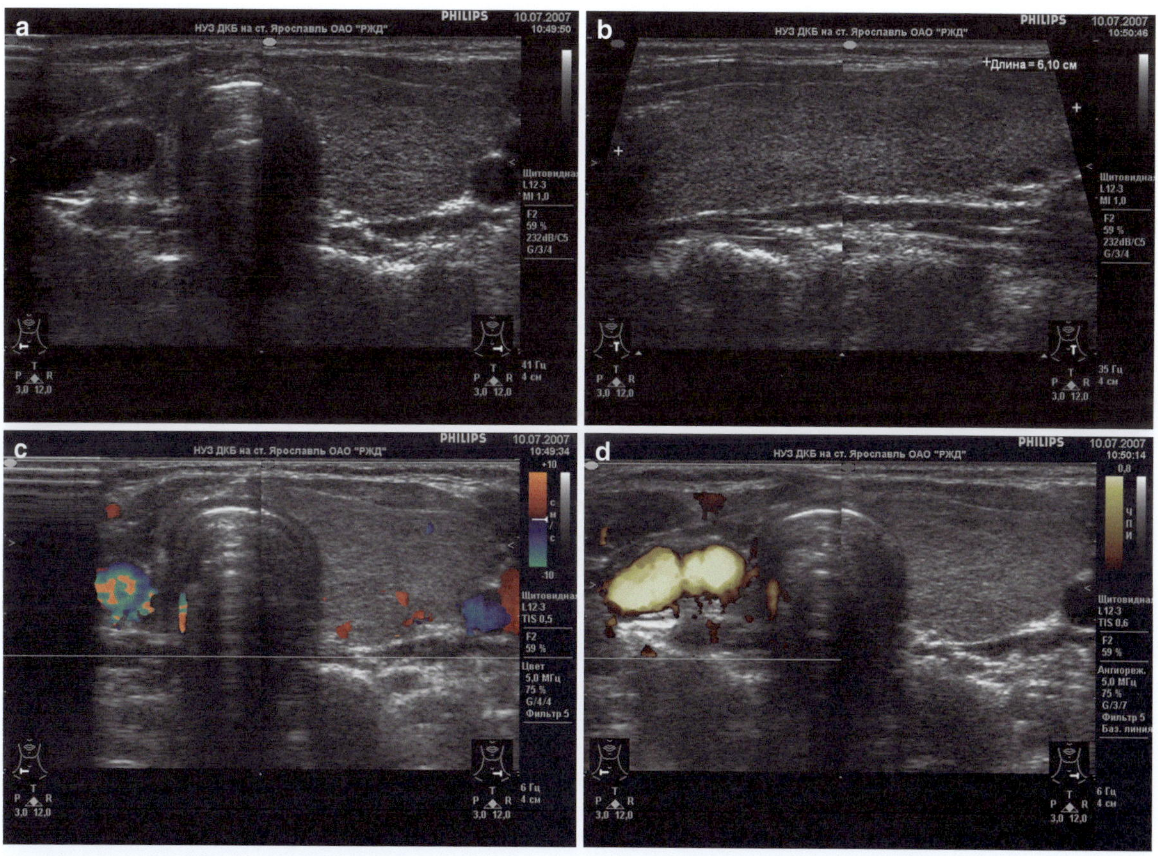

Fig. 7.3 (**a–d**) Status three months after hemithyroidectomy. Grayscale, CDI, and PDI

Fibrotic changes are often seen in the bed of the removed lobe. The remnants of organized hematomas may be detected in rare cases as dense heterogeneous inclusions with indistinct contours, calcifications, suture granulomas, or individual cysts. The vascular bundle on the operated side is displaced medially towards the trachea (Fig. 7.4).

Central neck dissection leads to specific changes in sonograms. The trachea contours appear indistinct, and vascular bundles migrate superficially close to the trachea. Fibrous changes in the tissues adjacent to the thyroid bed are prominent.

Several operations for thyroid cancer and malignant tumors of the head and neck require the removal of different neck structures. In some cases, cervical and supraclavicular lymph nodes, the submandibular salivary gland, sternomastoid and omohyoid muscles, or the internal jugular vein is/are excised, resulting in corresponding sonographic changes.

Five years or more after the resection of more than half of the thyroid lobe, its volume usually remains unchanged; in the case of the resection of one-half to one-third of the thyroid lobe, it usually recovers to its full size as a rule. The thyroid remnant shows well-defined margins, normal or slightly increased echodensity, and possible heterogeneity. A decreased or normal parenchymal blood flow pattern is seen in CDI, PDI, and 3DPD.

In some patients who have undergone total thyroidectomy, the thyroid bed may subsequently display thyroid remnants of various sizes, shapes, and vascularities upon US and radionuclide scans. According to Salvatori et al. (2007), scintigraphy after total thyroidectomy and radioiodine therapy did not detect any residual thyroid tissue in the thyroid bed in only 7% of patients.

Radioiodine (^{131}I) treatment and remote gamma therapy after thyroidectomy lead to some distinctive sonographic features. The thyroid remnant, if any, after the treatment is poorly differentiated from the surrounding tissues (Fig. 7.5). It appears to have indistinct and irregular margins, heterogeneous hypoechoic echostructure, and decreased vascularity. Areas of

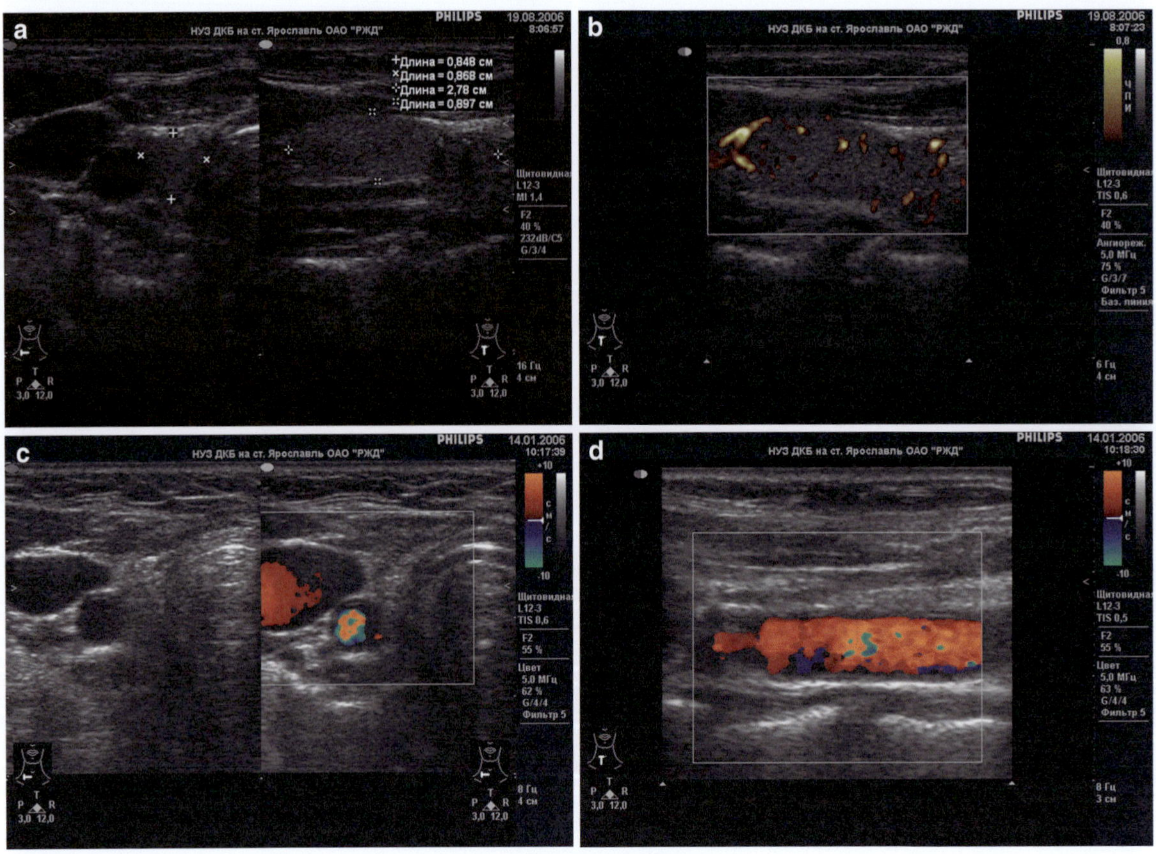

Fig. 7.4 (**a–d**) Status one year after thyroid surgery. Grayscale, CDI, and PDI

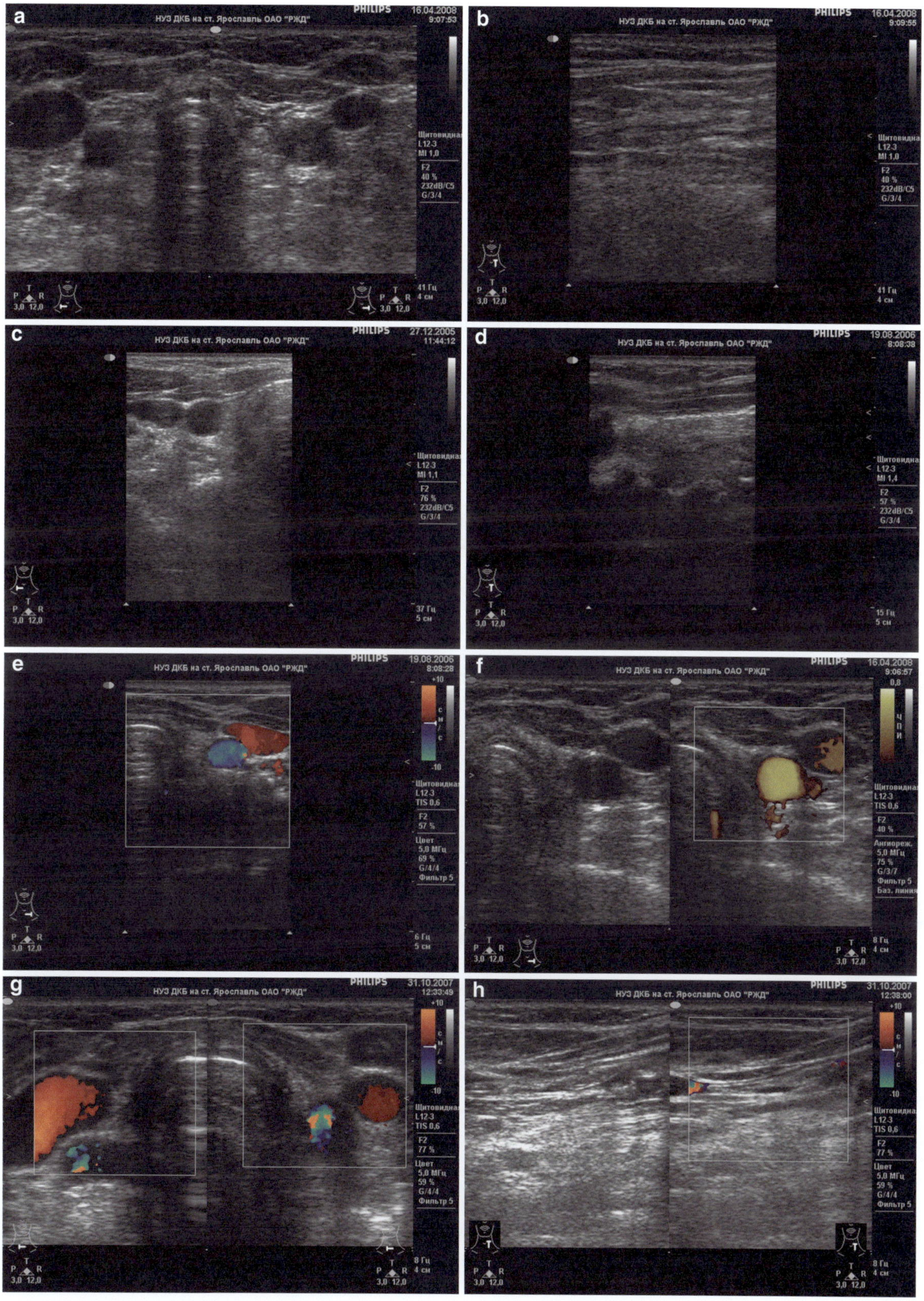

Fig. 7.5 (**a–h**) Status one year after radioiodine (^{131}I) treatment. Grayscale, CDI, and PDI

increased echodensity and fibrous changes in the surrounding tissues may arise (Altunina 1996).

Patients who have been operated on for thyroid malignancy should be examined sonographically at the following intervals:

- Once every three months during the first postoperative year
- Once every six months for the next five years
- Once a year after that

After surgery for benign thyroid diseases, patients should undergo thyroid US at three, six, and twelve months after the operation during the first year, and once a year after that.

Each scheduled US follow-up permits the precise characterization of the thyroid bed and residue, allowing the potential for future recurrence to be determined.

The example of US report in postoperative neck

First name, middle initial, last name:
Age:
Date:
The number of case history:
US scanner:
The thyroid is operated on (the surgery – 2000, September; histology – unknown).

The **isthmus** is removed	
Right lobe	**Left lobe**
Depth 20 mm Width 19 mm Length 42 mm	is removed. Thyroid tissue, cystic, and solid lesions are not detected in the bed of the lobe. The bed echodensity is slightly diffusely increased with relatively homogeneous structure.
Volume 8.0 cm^3	

The total volume 8.0 cm^3 does not exceed the upper limit for the endemic region and the WHO recommendations.
The echodensity of parenchyma of the thyroid residue is slightly diffusely decreased, locally heterogeneous with hypoechoic areas of different shape and size. The lesions are not detected. Vascular pattern intensity of the parenchyma is slightly decreased in CDI and PDI. CPD is up to 5-10 %. The left vascular bundle is moderately displaced medially.
The lymph nodes in the neck and supraclavicular areas are not enlarged.
CONCLUSION: The status after hemithyroidectomy. No recurrence is determined.
US specialist:

Recurrent Thyroid Lesions

8

Postoperative recurrent goiter is characterized by the reappearance of thyroid pathology in patients who have previously been operated on for this condition. Recurrence is considered to be the thyroid disease that was observed prior to the surgery and was the reason for the operation. According to Akinchev et al. (2005), 89% of the diseases in a thyroid remnant are primary thyroid diseases. However, diseases that are different from the preoperative abnormality arise in some patients. Such cases should be considered new diseases of the thyroid remnant. The rates of recurrence for various thyroid diseases are as follows: multinodular euthyroid goiter 54.7%, Graves' disease 14.5%, nodular euthyroid goiter 13.1%, multinodular toxic goiter 6.8%, thyroid cancer 1.3%, cancer with another pathology 2.8%, AITD 2.3%, nodular toxic goiter 1.7%, and undifferentiated thyroid cancer 0.8% (Akinchev et al. 2005).

Some authors differentiate between false and true recurrences (Goch 1994). False recurrences are detected soon after surgery. A false recurrence is actually associated with inadequate revision during the operation, which results in some remnant of the lesion being left in the thyroid gland. True recurrence appears much later, in the unchanged tissue of the thyroid residue, and has the same causes as the primary lesion (Shuhgalter 1990).

US is the main visualizing method used for the early diagnosis of recurrent goiter.

The most frequent US features of recurrent nodular goiter are as follows (Figs. 8.1 and 8.2; Table 8.1):

- Lesion in the thyroid bed or thyroid residue
- Roundish or oval shape of lesion
- Hyper-, hypoechodensity
- Heterogeneous echostructure
- Regular, well-defined margins
- Additional lesions during the course of lymphatic drainage of the neck (in cases with thyroid cancer recurrence and metastases)
- Different types of vascularity in CDI, PDI, and 3DPD

It is not correct to use the term "recurrence" in relation to AITD and Graves' disease, because autoimmune diseases initially affect the whole thyroid gland, so the part that remains after the surgery is sure to be affected (Fig. 8.3), as surgical treatment does not interrupt the pathogenesis of the disease.

Cancer in the thyroid residue and metastases in regional lymph nodes that are detected within three months of surgery, and remote metastases found within six months of surgical treatment are regarded as cancer recurrences (AJCC).

The frequency of long-term recurrent nodular goiter (relative to all operated patients) after surgery is 1.8–88%. The incidence of thyroid cancer in recurrent goiter is 10–31.7%, including 6.8–30% for well-differentiated cancer and 30–88% for poorly or undifferentiated cancer (Goch 1994; Paches et al. 1995; Altunina 1996). According to Akinchev et al. (2005), the frequency of new cases of thyroid cancer in recurrent goiter is about 4.9%.

Thyroid cancer recurrence is usually diagnosed 2–10 years (up to 30%) after the operation, with the ratio of men to women affected is 1:4, with an average age of 31–60 years (Sencha 2001). It is usually seen on the side of the primary lesion (43.8%), on the opposite side in 30.2%, and on both sides in 26%.

Recurrent cancer is usually characterized by the same US features as the primary tumor (Figs. 8.4–8.6).

V.P. Kharchenko et al., *Ultrasound Diagnostics of Thyroid Diseases*,
DOI: 10.1007/978-3-642-12387-0_8, © Springer-Verlag Berlin Heidelberg 2010

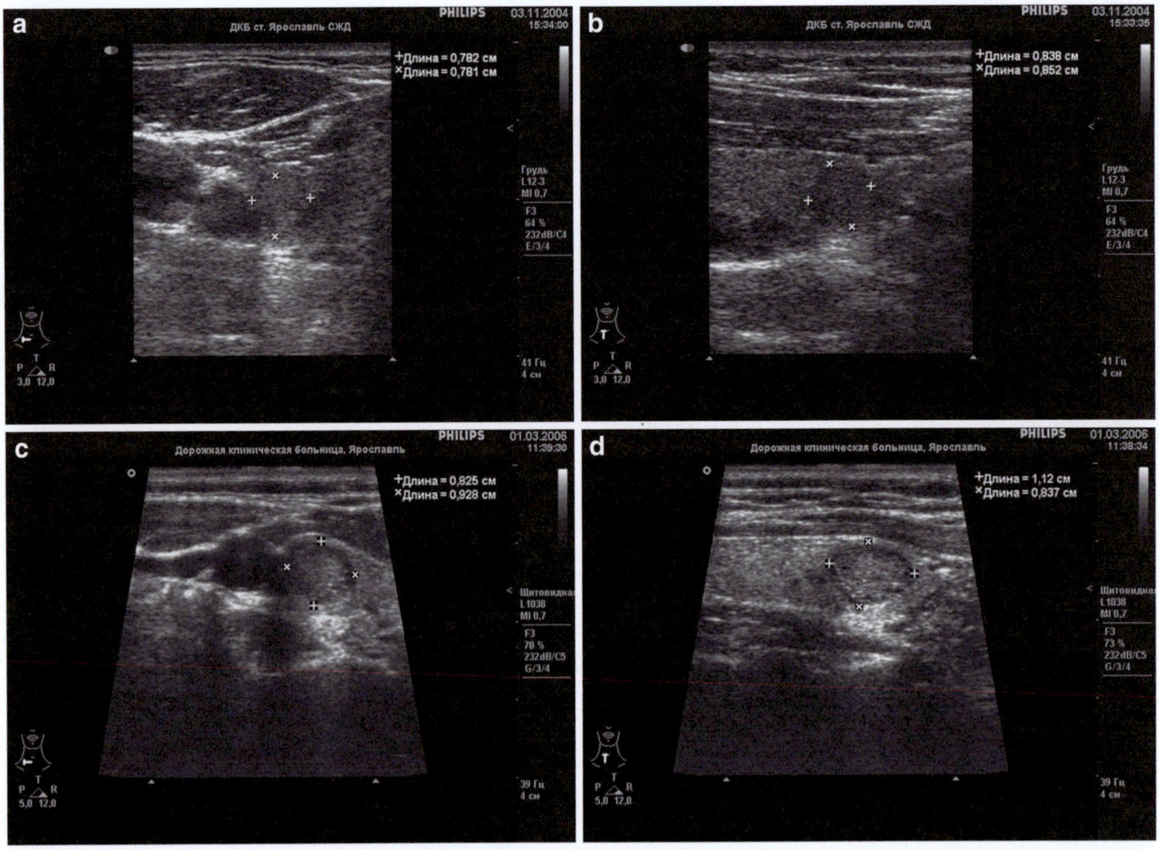

Fig. 8.1 (**a–d**) Status after thyroid surgery. Recurrent nodular goiter. Gray scale

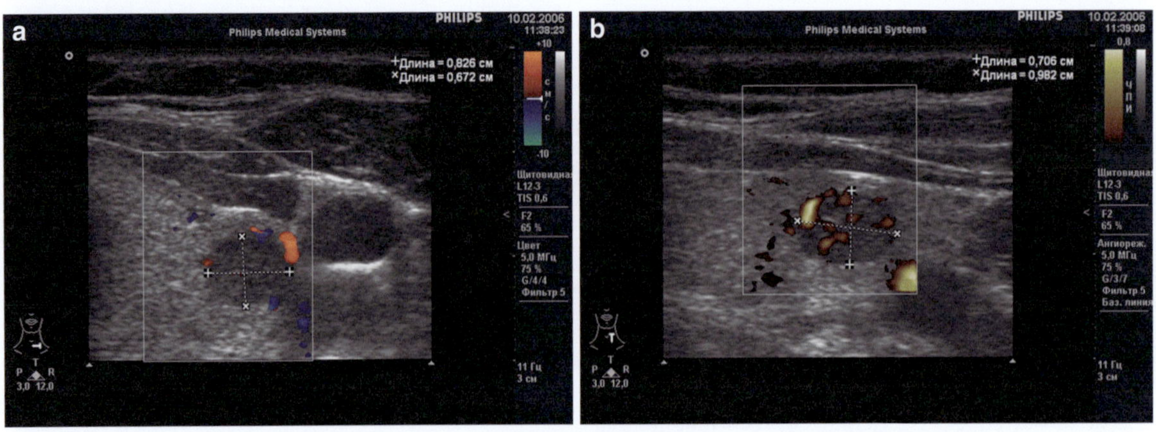

Fig. 8.2 (**a**, **b**) Status after thyroid surgery. Recurrent nodular goiter. CDI and PDI

However, it exhibits rare calcifications, often an increased vascular pattern, and invasion into the surrounding organs (Table 8.1).

Recurrent thyroid cancer is represented by the following histological types: papillary, 50–80%; follicular, 15–40%; poorly or undifferentiated carcinoma, 2–5% of cases (Samaan et al. 1992;).

The diagnosis of thyroid cancer in recurrent goiter is extremely complex and demands the use of a combination of all diagnostic options and technologies. The sensitivity of US to local recurrence of thyroid cancer is 83–93.6%; its specificity is 90.2–92% and its diagnostic accuracy is 90–91% (Agapitov 1996; Sencha 2008).

Table 8.1 Sonographic features of thyroid disease recurrence according to different authors

US features	Recurrent thyroid cancer		Recurrent thyroid goiter
	Altunina (1996) $n=73$Tsyb (1997)	Own data $n=51$	Own data $n=21$
Thyroid volume increase:			
Present	–	37.25	23.8
Absent	–	62.75	76.2
Shape:			
Spherical	32.8	15.7	42.9
Oval	12.3	19.6	52.4
Irregular	54.9	64.7	4.7
Margins:			
Smooth	–	37.25	71.4
Irregular	–	62.75	28.6
Contours:			
Well-defined	46.6	7.8	76.2
Blurred	53.4	92.2	23.8
Echodensity:			
Hyper-	1.4	92.2	61.9
Iso-	–	5.8	4.75
Hypo-	83.6	2.0	28.6
An-	–	–	4.75
Echostructure:			
Homogeneous	45.2	9.8	57.1
Heterogeneous	54.8	90.2	42.9
Calcifications or hyperechoic inclusions:			
Present	12.3	5.9	9.5
Absent	87.7	94.1	90.5
Fluid collections:			
Present	2.7	19.6	4.8
Absent	97.3	80.4	95.2
Relation to thyroid capsule, CCA, and IJV:			
Not adjacent	49.3	33.3	66.7
Adjacent	42.5	56.9	33.3
Invasion	8.2	9.8	–
Vascularity:			
Avascular	–	15.7	52.4
Hypovascular	–	19.6	23.8
Hypervascular	–	64.7	23.8
Neck lymph node enlargement:			
Absent	–	35.3	81.0
Present:	–	64.7	19.0
Unilateral	–	41.2	14.3
Bilateral	–	23.4	4.7

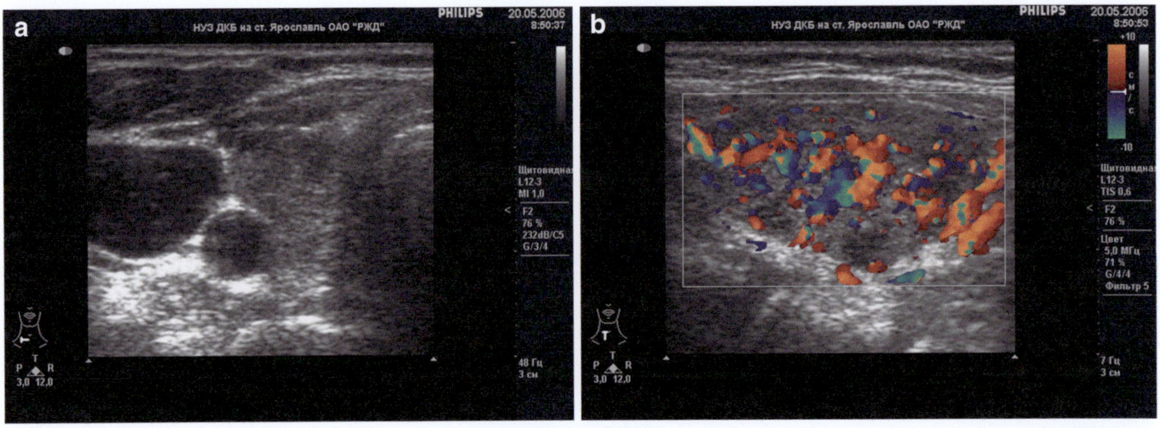

Fig. 8.3 (**a**, **b**) Status after thyroid surgery. AITD. Grayscale and CDI

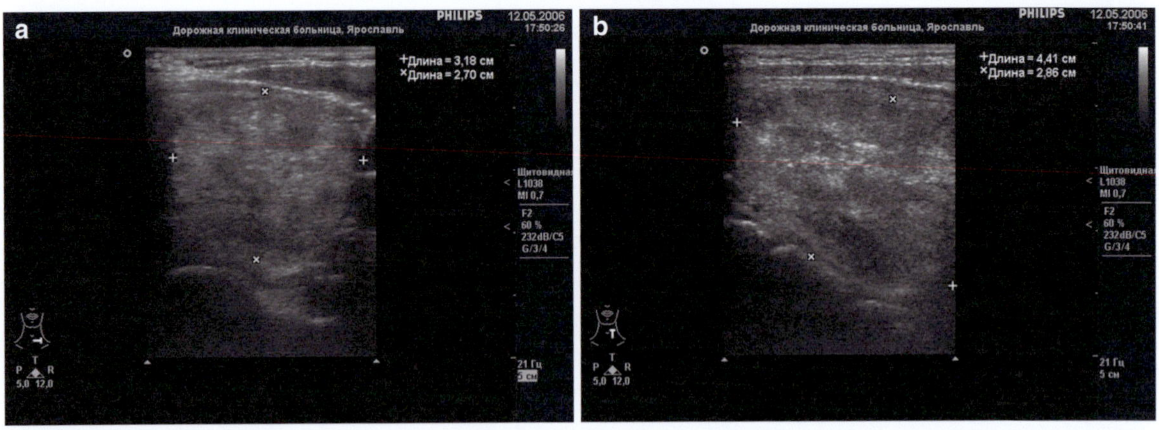

Fig. 8.4 (**a**, **b**) Status after thyroid surgery. Recurrent thyroid cancer. Grayscale sonography

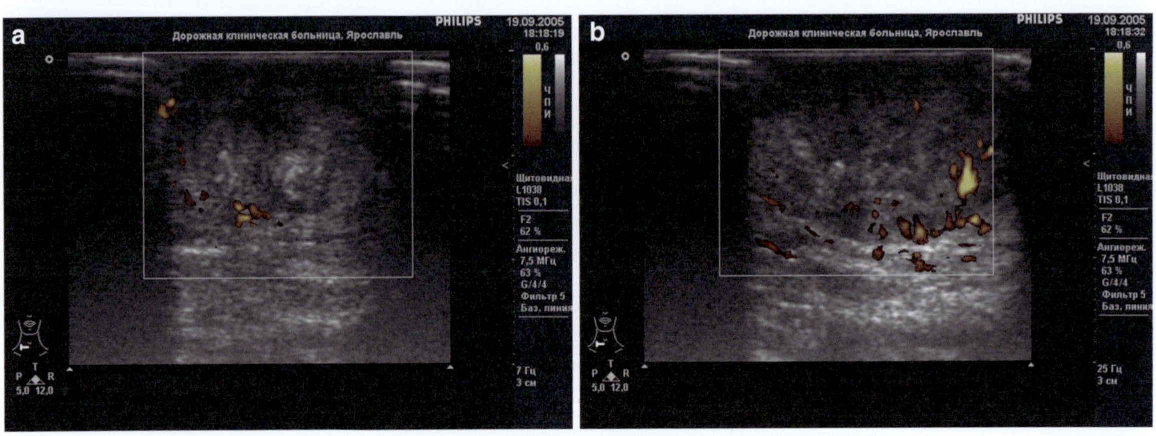

Fig. 8.5 (**a**, **b**) Status after thyroid surgery. Recurrent thyroid cancer. PDI

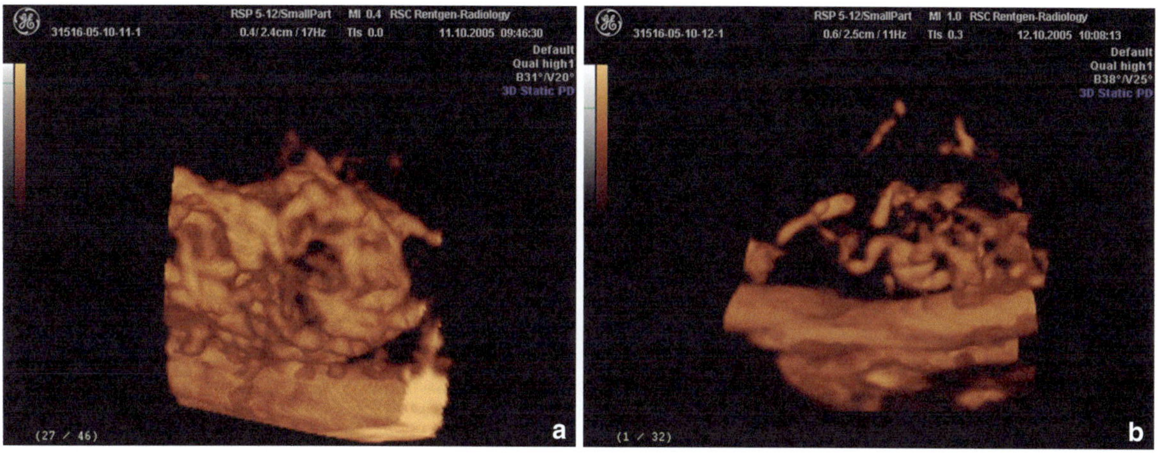

Fig. 8.6 (**a**, **b**) Status after thyroid surgery. Recurrent thyroid cancer. 3DPD

The example of US report in recurrent nodular goiter

First name, middle initial, last name:
Age:
Date:
The number of case history:
US scanner:
The thyroid is operated on (the surgery – 1992; histology – colloid goiter).

The **isthmus** is removed	
Right lobe	**Left lobe**
Depth 17 mm Width 22 mm Length 48 mm Volume 9.0 cm^3	is removed. Thyroid tissue, cystic, and solid lesions are not detected in the bed of the lobe. The vascular bundle is moderately displaced medially.
The total volume 8.0 cm^3 does not exceed the upper limit for the endemic region and the WHO recommendations.	
Two isoechoic heterogeneous avascular nodules of 0.6x0.5x1.0 cm and 0.6x0.9x1.0cm in size with well-defined regular margins are located in the middle compartment of the lobe.	

The vascular pattern of the parenchyma of the thyroid residue in CDI and PDI is unchanged.
Bilateral lymph nodes along IJV of 0.3x0.8cm in size with unchanged differentiation are detected.
The lymph nodes in supraclavicular areas are not enlarged.
CONCLUSION: The status after hemithyroidectomy. Nodules in the right thyroid lobe (recurrent thyroid goiter is probable).
US specialist:

The example of US report in recurrent thyroid cancer

First name, middle initial, last name:
Age:
Date:
The number of case history:
US scanner:
The thyroid gland is removed (the surgery – 2000; histology – papillary carcinoma).
A heterogeneous hypoechoic lesion of 2.3x2.2x3.6cm in size of irregular shape, with indistinct margins and small anechoic areas, hypervascular in CDI and PDI is located in the right thyroid lobe bed. An anechoic avascular lesion of 0.3x0.5x0.6 with well-defined irregular margins is located adjacent to the previous one with the tendency to merging.
No lesions are detected in the left lobe bed and isthmus site.
The left vascular bundle is displaced medially.
Bilateral enlarged lymph nodes along IJV are located: at the right side up to 0.6x1.9cm hypoechoic, heterogeneous, avascular; at the left side up to 0.7x2.4cm, hypoechoic, heterogeneous, hypovascular with moderate chaotic vascularity throughout the cortex, of irregular shape with the tendency to merging. The lymph nodes in supra- and infraclavicular areas are not enlarged.
CONCLUSION: The status after thyroid surgery. The image suggests thyroid carcinoma recurrence. Suspicion for bilateral metastases into the lymph nodes of the neck.
US specialist:

9 Ultrasound Examination of Regional Lymph Nodes

An examination of the lymph nodes of the neck is an essential part of thyroid US. In some cases the appearance of metastatic lymph nodes is the first clinical sign of thyroid cancer (Mack et al. 2008). The main problem with the US assessment of regional metastases of thyroid malignancies is the large number of diseases that are accompanied by lymph node enlargement, and thus the difficulties involved in the differential diagnosis of the origin of the enlargement (Esen 2006). Lymphadenopathies show benign character in 80% of patients younger than 30 years, although only 40% of enlarged lymph nodes appear to be benign in patients over 50 years old (Zabolotskaya 1999).

Sonography of the lymph nodes of the neck is performed in the standard position of the patient for thyroid scanning: supine with a bolster under the shoulders and the head thrown back (Fig. 9.1). To facilitate the examination of the right half of the neck, the patient may be asked to turn their head to the left and vice versa. Abbasova et al. (2005) suggest dorsal access to visualize the upper neck lymph nodes when the patient lies on their stomach with head flexion. A linear US probe with a frequency of 7.5–15 MHz is utilized.

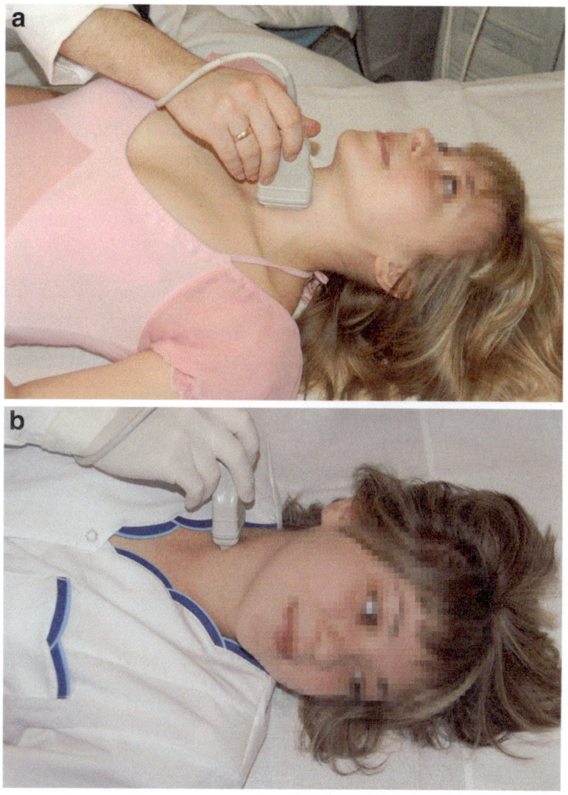

Fig. 9.1 (**a**, **b**) Position of the patient while examining the lymph nodes of the neck

Neck lymph nodes are divided into groups according to their sites. The American Joint Committee on Cancer (AJCC) classification of cervical lymph nodes is commonly used, especially by surgeons and oncologists. As the AJCC classification is not specific to ultrasound examination, some lymph nodes in the classification, such as the prelaryngeal, paratracheal and upper mediastinal nodes, may not be accessible with ultrasound. Some other classifications of cervical lymph nodes have been established that to some extent correspond to the AJCC classification. For instance, Hajek et al. (1986) suggested a classification for ultrasound examinations. The cervical lymph nodes were classified into the following eight regions according to their location in the neck: submental, submandibular, parotid, upper cervical, middle cervical, lower cervical, supraclavicular, and posterior triangle (accessory chain). The upper cervical group of lymph nodes is located within the upper one-third of the neck above the CCA bifurcation (or hyoid bone), the middle cervical at level of the CCA bifurcation and 3 cm below it (between the level of the hyoid bone and cricoid cartilage), and the lower cervical in the inferior one-third of

V.P. Kharchenko et al., *Ultrasound Diagnostics of Thyroid Diseases*,
DOI: 10.1007/978-3-642-12387-0_9, © Springer-Verlag Berlin Heidelberg 2010

the neck. These comprise the internal jugular chain (Figs. 9.2–9.4).

US characterization of the lymph nodes of the neck involves evaluating the following aspects:

- Site, according to anatomical area
- Number
- Dimensions (in three planes)
- Short/long axis in transverse view
- Similarity of changes
- Shape (flat, oval, spherical, or irregular)
- Echodensity of the lymph node in general (increased, medium, or decreased)
- Differentiation of lymph node parts (present/absent)
- Differentiation of the hilum (present/absent)
- Core echodensity (high, low, or isoechoic)
- Status of the cortex of the lymph node (narrow/wide)
- Mobility upon compression with the probe
- Vascularity

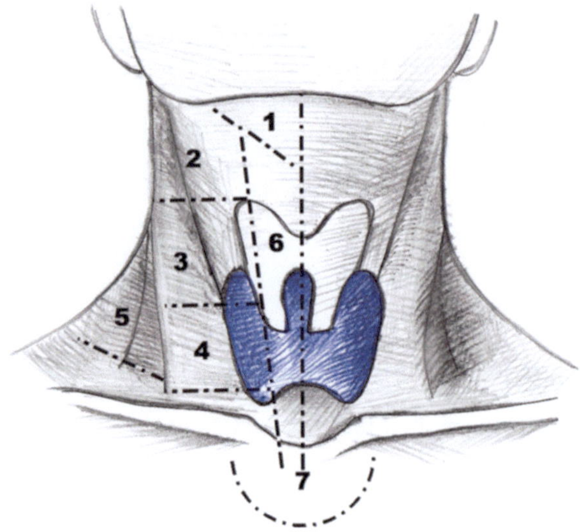

Fig. 9.3 Classification of cervical lymph nodes (Moley and Spiro 1994). *1*, Submandibular and mental groups; *2*, superior jugular, jugulodigastric, and accessory nerve groups, *3*, middle jugular, *4*, inferior jugular and jugulo-omohyoid groups; *5*, nodules of the back triangle of the neck (the inferior group of lymph nodes in the accessory nerve region), *6*, pretracheal and paratracheal nodes; *7*, lymph nodes of the supraclavicular group and anterior mediastinum ("thymic")

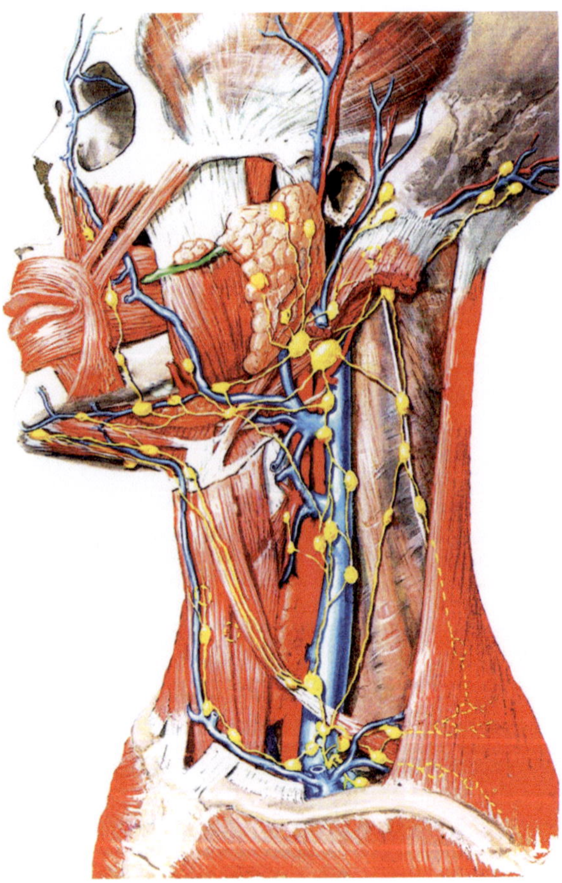

Fig. 9.2 Neck lymph nodes (Netter 2003)

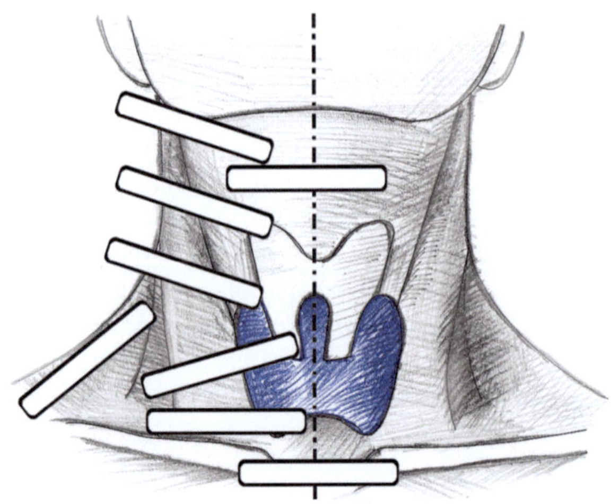

Fig. 9.4 US probe location during US scanning of lymph nodes of the neck (*right side*)

Normal lymph nodes of the neck demonstrate the following sonographic features (Fig. 9.5):

- Oval (or bean-like, tape-like) shape, close proximity to neck vessels, more often near large veins
- Length smaller than 10 mm
- Regular, well-defined contours

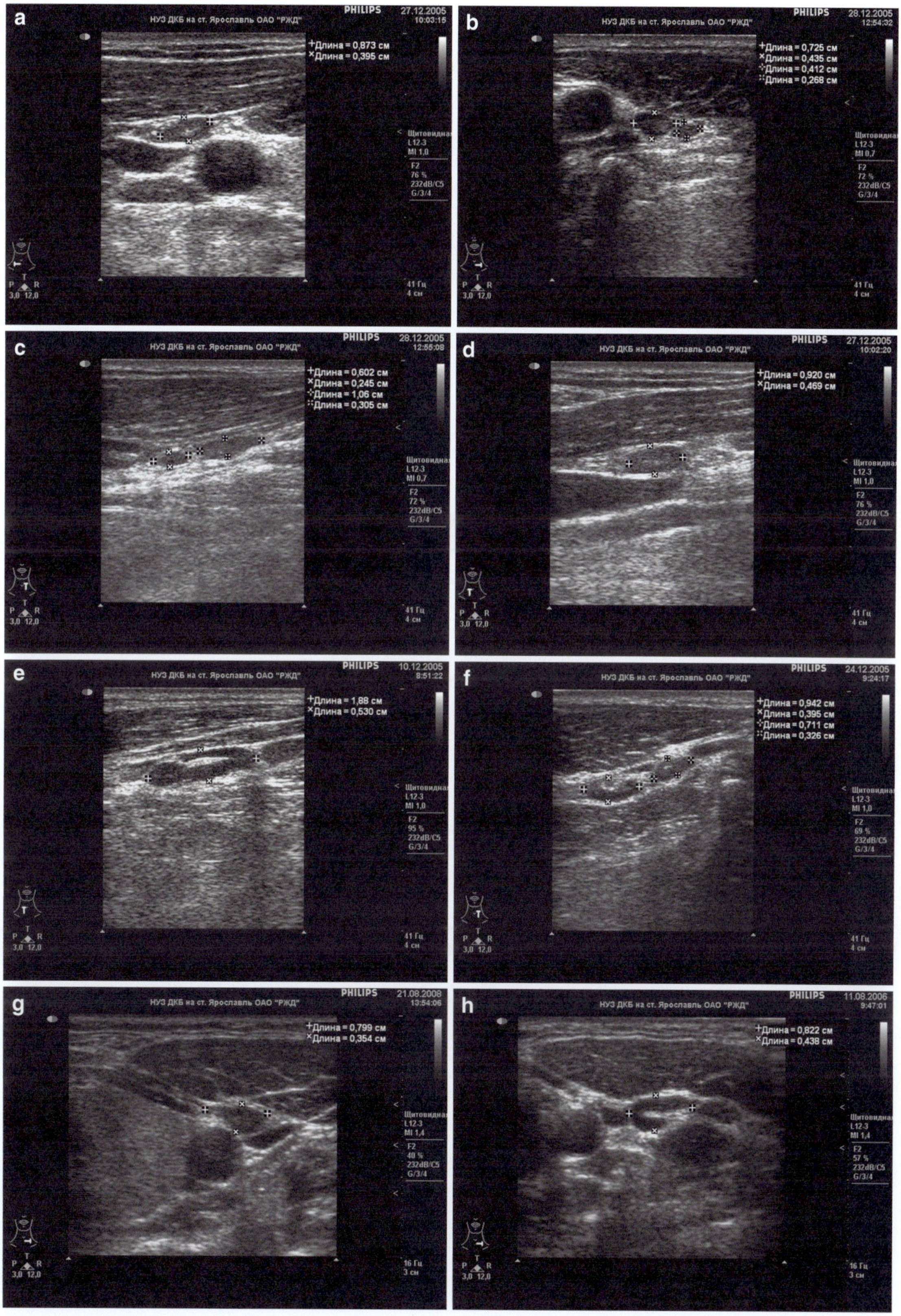

Fig. 9.5 (**a–h**) Normal lymph nodes of the neck. Grayscale sonography

- Hypo- or isoechoic peripheral part and hyperechoic central part
- Painless, moderately mobile upon compression with the US probe
- Avascular or hypovascular in CDI, PDI, and 3DPD, with predominant vascularity of the hilum

According to Zabolotskaya (1999), a normal lymph node has a width of up to 10 mm on transverse scan, although, according to a number of authors, the dimensions of normal lymph nodes vary significantly. However, normal jugulodigastric lymph nodes can exceed this limit.

The Solbiati index (SI), which is the ratio of the largest to the smallest diameter of a lymph node, is normally 2.9 ± 0.13 in adults, and 2.4 ± 0.05 or above in children.

The assessment of vascularity with CDI and PDI supplies additional data for the differential diagnosis of the origin of an enlarged lymph node (Fig. 9.6). Vessels, if any are detected, are usually located within the hilum in normal or reactive lymph nodes. Even in large benign hyperplastic lymph nodes, the vascular pattern remains regular. Vessels are normally observed along the capsule and radially from the hilum to the periphery (Trofimova 2008).

Giovagnorio et al. (1997) distinguish hilar and peripheral patterns of lymph node vascularity. The hilar pattern is further subdivided into two subpatterns: a "normal hilar" (type I, with evidence of a single vascular pole; small, regular branches may also be visible), and a "hypertrophic hilar" (type II; here, the main hilar feeding artery is almost double its normal diameter and length, and there is evidence of two or more regular branches). The "peripheral" pattern is defined as "mainly peripheral vascularity, with three or more vascular branches perforating the capsule peripherally and directed toward the center of the node" (type III). The "normal hilar" pattern is associated with chronic inflammation with a sensitivity of 85% and a specificity of 90%, the "hypertrophic hilar" pattern was associated with acute inflammation with a sensitivity of 68% and a specificity of 55%, and the "peripheral" pattern was associated with metastasis with a sensitivity of 47% and a specificity of 91%.

Abbasova et al. (2005) classify the vascular pattern of the lymph node into the following four categories:

1. Hilar: individual arterial and/or venous flow signals without diffusion to the parenchyma of the lymph node and without branching
2. Activated hilar (central) type: venous and arterial flow signals branching radially within the hilum and medulla
3. Peripheral: flow signals along the periphery of the lymph nodes without subcapsular branches arising from the hilar vessels
4. Mixed: presence of hilar and peripheral flow signals
   (a) One large artery in the hilum with individual dot-shaped color signals in the periphery
   (b) Fragments of afferent artery and chaotic flow signals within the solid component of the lymph node

Several authors refer to an additional "spotted" type of vascular pattern. Wu et al. (1998) reports that malignant (as opposed to benign) lymphadenopathies dominate in spotted (72%), peripheral (60%), and mixed (80%) types.

Doppler data, according to Abbasova et al. (2005), do not affect the differential diagnosis of enlarged lymph nodes.

Enlargement of a lymph node of the neck may appear as a manifestation of a variety of diseases, such as specific or nonspecific inflammation of head and neck organs, metastases, and hemoblastoses (e.g., Hodgkin's disease).

Nonspecific types of lymphadenitis are divided into the following groups (Trofimova 2008):

1. According to disease severity
   - Acute
   - Subacute
   - Chronic
2. According to dispersion
   - Isolated
   - Regional (in groups)
   - Extended
   - Generalized

Individual and multiple lymph nodes as well as lymph node conglomerations can be also described.

Lymph node pathology may be sonographically interpreted as reactive hyperplasia, metastasis, or malignant lymphoma.

Reactive hyperplasia of lymph nodes may result from different pathological processes (an inflammatory

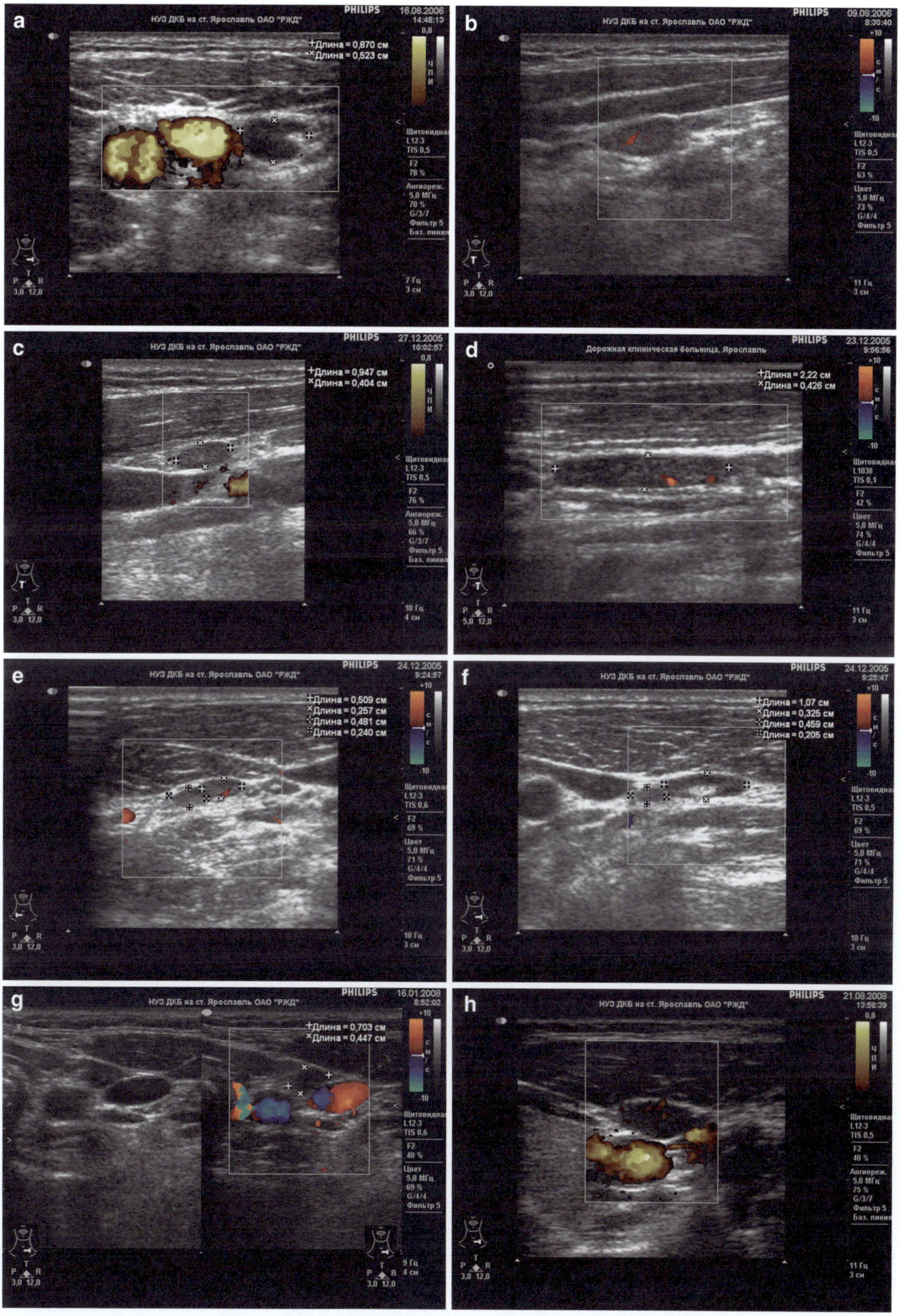

Fig. 9.6 (**a–h**) Normal lymph nodes of the neck. CDI and PDI

process, vaccination, injections, etc.). Expression depends on individual reactivity, the status of the immune system, how aggressive the infection is, and other factors. Lymph nodes that are close to a tumor, can also present a nonspecific reaction of inflammatory character (Trofimova 2008). Abbasova et al. (2005) differentiate the following types of US image for inflammatory processes in lymph nodes (Figs. 9.7 and 9.8):

1. Reactive hyperplasia (minimal sonographic changes, accurate regular margins, distinct differentiation of the hilum, and activated hilar type of blood flow)
2. Subacute lymphadenitis (multiple enlarged lymph nodes of decreased echodensity, indistinct differentiation of echostructure, morbidity upon compression with the probe, and activated hilar type of blood flow, often with branching)
3. Acute lymphadenitis (enlargement of lymph nodes with roundish shape, significant decrease in echodensity, sharp morbidity upon compression, disturbance of cortico-medullary differentiation, and activated hilar blood flow pattern)
4. Chronic lymphadenitis (enlargement of lymph nodes with roundish shape, decrease in echodensity, thickening of echogenic medulla and hilum, and hilar blood flow pattern)

Complex US is effective for monitoring how changes in lymph node develop. Inflammatory lymph nodes show fast dynamics. Even without therapy, they often sonographically disappear after 5–7 days (Zabolotskaya 1999). Treatment speeds up their involution, resulting in the restoration of the oval shape of the node and sharpness of margins, an increase in the general echodensity with more accurate cortico-medullary differentiation, and a decrease in blood flow intensity and morbidity upon compression.

Patients with metastases in lymph nodes of the neck with an unknown primary tumor are observed in 3–8% of cases (Karmazanovsky and Nikitaev 2005).

The incidence of metastases of thyroid cancer in regional lymph nodes is 9–90% (Pinsky et al. 1999) (Figs. 9.9 and 9.10). According to Mazzaferri (1993), unilateral lymph node affection is registered

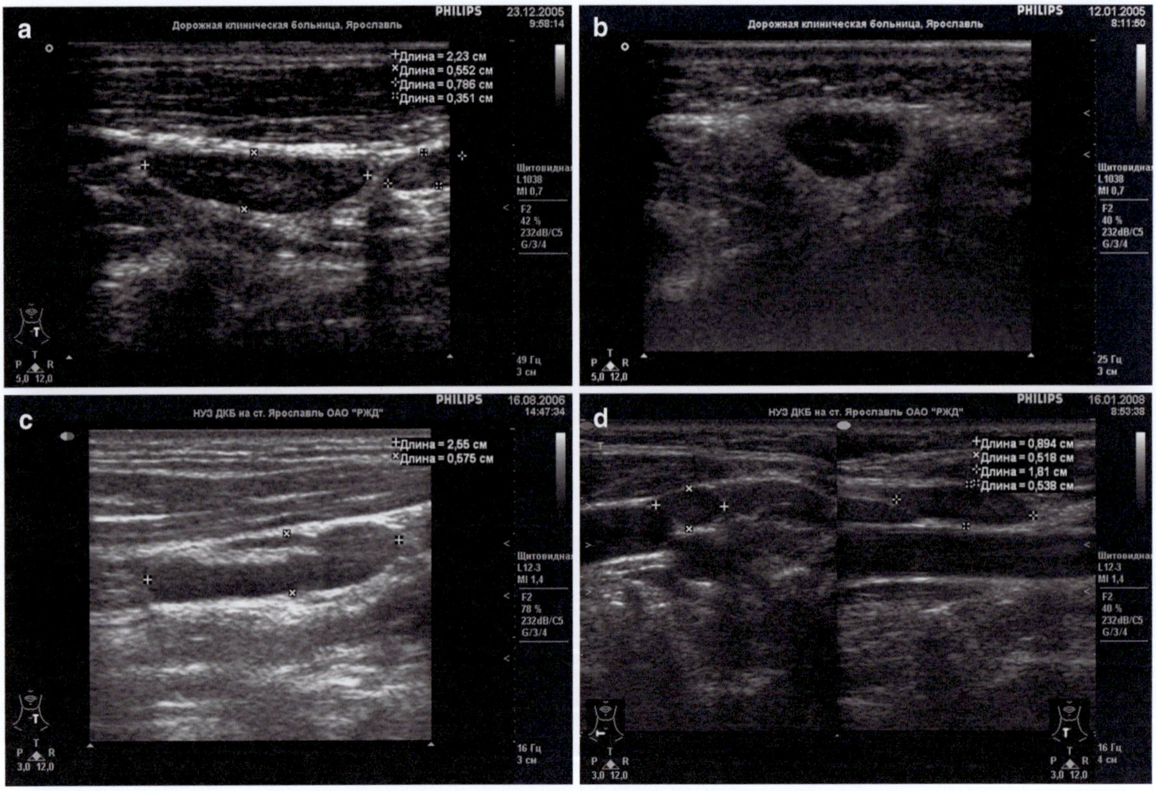

Fig. 9.7 (**a–j**) Reactive hyperplasia of the lymph node of the neck. Grayscale, CDI, PDI, and 3D reconstruction

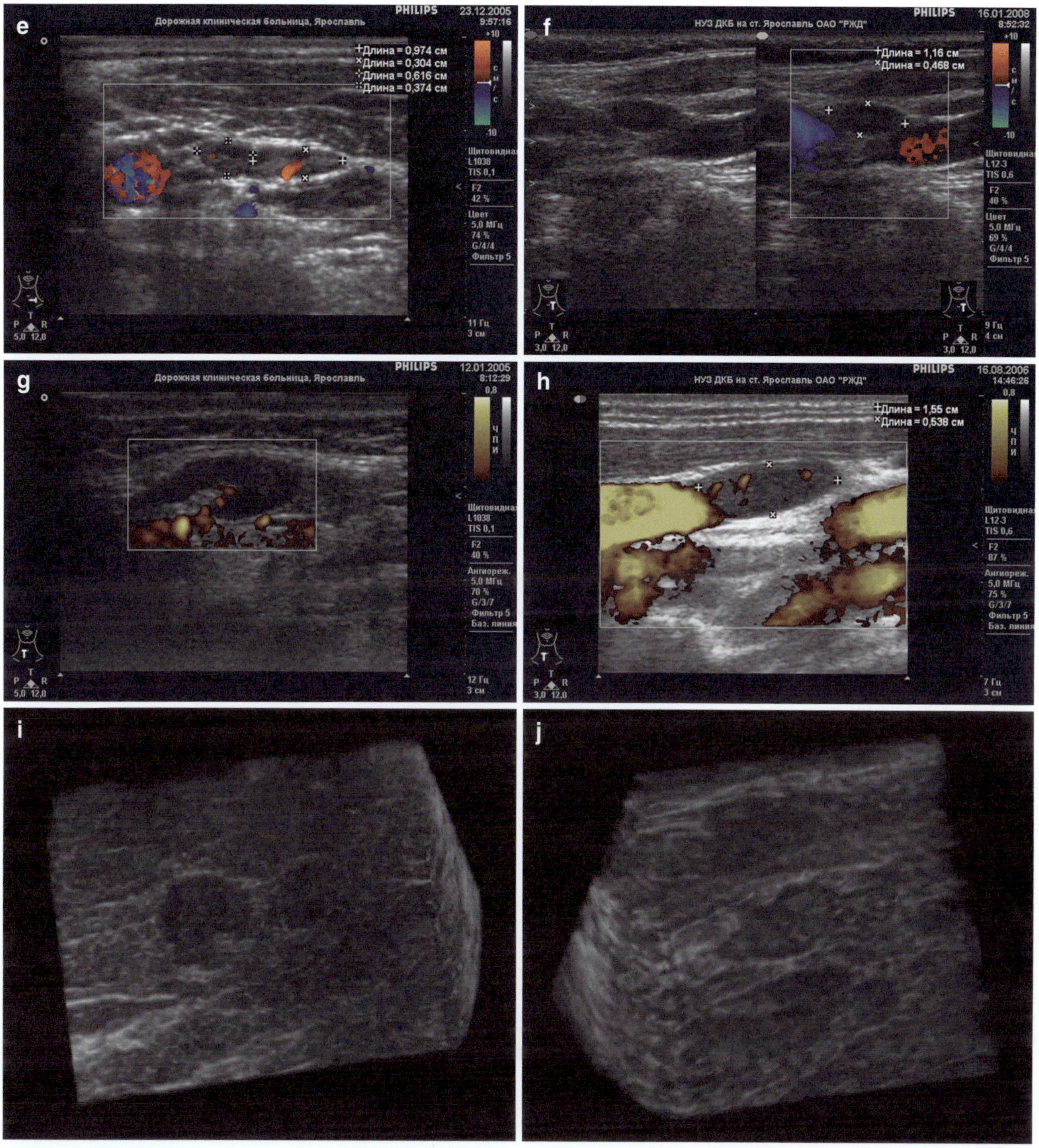

Fig. 9.7 (continued)

in 85% and bilateral metastases in 15% of cases. Regional metastases are most often observed in anaplastic cancer (32.3%). Papillary and medullary cancer have local metastasis rates of 18–36%, and the metastasis rate for follicular carcinoma is 7–17% of cases. According to Chiesa (2004), the frequency of metastases in neck lymph nodes with papillary thyroid cancer accounts for 32–57% of cases, about 10% of follicular cancer cases, 50–75% of medullary cancer cases, and 70–100% of anaplastic cancer cases.

Some US features that are suspicious for a malignant process in a neck lymph node are listed below (Table 9.1; Figs. 9.11 and 9.12):

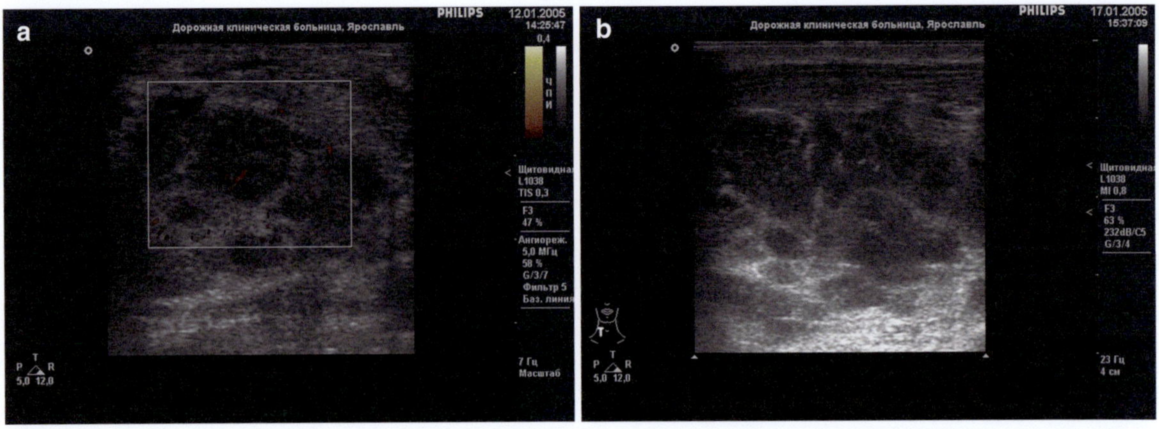

Fig. 9.8 (**a**) Acute neck lymphadenitis. (**b**) Purulent lymphadenitis (the same patient as in (**a**) five days later)

- Size of >10 mm
- Roundish shape
- Irregular blurred contours
- Decreased general echodensity
- Heterogeneous echostructure
- Pathological echogenic inclusions
- Anechoic component
- Dislocation or deformation of the hilum, indistinct image of the hilum of the lymph node up to its full disappearance
- Local thickening of the cortex of the lymph node in combination with dislocation of the hilar vessels
- Conglomerations of lymph nodes
- Immobility or limited mobility against the surrounding tissues
- Pathological vascular patterns in CDI, PDI, and 3DPD

The probability of malignancy increases if two or more of the features specified above are present. According to Kotlyarov et al. (2001), enlarged regional lymph nodes in the case of proven thyroid cancer are indicative of a metastatic origin with an accuracy of 95–100%.

The site of the metastasis does not directly correspond to the location of the primary tumor. Metastases are more often observed on the same side of the neck as the primary tumor. Bilateral affection is seen less often. According to Sencha (2008), in 76% of cases of verified thyroid cancer, metastases affect only the jugular group, and are combined with other groups of lymph nodes in 24%. A combination of metastases in jugular lymph nodes and submandibular or submental lymph nodes was detected in 12%, with

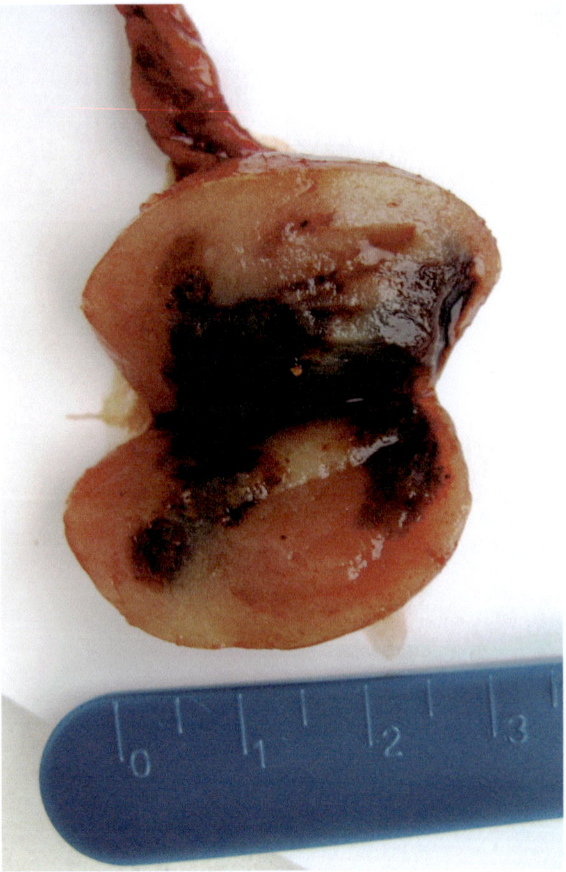

Fig. 9.9 Metastasis of thyroid cancer in a neck lymph node. Macroscopic view

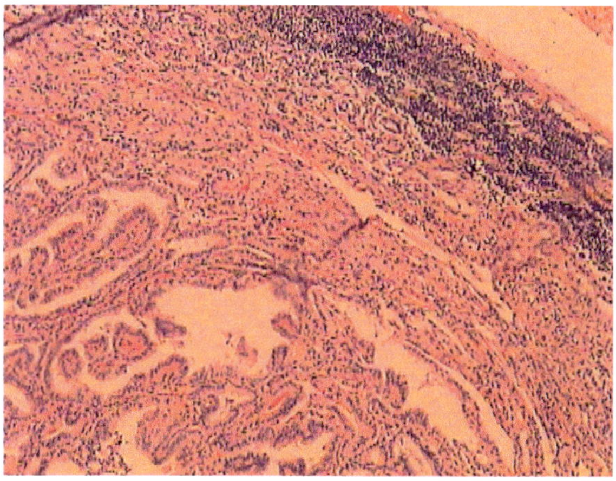

Fig. 9.10 Metastasis of thyroid cancer in a neck lymph node (hematoxylin and eosin stained smears; original magnification, ×200)

Table 9.1 Sonographic features (frequency, %) of normal and metastatic neck lymph nodes

US features	Lymph nodes in cases with a normal thyroid ($n=300$)	Lymph nodes in cases with thyroid cancer ($n=144$)
Maximal size of lymph nodes (mm):	5.3±1.2	15.4±3.1
Shape:		
Spherical	20	18.1
Oval	76	50.0
Irregular	4	31.9
Margins:		
Smooth	95.7	70.1
Irregular	4.3	29.9
Contours:		
Well-defined	92.0	74.3
Blurred	8.0	25.7
Echodensity:		
Hyper-	–	2.1
Iso-	85	34.0
Hypo-	15	58.3
An-	–	5.6
Echostructure:		
Homogeneous	95.0	44.4
Heterogeneous	5.0	55.6
Calcifications or hyperechoic inclusions:		
Present	–	2.1
Absent	100	97.9
Fluid collections:		
Present	–	6.3
Absent	100	93.7
Vascularity:		
Avascular	85.0	45.8
Hypovascular	10.0	45.8
Hypervascular	5.0	8.3

posterior neck lymph nodes in 8%, and with supraclavicular or anterior mediastinum lymph nodes in 4% of cases.

Choi et al. (1995) consider that assessing EDV in lymph nodes with PW Doppler interrogation may help to differentiate between a hyperplastic and a metastatic origin. The authors suggest that this parameter is of high diagnostic value. They also underline that increased blood flow velosity may be also sometimes registered in lymph node hyperplasia.

According to Tschammler et al. (1999), avascular areas and additional peripheral vessels in CDI and PDI are indicative of lymph node malignancy. Allahverdieva et al. (2005) report that metastatic lymph nodes in cases of papillary thyroid carcinoma are characterized by a diffuse distribution of vessels (a "glowing" lymph nodule). According to Ahuja et al. (2000), CDI and PDI do not supply any significant information for the differential diagnosis of enlarged lymph nodes of the neck (Figs. 9.12 and 9.13).

Extracapsular expansion of the metastases in lymph nodes often leads to the integration of several affected lymph nodes into amorphous conglomerations that merge into surrounding structures. The basic US feature of invasion is indistinct contour of the lymph node.

Remote metastases are observed in 6–55.5% of patients with thyroid cancer (Altunina 1996). They are most often detected in lungs (62.5%), bones (20%), and mediastinal lymph nodes (7.5%). US often fails to visualize metastases within the thorax, so other radiological methods are preferable.

The sensitivity of US for the detection and differential diagnosis of lymph nodes in thyroid cancer is 30–86.65%, with a specificity of 57–84.2% and a diagnostic accuracy of 56–81.48%. These figures appear to be highly dependent on the quality of the equipment as well as the skill and experience of the operator (Zabolotskaya 1999), especially in cases with small local metastases within lymph nodes (Fig. 9.14).

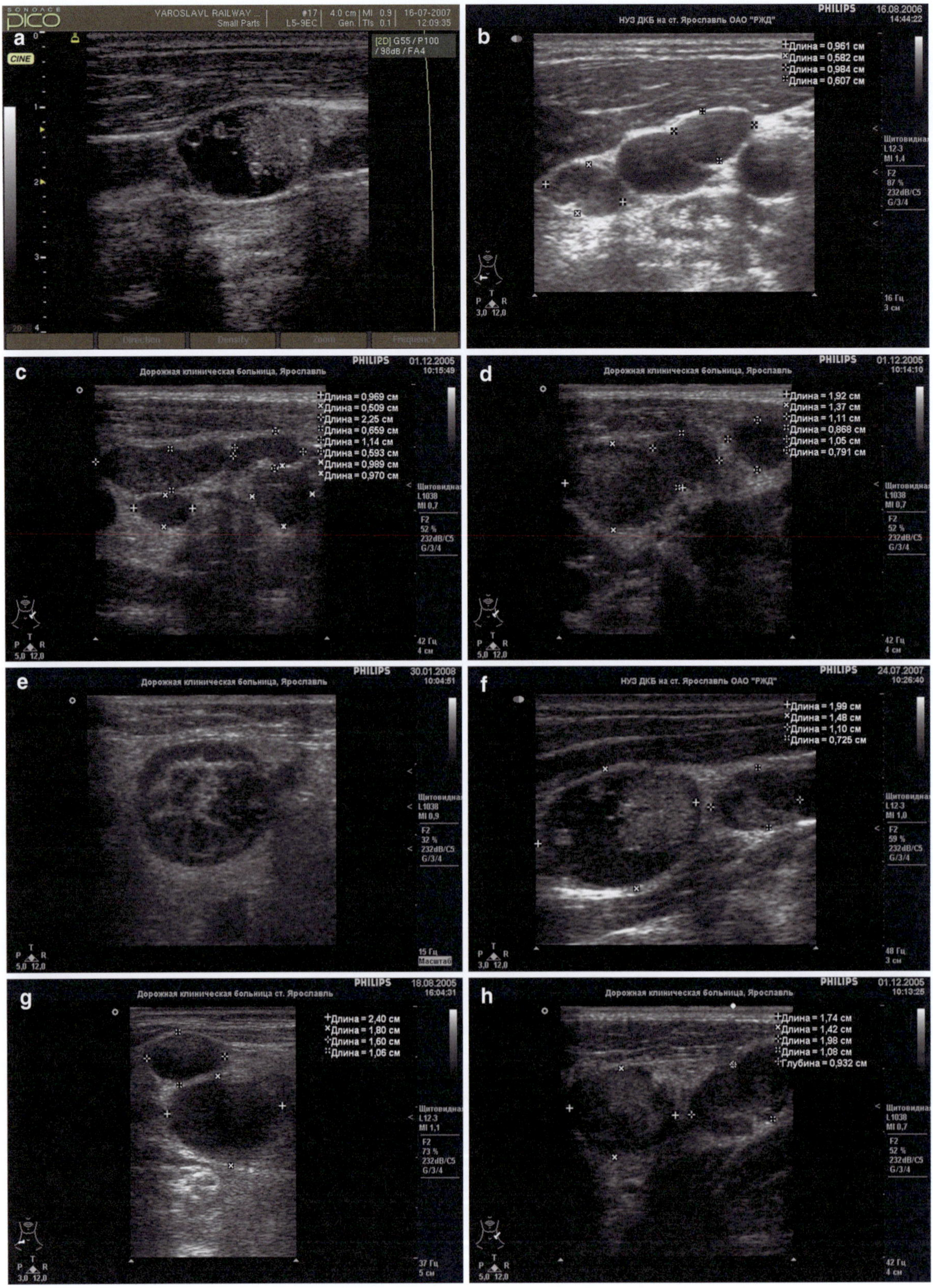

Fig. 9.11 (**a–p**) Metastases in neck lymph nodes. Grayscale

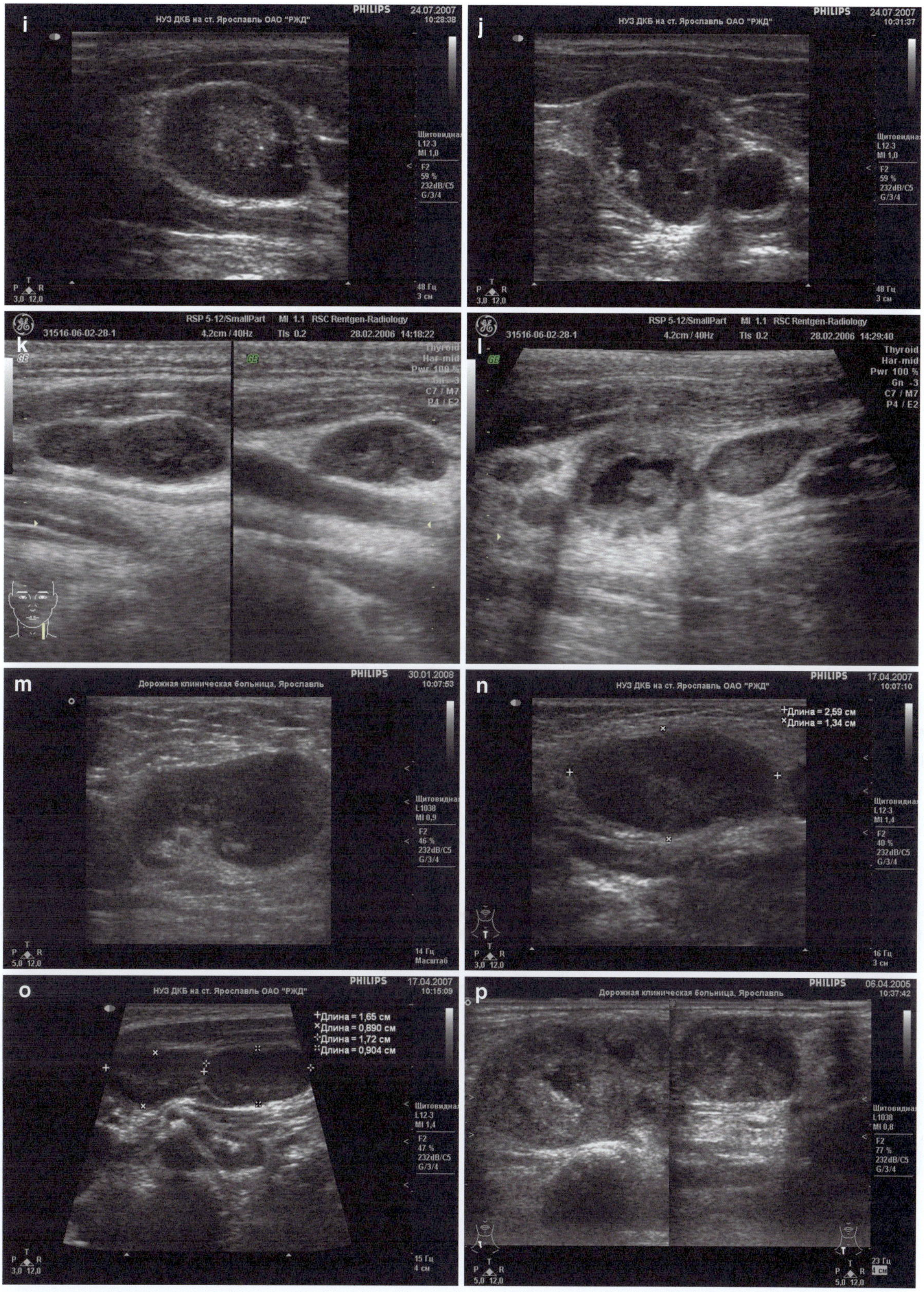

Fig. 9.11 (continued)

Most authors agree that, in many cases, sonography does not allow the ultimate definition of the nature of the lymph nodes of the neck, although it does detect indirect features that facilitate further diagnostics. US-guided FNAB with definition of the thyroglobulin level and cytological examination is feasible.

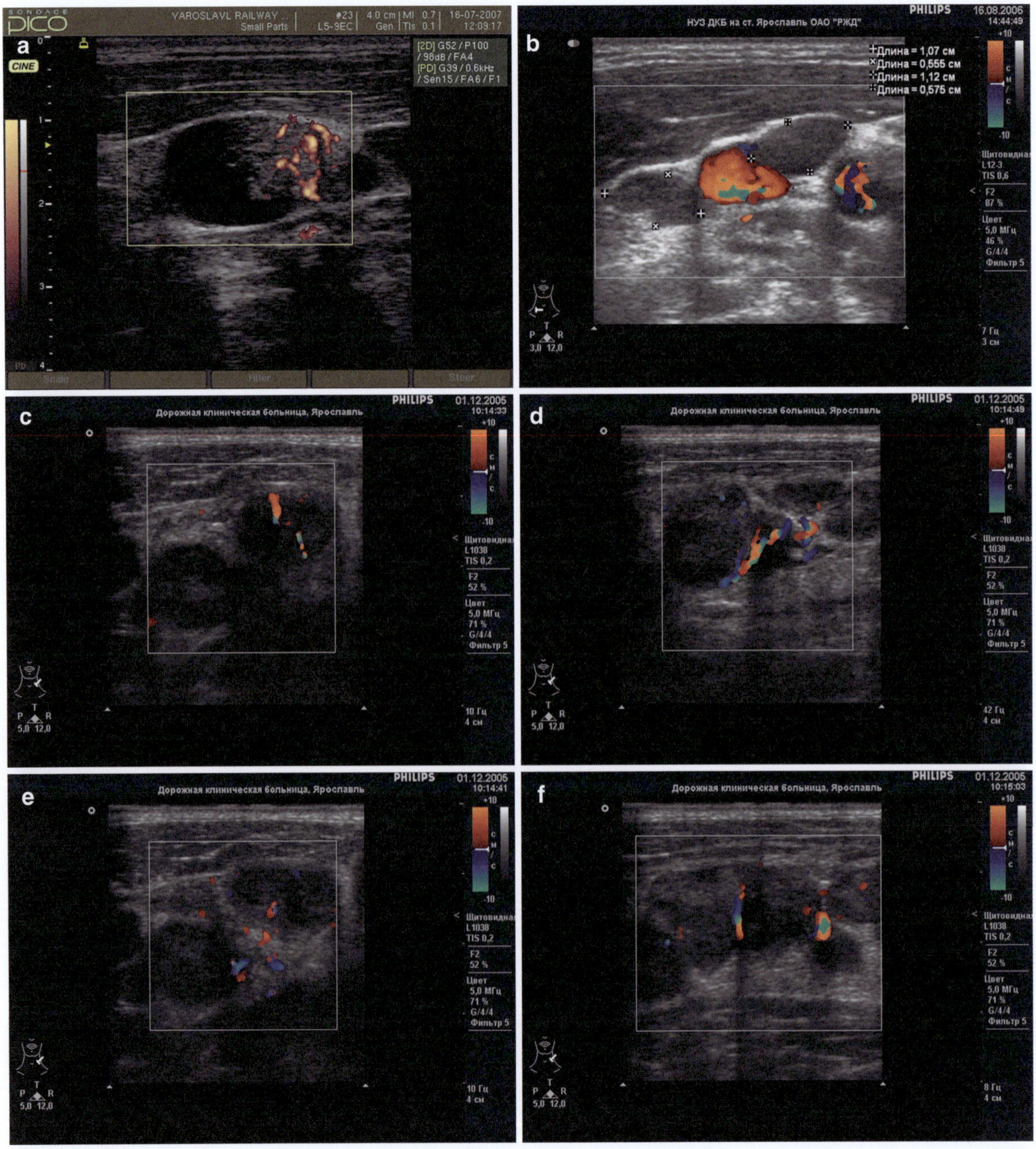

Fig. 9.12 (**a–p**) Metastases in neck lymph nodes. CDI and PDI

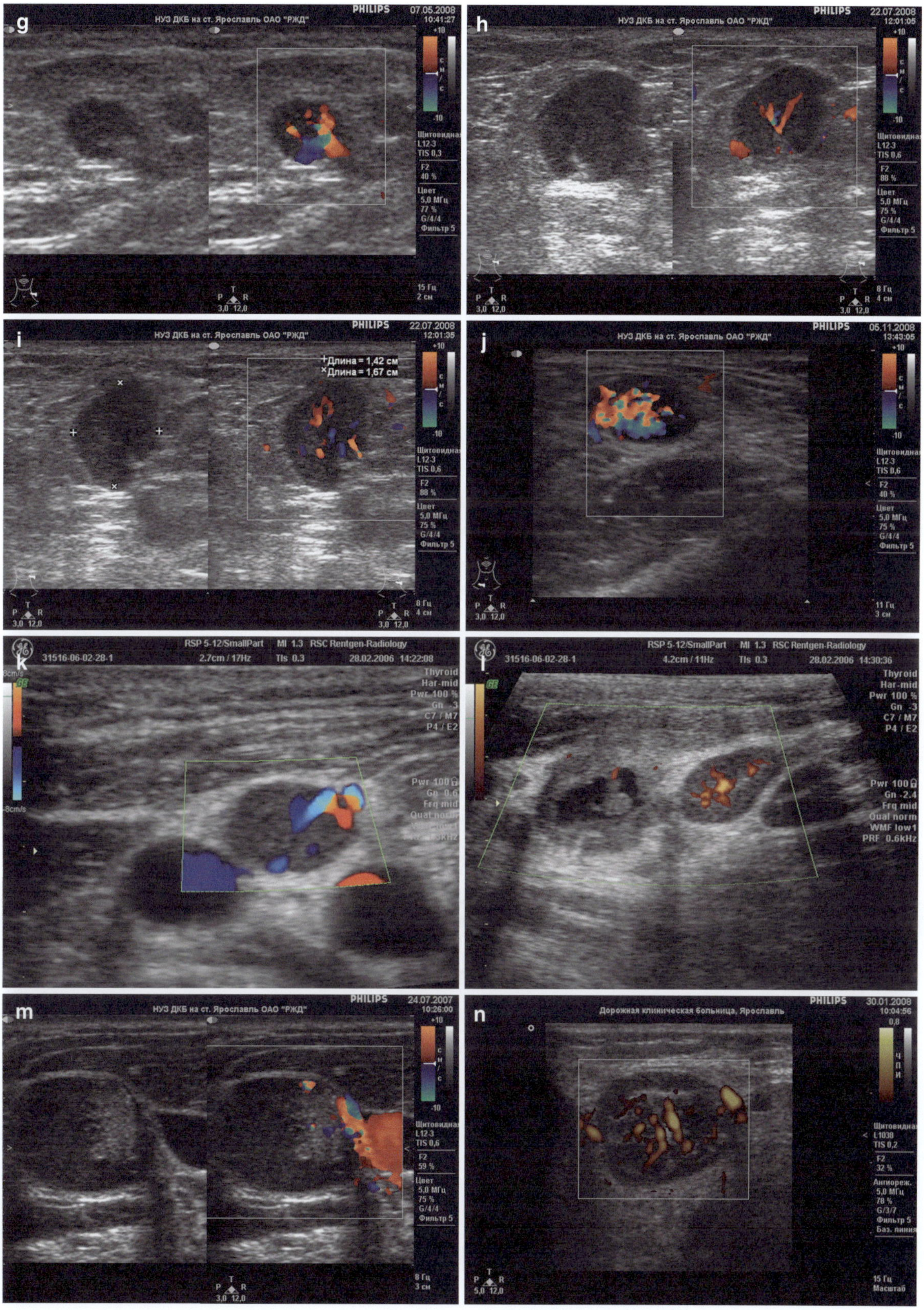

Fig. 9.12 (continued)

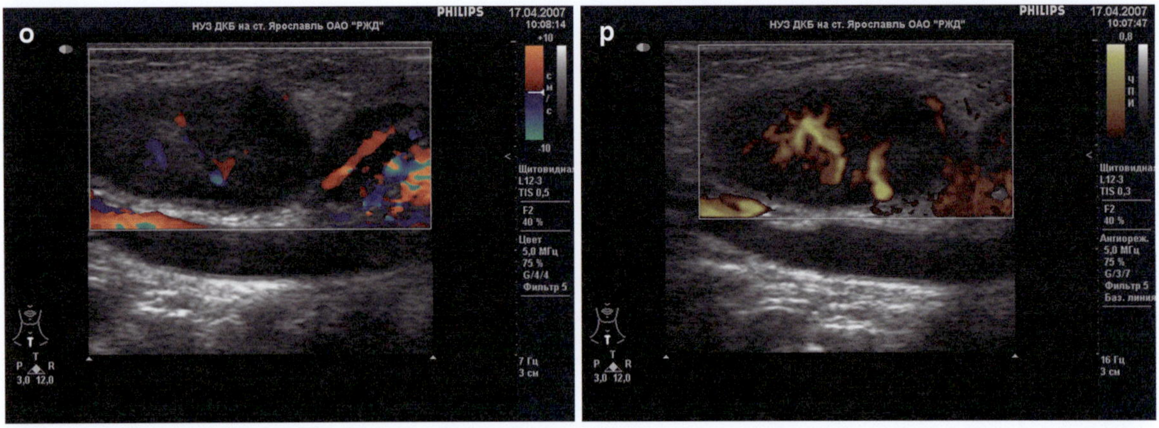

Fig. 9.12 (continued)

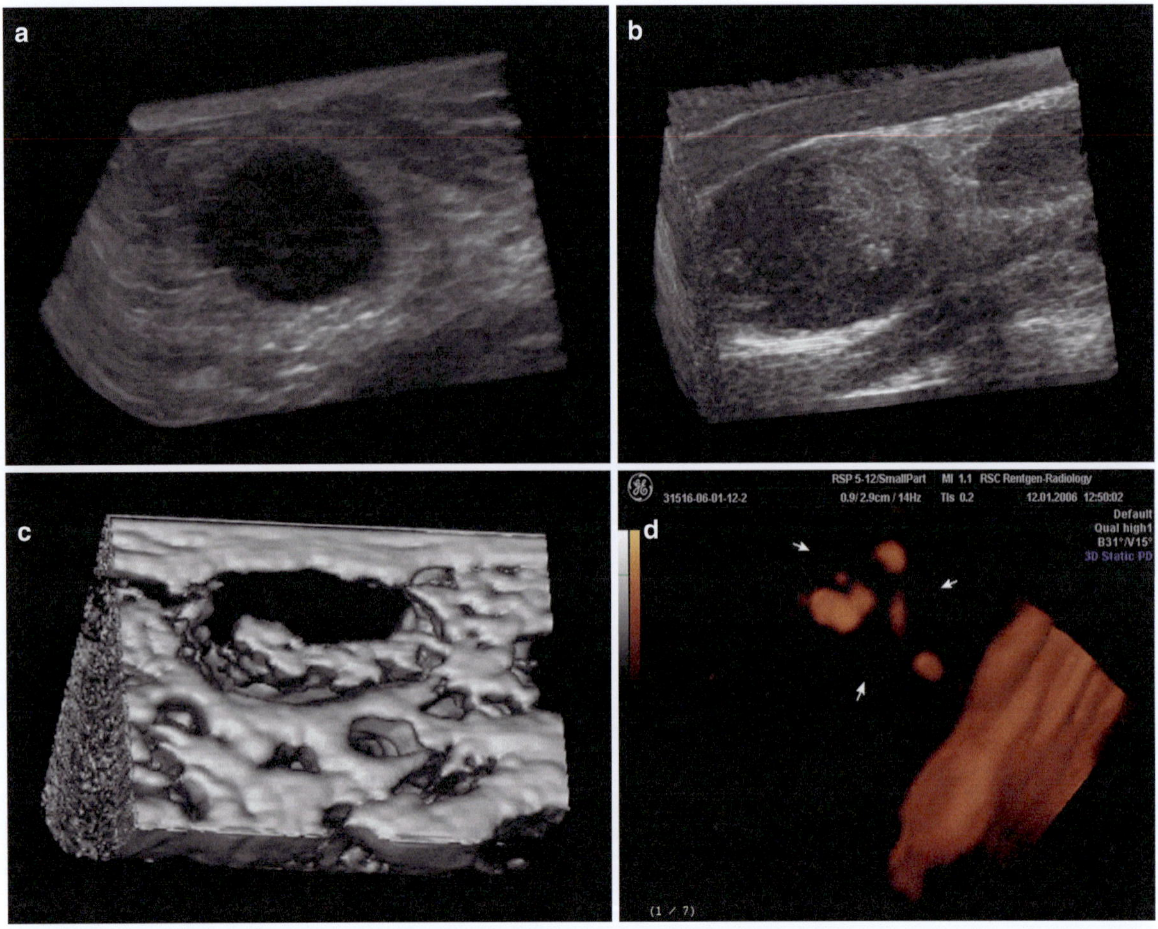

Fig. 9.13 (**a–d**) Metastases in neck lymph nodes. 3D reconstruction and 3DPD

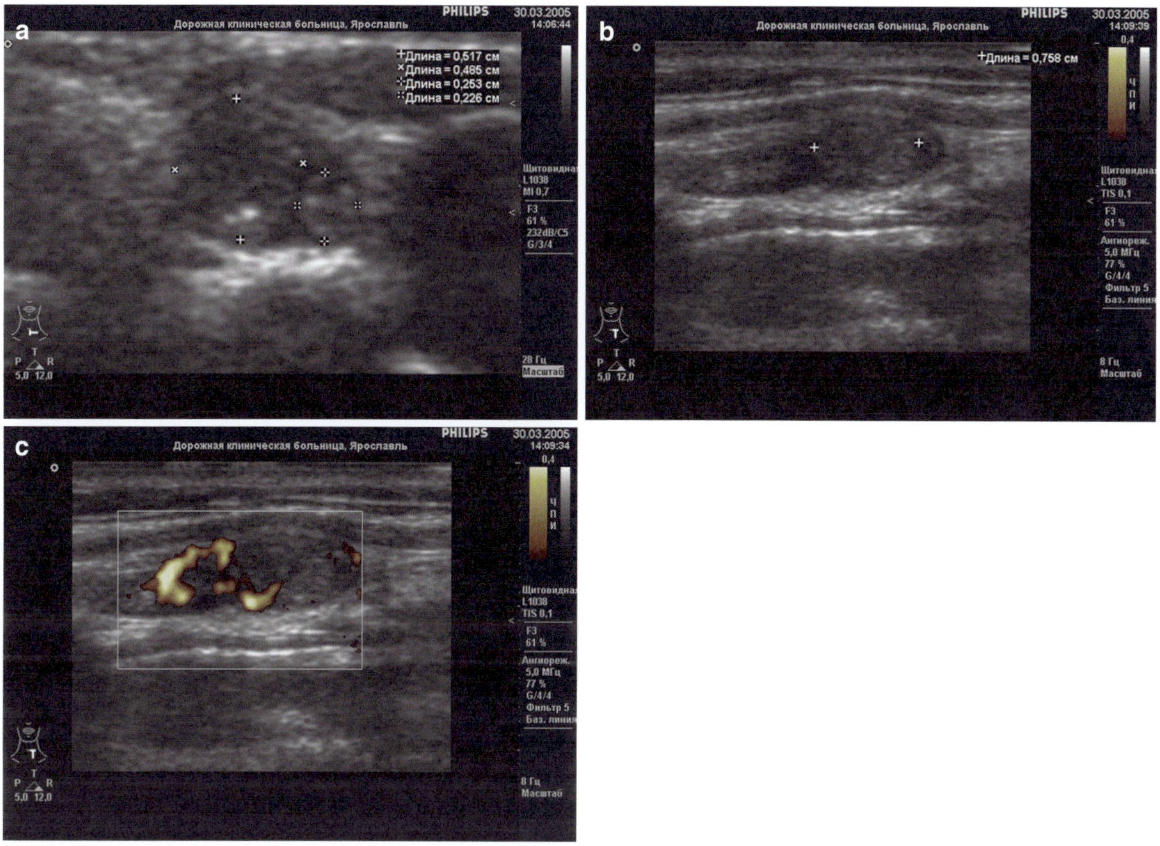

Fig. 9.14 (**a–c**) Local metastases within neck lymph nodes. Grayscale sonography and PDI

Substernal Goiter

10

The goiter is termed substernal when it is fully or partially located below the suprasternal fossa. Thus, part of the thyroid gland is localized in the thorax, mainly in the anterior mediastinum, or rarely in the upper-posterior mediastinum (Fig. 10.1). Several terms are used to describe a substernal goiter, such as a "retrosternal," "intrathoracic," "cervico-mediastinal," or "mediastinal" goiter. These all mean that more than 80% of the gland lies within the thorax. This thyroid site is often observed in elderly people. The main causes of the "descending" of the gland into the mediastinum are a wide superior thoracic aperture, especially in brachymorphic patients, increased weight of the organ due to the growth of the goiter, the sucking action of the thorax, and force from muscles on the anterior surface of the neck. Development of an intrathoracic goiter from an aberrant (ectopic) thyroid is possible (Vlasov 2006).

According to different authors, the frequency of substernal goiter in different countries ranges from 1 to 31% of the number of patients operated on for thyroid pathology (Cui et al. 2002; Sciume et al. 2005).

Substernal goiter is classified into the following five degrees:

1. The goiter tends to descend under the breast bone
2. The largest part of the gland is dislocated below the suprasternal fossa, but swallowing brings it back to the neck
3. The organ cannot be brought back to the neck completely with swallowing
4. Only the upper poles of the thyroid lobes may be defined
5. Complete intrathoracic location

Intrathoracic goiter accounts for 8–10% of all mediastinal lesions and about 5% of all cases of goiter (Vlasov 2006). According to Pinsky et al. (2005), thyroid cancer is detected more often in cases with substernal goiter than in cases with typical thyroid location.

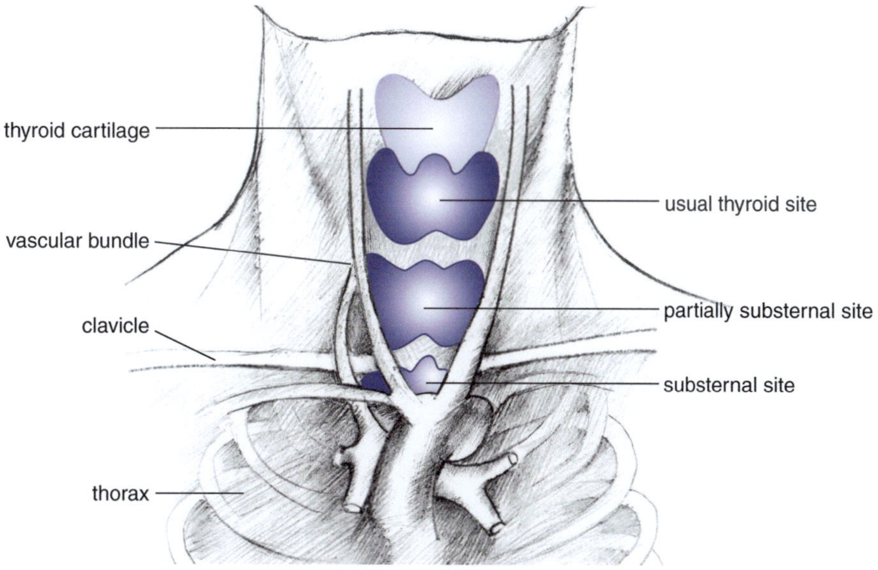

Fig. 10.1 Scheme of the location of the thyroid gland in substernal goiter

V.P. Kharchenko et al., *Ultrasound Diagnostics of Thyroid Diseases*,
DOI: 10.1007/978-3-642-12387-0_10, © Springer-Verlag Berlin Heidelberg 2010

The assessment of a “substernal location” is subjective to a certain degree due to the different positions of patients (upright or supine) and different degrees of patient head flexion during the examination. This naturally affects the thyroid site and appears clinically significant in cases of thyroid enlargement.

Substernal goiter shows symptoms related to the compression of the organs of the mediastinum, such as breathing difficulties in up to 39–65%, swallowing problems in up to 16% of cases, phonation disturbances, feelings of a lump in the throat, superior vena cava syndrome, and related complications (Cui et al. 2002; Ayache et al. 2006; Mackle et al. 2006). In 30–50% of cases, substernal goiter progresses asymptomatically and is discovered during medical examinations for other reasons (Dedov 1994; Ignjatovic 2001).

US, although successfully utilized to diagnose thyroid pathology at its typical site, exhibits significant limitations when applied to a substernal goiter. These result from the inability to achieve detailed visualization of the compartments of the gland that are located deeply in the mediastinum. Nevertheless, sonography may be effective in depicting a partially substernal goiter localized in the upper mediastinum (Fig. 10.2).

The sonographer faces several difficulties when utilizing high-frequency linear probes of 7.5–15 MHz to examine a substernal thyroid. First, acoustic access to the substernal part of the gland is technically complex. A “short neck” prevents inclination of the probe, thus limiting the effective scanning range. To improve the situation, the patient is asked to throw their head back and turn it to the opposite side. This significantly extends the area available for manipulating the probe and elevates the deeper part of the thyroid lobe. It increases the efficacy of scanning and enables the larger part of the thyroid to be examined. However, if the retrosternal part of the gland has significant volume, the operator must use lower-frequency probes. Thus, a second problem inevitably arises: a decrease in the quality of the image, which does not allow the echostructure to be assessed with the desired precision. In such cases it is often impossible to differentiate the lesions with the grayscale scan or with

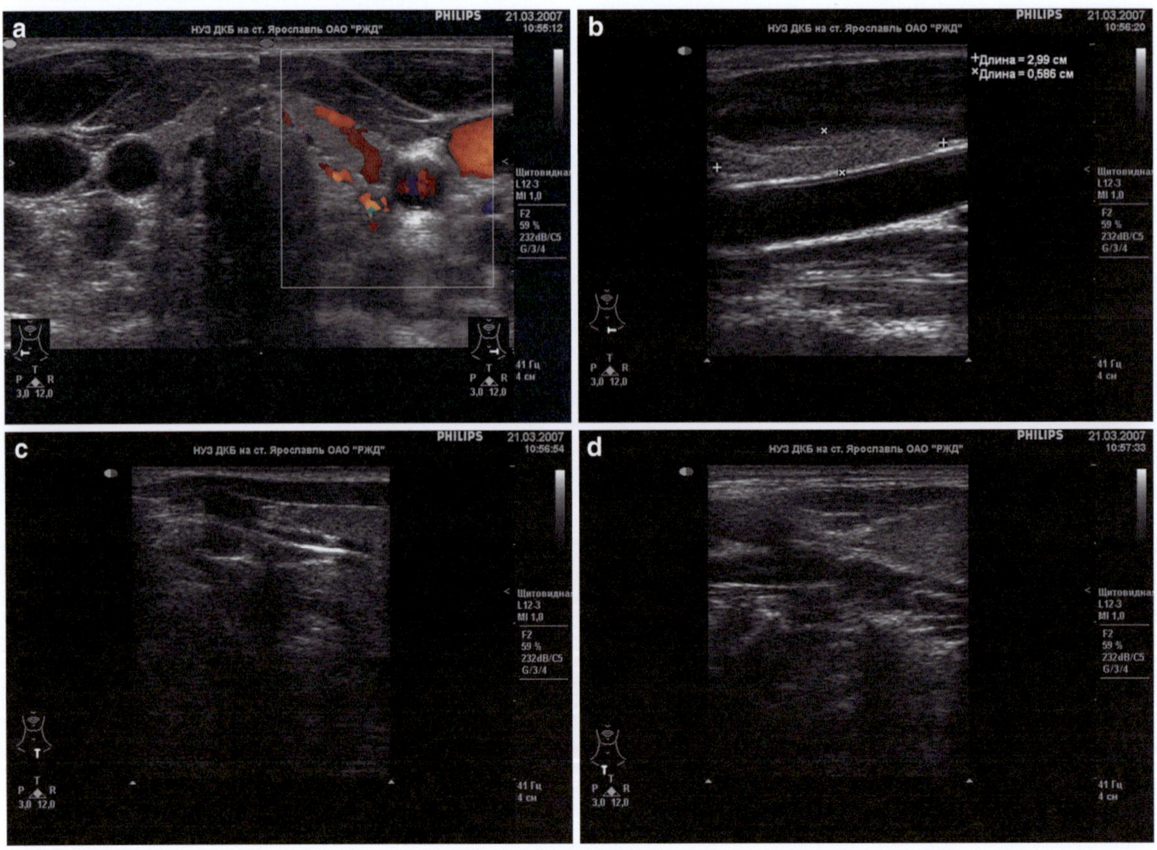

Fig. 10.2 (**a–d**) US visualization of the thyroid in substernal goiter

Doppler mapping options (due to motion artifacts). Nevertheless, US supplies required information on thyroid size. Abnormal thyroid tissue can be identified well enough with low-frequency probes against the fat and mediastinal organs. Sonography with microconvex or sector probes in the suprasternal fossa and intercostal parasternal access near to adjacent pulmonary tissue is useful. It is often possible to measure the anteroposterior and craniocaudal dimensions of the thyroid. The transverse dimension is often measured inaccurately because of wide acoustic shadowing posterior to the breast bone.

There are individual publications about the use of US to examine the intrathoracic component of a thyroid mass. They report that US permits the visualization of the mediastinum and the intrathoracic component of the thyroid, the definition of its location (anterior, posterior mediastinum, or mixed location), and the differentiation of an intrathoracic goiter from tumors with other origins and metastases in lymph nodes.

Kazakevich (2007) recommends US under the following circumstances:

- Suspicion for intrathoracic expansion of a tumor according to clinical examination or chest X-ray
- Dilation of the mediastinum of unknown genesis or suspicion of dilation of the mediastinum according to X-ray
- Detection of the substernal component of a tumor during standard thyroid US
- Widespread metastatic affection of cervical lymph nodes
- Malignant tumor in the inferior segments of the thyroid
- As a follow-up method after surgery for a tumor in the inferior compartment of the thyroid gland, the intrathoracic component of thyroid neoplasm, or widespread metastases in cervical or mediastinal lymph nodes

US of the mediastinum is performed with 3–5 MHz convex probes with a small scanning radius through the suprasternal, supraclavicular, and parasternal areas at the level of the first four intercostal spaces.

Computed tomography is more often the method of choice for exactly assessing the structure of the mediastinum and for differential diagnosis between substernal goiter, lymphomas, and other masses of the thorax. The sensitivity of CT for mediastinal neoplasms is about 98.8%, with a diagnostic accuracy of 92.7% (Pishchik 2008).

Chest radiography including X-ray of the mediastinum with contrasted esophagus and radionuclide scan are often mandatory (Figs. 10.3 and 10.4).

MRI, PET (more often in carcinomas), and SPECT also supply additional data in cases of substernal goiter. Puncture biopsy is readily available and is of high diagnostic value. Nevertheless, it is not recommended by most authors due to the high risk of complications relating to damage to the large vascular structures and

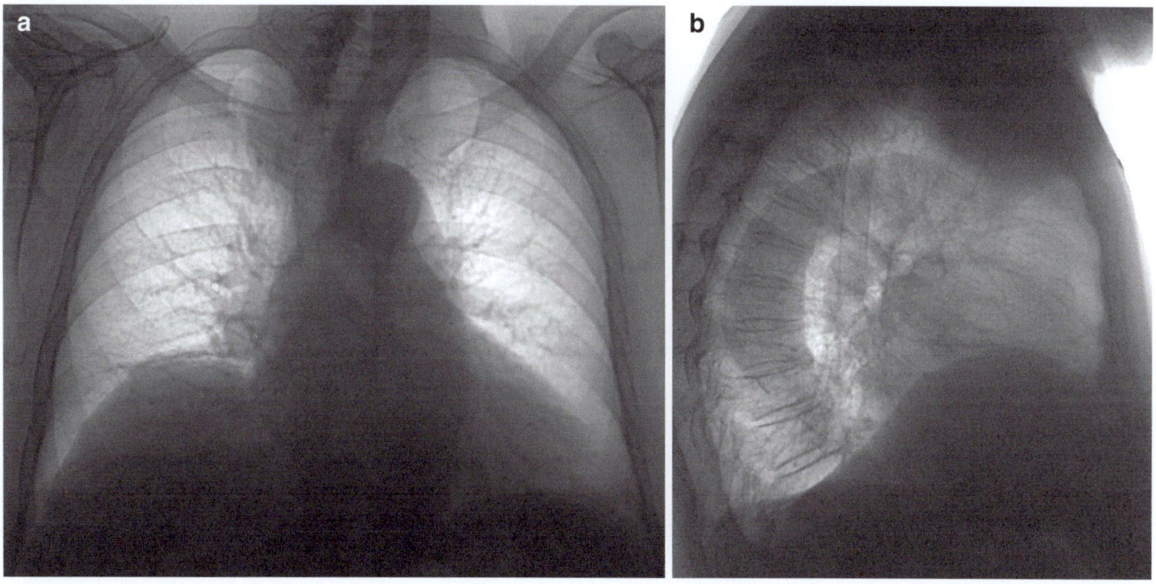

Fig. 10.3 (**a**, **b**) Substernal goiter. Chest X-ray

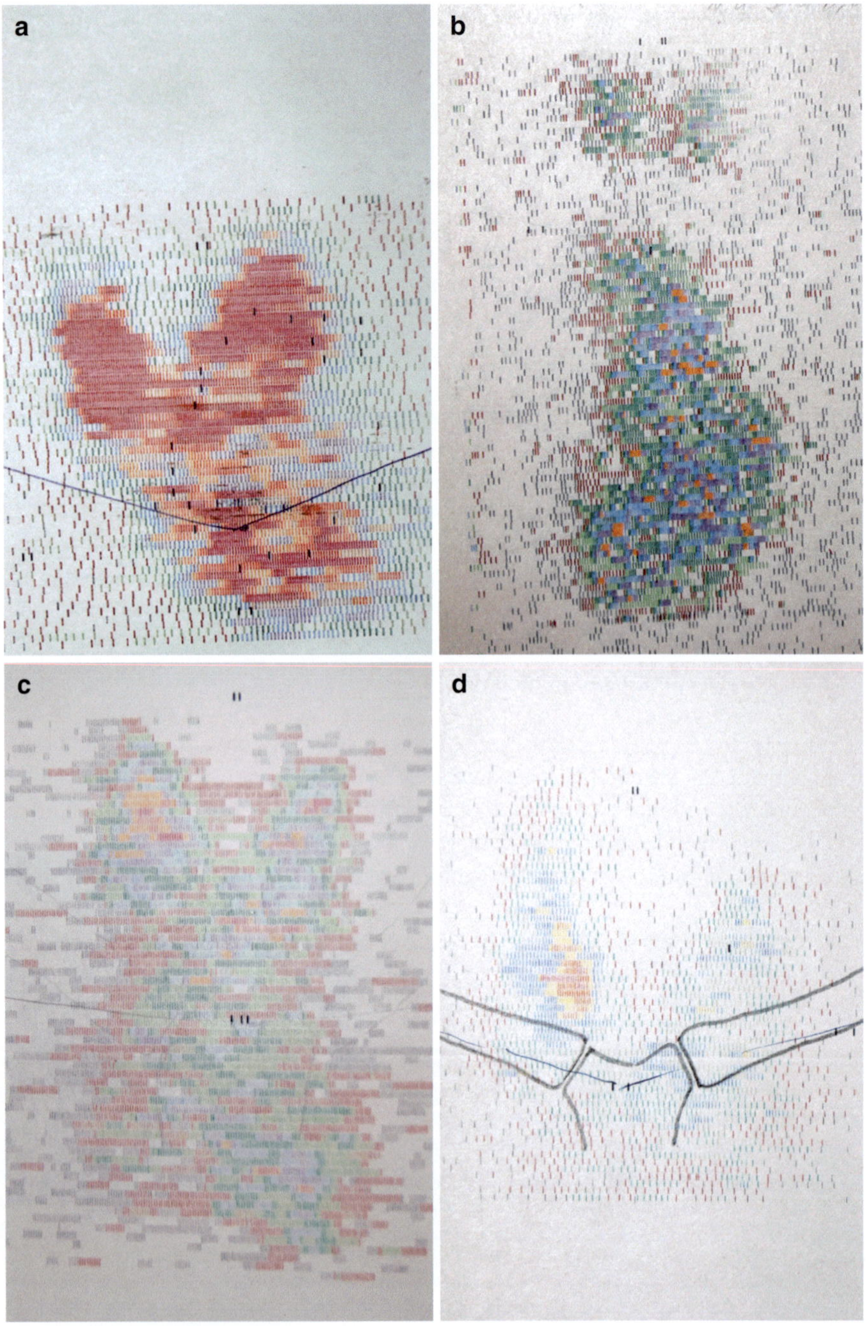

Fig. 10.4 (**a–f**) Substernal goiter. Radionuclide scan with ^{131}I

Fig 10.4 (continued)

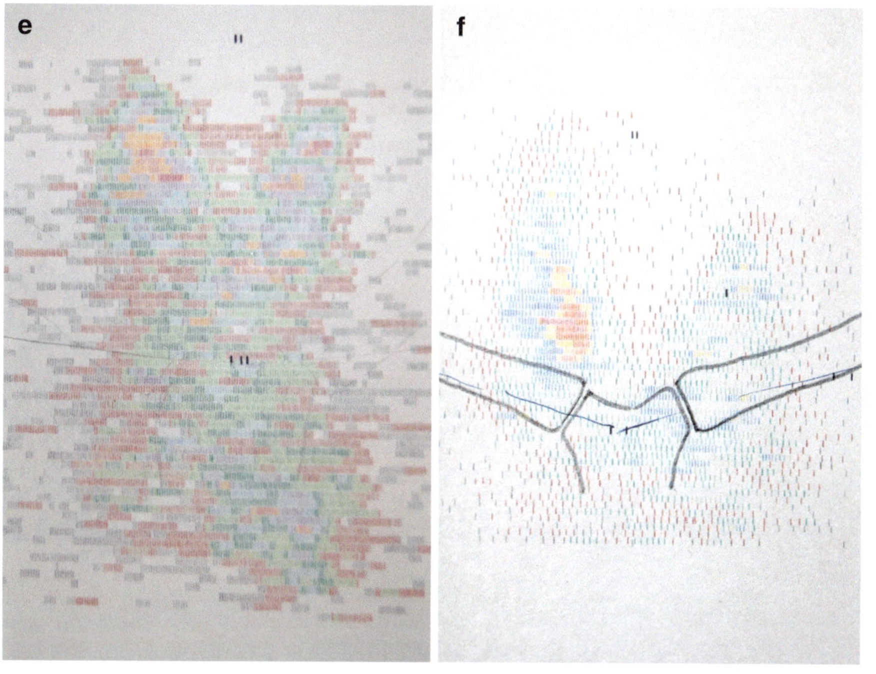

organs of the thorax. Substernal goiter is usually represented by a large mass. Therefore, the material obtained for biopsy cannot supply complete information on all areas of the lesion so that malignancy can be ruled out. According to Ignjatovic (2001), complete correct diagnosis appears impossible to achieve in 20% of cases.

11 Ultrasound of the Parathyroid Glands

The diagnosis of parathyroid diseases is a complex and equivocal problem. Parathyroid gland pathologies are the third most common of all endocrine diseases. The incidence of primary hyperparathyroidism (HPT) in a particular country directly depends on whether social programs aimed at its early diagnosis are being implemented in that country. It ranges from 1:500 to 1:2,000 within the population depending on age and gender, with a ratio of men to women of 1:4. In Sweden, the implementation of careful examinations has resulted in a morbidity of 1:200 (Cristensson et al. 1976). At the same time, patients who are diagnosed early with primary HPT constitute less than 10% of all those with the actual morbidity. According to Kotova (2003), primary HPT is practically undiagnosed in many regions. In some cases, nephrocalcinosis, nephrolithiasis, cholelithiasis, stomach or duodenal ulcers, or osteoporosis appear to be consequences of HPT rather than independent diseases.

Methods of visualizing parathyroids may be classified as either noninvasive or invasive, and preoperative or intraoperative:

1. Noninvasive preoperative methods
   - Radionuclide scan with ^{99m}Tc-sestamibi and ^{131}I (^{123}I) or ^{99m}Tc-pertechnetate
   - Radionuclide scan with ^{201}Tl and ^{99m}Tc-pertechnetate
   - Two-phase scintigraphy with ^{99m}Tc-Sestamibi
   - SPECT
   - US
   - CT
   - MRI
   - PET
   - Thermography
2. Invasive preoperative methods
   - FNAB with cytological examination
   - Selective arteriography
   - Subtraction angiography
   - Selective blood sampling from veins to define the PTH level
   - Selenium methionine administration
3. Intraoperative methods
   - Intraoperative US
   - Intravenous administration of toluidine or methylene blue
   - Quick PTH assay
   - Intraoperative gamma detection

The preoperative detection of pathological parathyroids involves the use of "functional" and "anatomical" methods. Globally, radionuclide scan is thought to be preferable. It is the method of choice for localizing parathyroid adenomas (Table 11.1).

Indications for radionuclide scan to diagnose HPT are as follows:

- HPT proved by laboratory data
- Recurrent or persistent HPT
- Differential diagnosis of mediastinal mass
- Planning or follow-up of surgery for HPT
- Differential diagnosis of primary and secondary HPT
- Suspicion of multiple abnormal parathyroids

When an abnormal parathyroid is identified, the second visualization procedure should be chosen based on the data obtained. As a rule, a combination of two localizing modalities is utilized (scintigraphy with ^{99m}Tc-sestamibi and US, SPECT and MRI, PET and CT, and other combinations). Modern radiological methods permit the precise detection of abnormal parathyroids in 22–90% of cases. Additionally, combining different modalities increases the accuracy of localization up to 95%.

The efficacy of sonography for primary HPT was first assessed by Edis and Evans (1979). Good results were

V.P. Kharchenko et al., *Ultrasound Diagnostics of Thyroid Diseases*,
DOI: 10.1007/978-3-642-12387-0_11,

Table 11.1 Characteristics of noninvasive methods of localization in primary HPT (according to Gonzalez and Paricio 1997)

Features	US	CT	MRI	Scintigraphy with ^{201}Tl/^{99m}Tc	Scintigraphy with ^{99m}Tc-sestamibi
Sensitivity (%)	22–82	47–76	50–80	45–68	70–90
Economic expense	+	+++	++++	++	++
Operator dependence	+++	+	++	–	–
Radiation dose	–	++	–	+	+
Site of best visualization	Close to the thyroid gland	Ectopia	Ectopia	Close to the thyroid gland	All sites
Site of poor visualization	Mediastinum	Thyroid gland	–	Mediastinum, deep neck compartments	–

obtained in cases of "typical" parathyroid location. This led to the suggestion that US could be used to test for the first stage of primary HPT (Taillandier 1994). This point of view was later revised and withdrawn due to large number of false-positive and false-negative results. US is, however, successfully applied as an auxiliary method for visualizing abnormal orthotopic parathyroid glands (Quiros 2004). Sonography may also be utilized as an alternative method in cases where other techniques are inefficient or limited (2–5% of all cases).

Parathyroid US is absolutely indicated in patients with primary HPT during the localization stage under the following circumstances:

- Parathyroid tumor that does not accumulate ^{99m}Tc-sestamibi
- Concomitant pathology of the parathyroid and thyroid glands, to choose the type of surgery
- Concomitant pathology of the parathyroid and neck lymph nodes
- Persistent and recurrent primary HPT
- Several foci on radionuclide uptake in a patient with primary HPT
- Secondary HPT in patients with chronic renal failure on chronic program hemodialysis
- Differential diagnosis of secondary and tertiary HPT
- Intrathyroid parathyroid tumor
- Multiple parathyroid lesions
- Prior to minimally invasive US-assisted methods of treatment of parathyroid diseases
- Impossibility of scintigraphy with ^{99m}Tc-sestamibi
- Refusal of the patient to undergo radionuclide scan with ^{99m}Tc-sestamibi (radiophobia)
- Syndromes of multiple endocrine neoplasia (MEN I, MEN II)
- Familial primary HPT

The technology used in parathyroid US is the same as that used for examinations of the thyroid gland. Special preparation for parathyroid sonography is not required. The patient is positioned supine on the examination couch, with the neck hyperextended. A pillow or triangular soft pad is placed under the patient's shoulders and lower neck for support. US may be sometimes performed in the sitting position, with the head thrown back in seriously ill patients. US probes of 7.5–15 MHz are used. The probe is positioned on the anterior surface of the neck and moved consistently from the submandibular area to the suprasternal fossa and supraclavicular area. Special attention should be paid to the dorsal aspects of thyroid lobes and the fat close to the inferior poles of thyroid lobes between ITA branches (orthotopic sites of the parathyroids). A prior radionuclide scan facilitates the search.

US report should contain the following data:

1. Number of lesions
2. Location in relation to the thyroid, neck vascular bundles, trachea, esophagus, larynx, or hyoid
3. Dimensions (in three mutually perpendicular planes) and volume
4. Shape (spherical, oval, or irregular)
5. Borders (smooth or irregular)
6. Contours (accurate or indistinct)
7. Echodensity
8. Echostructure

9. Calcifications (dimensions, location, and posterior acoustic shadowing)
10. Fluid component (dimensions and fluid/solid ratio)
11. Posterior echo pattern (enhancement or shadowing)
12. Vascularity

11.1 Normal Parathyroid

US is a valuable method in cases where the parathyroid glands are in their typical locations, and also for the diagnosis of concomitant thyroid pathology. Sonography is of low value for abnormal parathyroids located behind the trachea, larynx, pharynx, esophagus, and in the postoperative neck. It is not informative in ectopic mediastinal parathyroids (Eigelberger and Clark 2000). Normal parathyroids do not show sufficient functional activity to be seen by scintigraphy or SPECT. Therefore, modalities that are focused on determining functioning tissue detect only thyroid tissue and do not see normal parathyroids. Much depends on the histological structural features.

Eighty-four percent of people have four parathyroids (two on each side). Five to six glands are observed in 3–13% of cases, 2–3 glands in 1–7%, and in rare cases up to 12 parathyroids may be observed (Wang 1977) (Fig. 11.1). The length of each gland is 2–7 mm, its width is 2–4 mm, its thickness is 0.5–2 mm, and its weight is 35–55 mg (Netter 2003). Parathyroids can have different shapes. Wang (1977) described eight shape variants of normal parathyroids, ranging in dimensions from 2 to 10 mm, based on the results of morphological examinations.

Twin superior and inferior parathyroids are located on the back surfaces of the thyroid lobes. Superior

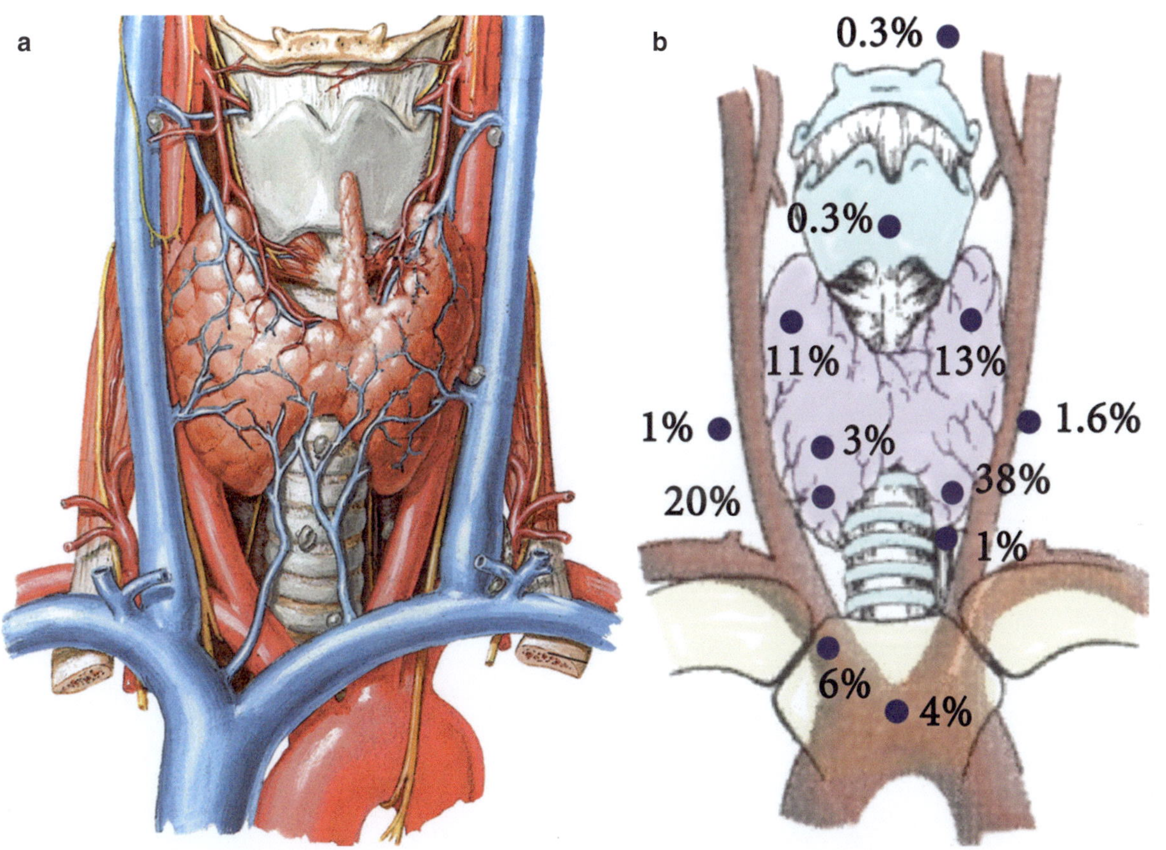

Fig. 11.1 (**a**, **b**) Location of the parathyroid glands (according to Netter 2003). Incidences for different sites (LiVolsi and Hamilton 1993)

parathyroids are normally detected in the middle of the posterior margin of the thyroid lobes and are projected at the level of the cricoid plate. About 80% of all superior parathyroids can be found within a circle 2 cm in diameter that is shifted 1 cm cranially from this site (Randel et al. 1987). Inferior parathyroids are usually located near the inferior poles of the thyroid lobes close to the ITA (as a rule, dorsally from it). However, their location is more variable than that of the superior parathyroids. They may be detected deep in the thyroid parenchyma, between two capsules, outside the surgical capsule of the thyroid gland, close to the CCA bifurcation, or in the upper mediastinum. Ectopic parathyroid glands occur in 15–20% of patients. They may also be found in a number of unusual locations.

Every parathyroid is surrounded by a fibrous capsule, the interior of which contains gland septa carrying blood vessels and vasomotor nerve fibers. As a rule, the parathyroids are surrounded by a compact layer of fat. They are normally supplied with arterial blood from the inferior thyroid artery. The venous blood is drained via the veins of the thyroid, trachea and esophagus.

The possibility of and the reliability of the visualization of normal parathyroid glands are somewhat dubious. Normal adult parathyroids contain a large amount of adipocytes. Thus, unlike thyroid parenchyma, they are practically invisible against the surrounding fatty tissue. According to most authors, they are normally not detected by anatomical visualizing modalities (US, CT, or MRI). However, according to other authors, high-quality US scanners with high-frequency probes (7.5–15 MHz) sometimes (in 10–20% of cases) permit the visualization of normal parathyroids (Gooding 1993; Solbiati et al. 1993; Harchenko et al. 2007). The inferior normal parathyroid gland may be detected more often.

A normal parathyroid can be identified as a structure with the following attributes (Fig. 11.2):

1. Structure, more often adjacent to the inferior segment/pole of thyroid lobe or to the dorsal surface of the middle segment of the thyroid lobe, sometimes partially or completely within the thyroid (Fig. 11.3)
2. Size of 0.2–0.7 cm

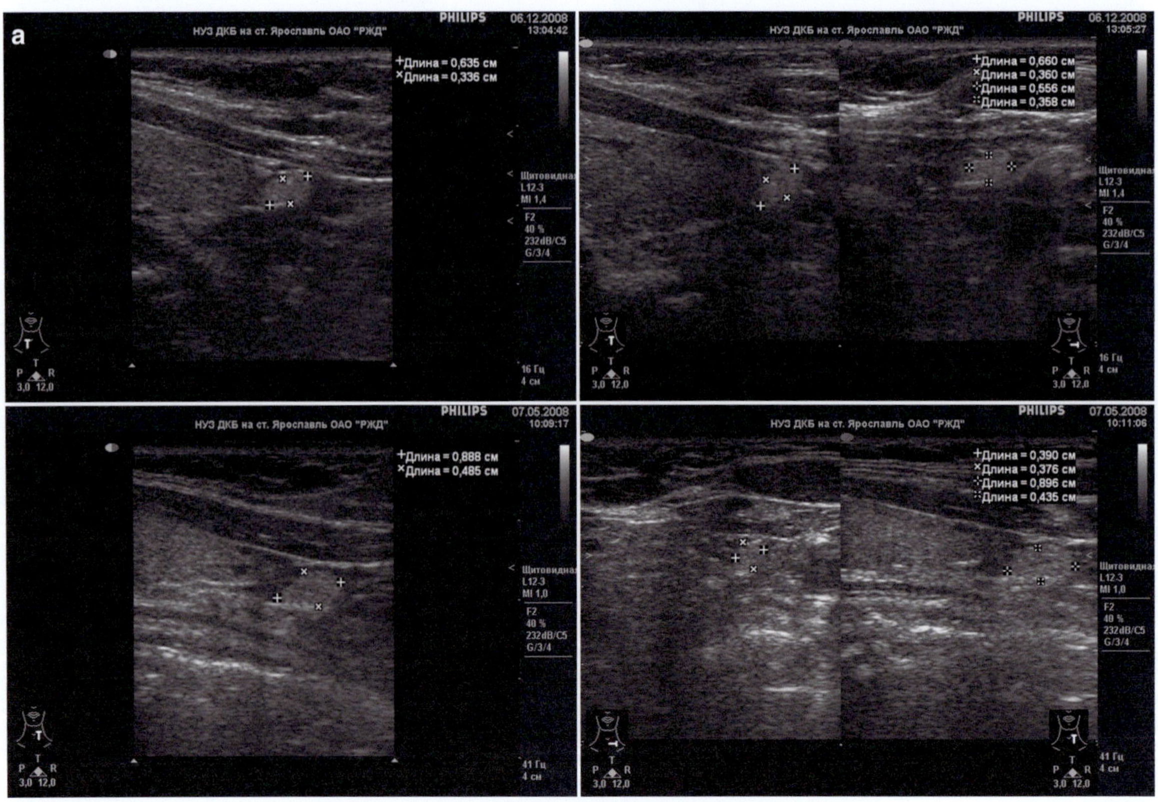

Fig. 11.2 Normal parathyroid. (**a**) Grayscale sonography. (**b**) CDI and PDI

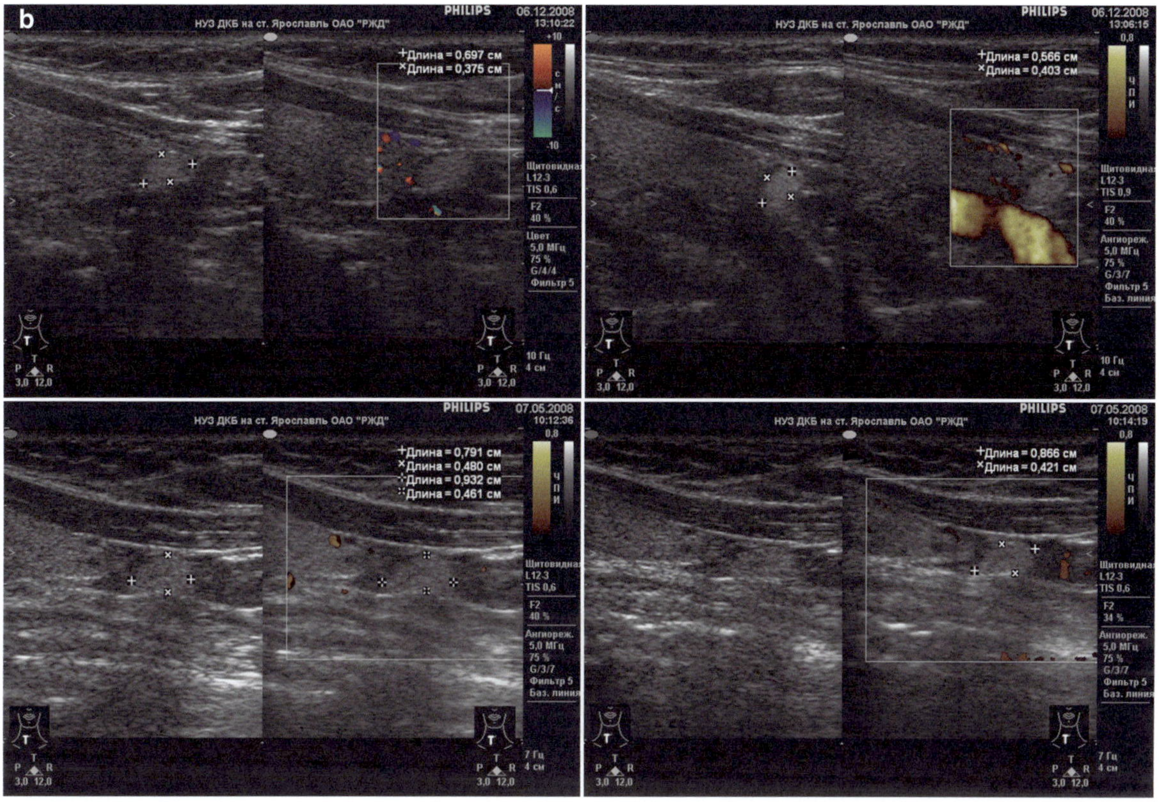

Fig. 11.2 (continued)

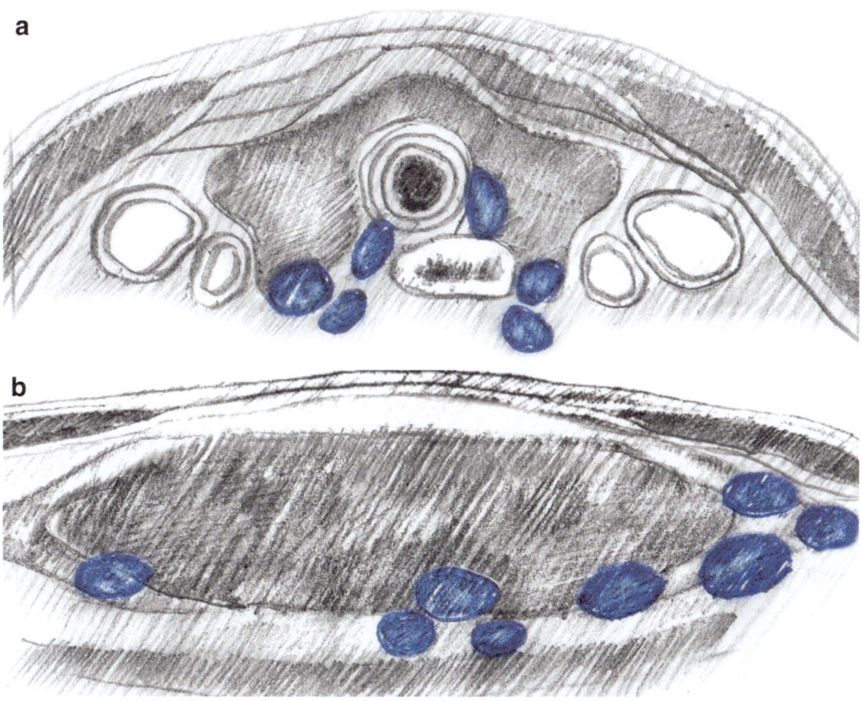

Fig. 11.3 Frequent sites of the parathyroids detected with US. (**a**) Transverse scan. (**b**) Longitudinal scan

3. Roundish or oval shape
4. Isoechoic or slightly increased echodensity
5. Homogeneous structure
6. Well-defined, regular margins
7. Avascular in CDI, PDI, and 3DPD

An abnormally enlarged parathyroid is often much more accessible to US visualization. According to Nazarenko et al. (2004), parathyroid lesions are found incidentally during thyroid US in 37% of cases. Focused searches reveal 63% of parathyroid lesions.

Parathyroid pathology is mainly observed in adults. A normal adult parathyroid contains up to 80% fat, so any hyperplasia of the main parathyroid cells results in a decrease in echodensity and better differentiation from the surrounding tissue. US has been proven to detect the following parathyroid abnormalities:

- Adenoma
- Cancer
- Hyperplasia
- Cyst

PTH hyperproduction is often a consequence of one (83%) or several (5%) parathyroid adenomas, in rather rare cases, or of parathyroid hyperplasia (11–20%) or malignant hormone-releasing parathyroid tumor (1%) (Nazarenko et al. 2004).

The sensitivity of sonography for the diagnosis of parathyroid abnormalities is 63–78%. It is 10% lower in cases with prior neck surgery (Gofrit et al. 1997). Its sensitivity to parathyroid hyperplasia is lower than it is for adenomas: 24–50% (Wakamatsu et al. 2003).

11.2 Parathyroid Adenoma

According to most experts, parathyroid adenomas are the cause of primary HPT in 80–85% of cases. The resulting change in histological structure, with a prevalence of chief and oxyphil cells and a decrease in adipose cells, leads to an improvement in parathyroid visualization with sonography (Figs. 11.4 and 11.5).

Adenoma of the superior parathyroid is usually detected with a longitudinal scan along the back margin of the middle segment of the thyroid lobe in the projection of the recurrent nerve and ITA branch. Adenoma of the inferior parathyroid is most often located below the inferior pole of the thyroid lobe or in the initial part of the thyrothymic ligament. Parathyroid adenoma is observed with a transverse scan dorsally from thyroid lobes, in paratracheal or paravasal (medially and dorsally from the CCA) sites.

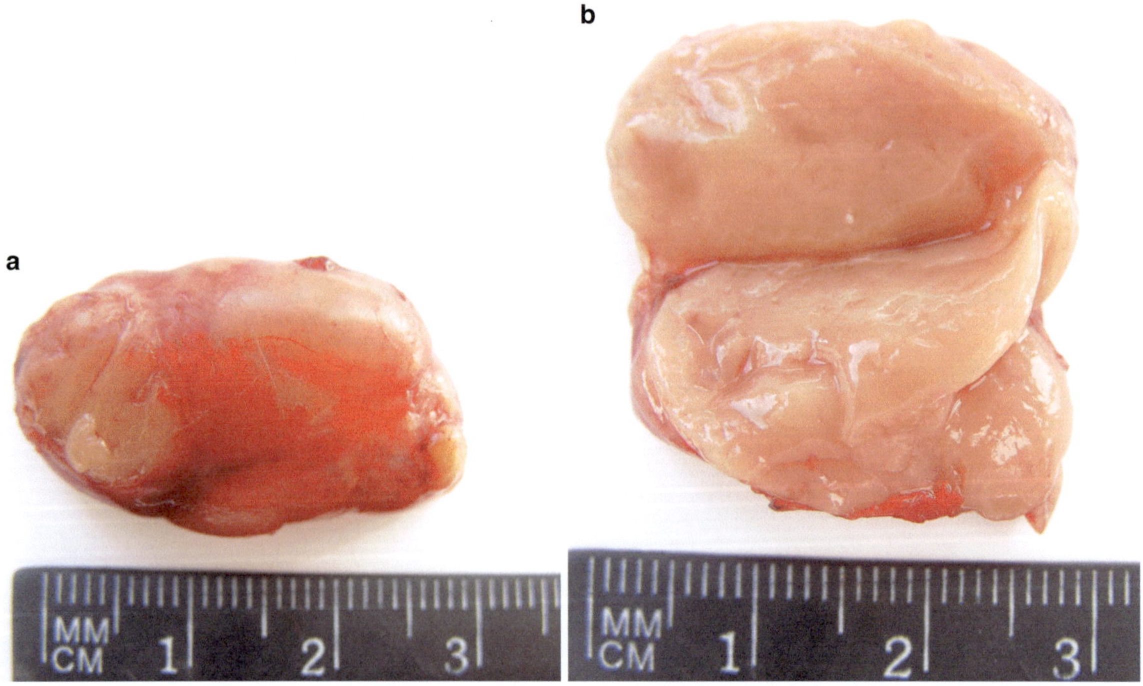

Fig. 11.4 (**a**, **b**) Parathyroid adenoma. Macroscopic view

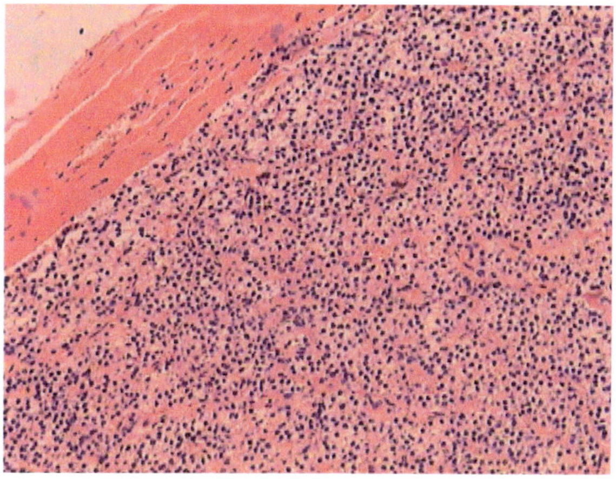

Fig. 11.5 Parathyroid adenoma (hematoxylin and eosin stained smears; original magnification, ×200)

According to Nazarenko et al. (2004), the dimensions of parathyroid adenomas range from 4 to 30 mm. Hara et al. (2001) report that the ratio of thickness to width in adenomas is about 0.64 (0.33–1.47).

Parathyroid adenomas are usually visualized as lesions of extended, triangular, dumbbell-like, or oval shape (Mitkov et al. 2005). They are most often hypoechoic in comparison with thyroid tissue and demonstrate relatively homogeneous echostructure (Fig. 11.6). In some cases the echostructure can be moderately or significantly heterogeneous due to small areas of increased echodensity, echogenic inclusions, or anechoic fluid collections. Their margins can be indistinct in cases of small adenomas. When the tumor is over 10 mm in size, the contours are, as a rule, well-defined and regular. Parathyroid adenomas of a small size (up to 10 mm) are oval or oblong in shape. During the process of enlargement, the tumor becomes more elongated and extended (Reading et al. 1982). A fluid component that is up to 5–80% of the tumor volume may be observed in parathyroid adenomas. The presence of this fluid component does not influence the expression of HPT (the level of PTH). It does not reflect the "age" of the adenoma either, and does not allow its development to be predicted.

CDI, PDI, and 3DPD often reveal an increased vascular pattern in parathyroid adenoma as compared with neck lymph nodes and most thyroid nodules (Fig. 11.7), and soft structure with sonoelastography (Fig. 11.8).

Parathyroid adenomas most often exhibit parenchymatous and mixed types of blood flow patterns (Mazzeo 1997; Nazarenko et al. 2004).

Graif et al. (1987) and Mazzeo et al. (1997) suggest that the following five types of vascular pattern can occur in parathyroid adenomas:

1. Focal perinodular ("vascular column")
2. Perinodular
3. Intranodular (parenchymatous type)
4. Mixed (peri- and intranodular)
5. Avascular

Lane (1998) considers that Doppler mapping should be an obligatory part of the US examination in patients with primary HPT, since it permits the specification of the parathyroid tumor location. An afferent artery penetrating into the gland (an ITA branch) may be observed in 83% of cases of parathyroid adenoma. According to Wolf (1994), a "vascular arch," which bends around the adenoma and covers 90–270 arc degrees, is a specific sign of parathyroid adenoma, and can be identified in 63% of patients.

In cases with a neck lesion, which is sonographically associated with parathyroid adenoma, it is still necessary to perform a careful examination of all possible sites of other parathyroids. This is due to the possibility of double parathyroid adenomas, which are poorly detected by scintigraphy with ^{99m}Tc-sestamibi. The detection of double parathyroid adenomas supplies additional information for the surgeon, thus influencing the type of operation. If this examination is not performed at the localization stage, it is necessary to do it prior to the surgery.

Difficulties arise in the localization of atypically located parathyroid adenomas within the neck in cases of intrathyroid, intrathymic, or paravasal location, or a location on the anterior thyroid surface. US fails to detect such adenomas in most cases. Neck lymph nodes, thyroid nodules, thymic granulomas, lipomas, or other lesions are interpreted as parathyroid adenomas in cases of proven HPT and in the absence of data from scintigraphy or SPECT. On the other hand, parathyroid adenomas of atypical location with unknown blood PTH and ionized calcium level can be misinterpreted as nodules, cystic or vascular structures of the thyroid gland, and so on. These errors result from incomplete utilization of the US options available, and the sonographer not being aware of HPT.

Intrathyroid parathyroids do not demonstrate evident capsules. This also complicates the diagnosis. Despite the problems listed above, US is advantageous in cases with intrathyroid and prethyroid

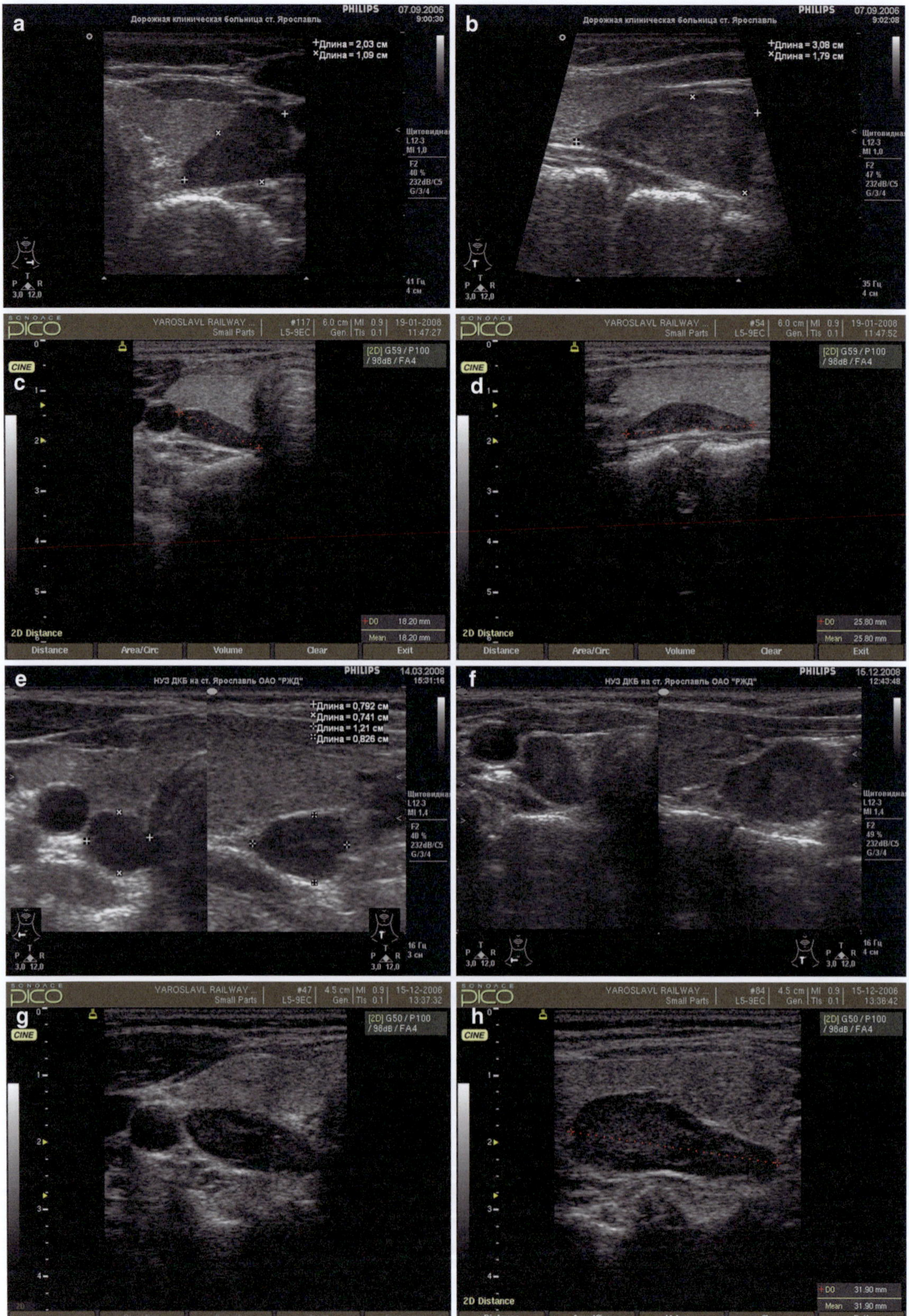

Fig. 11.6 (**a–h**) Parathyroid adenoma. Grayscale sonography

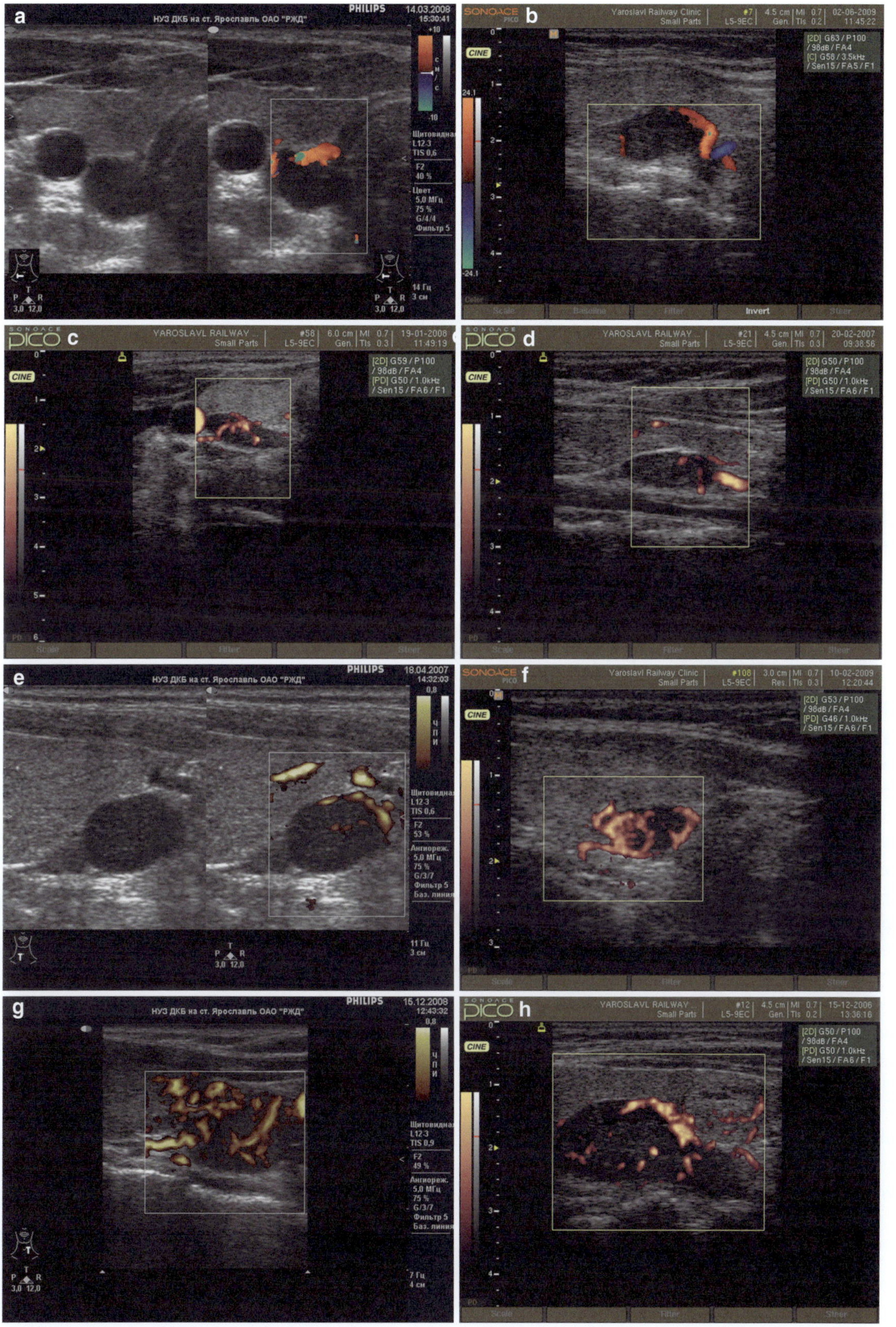

Fig. 11.7 (**a–h**) Parathyroid adenoma. CDI and PDI

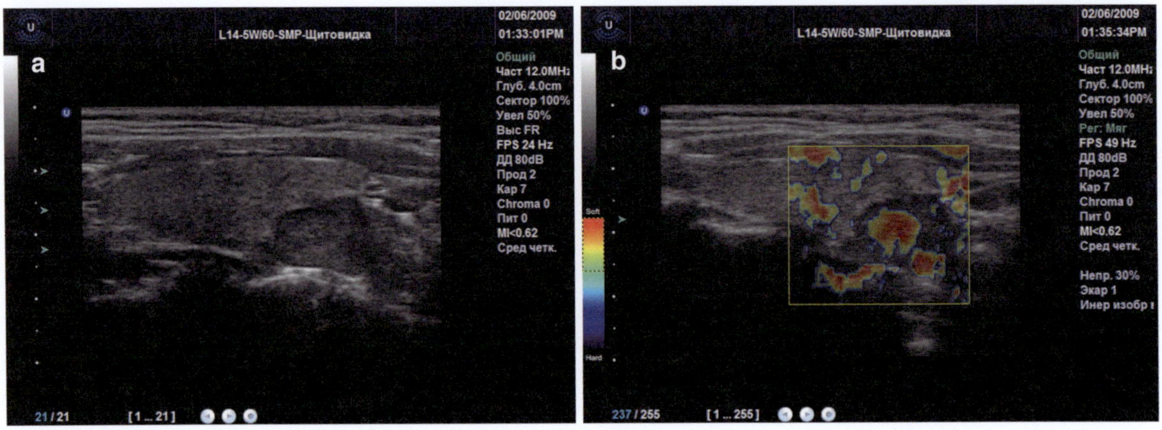

Fig. 11.8 (**a**, **b**) Parathyroid adenoma. Sonoelastography

locations of the parathyroid adenoma. Scintigraphy with ^{99m}Tc-sestamibi is more efficient for differential diagnosis in cases with paravasal and other atypical locations.

Difficulties with the differential diagnosis of parathyroid adenoma arise in cases of big lesions, which may be wrongly considered thyroid lesions. The detection of such a lesion during thyroid US by sonographers who are not accustomed to patients with HPT may result in a wrong diagnosis and lead to wrong tactics. In some cases the first recommendation is scintigraphy or SPECT. This is also a tactical error. The most reasonable approach is to conclude that a neck lesion is present, suggest a consultation with an endocrinologist, and prove HPT using laboratory assays (blood ionized calcium and PTH assays, etc.). Such parathyroid adenomas can displace adjacent organs (first of all the thyroid gland), taking their "typical" places. This complicates the diagnosis to such an extent that it may lead to wrong conclusions, even in positive scintigraphy with ^{99m}Tc-Sestamibi.

Difficulties with the US diagnosis of parathyroid adenomas occur in cases with prominent structural changes of the surrounding organs and tissues, first of all in nodular lesions of the thyroid gland, and also after neck surgery. False-positive results (6–15%) are mainly induced by thyroid nodules, enlarged lymph nodes, or pathology of the esophagus. A multinodular goiter which is characterized by several thyroid lesions with different echodensities can mask abnormal parathyroids. Additionally, an absence of clinical signs of HPT (asymptomatic primary HPT) and/or normal blood calcium (normocalcemic HPT) result in the lack of identification of some parathyroid adenomas.

In some cases, sonography does not permit the differentiation of a parathyroid adenoma from an enlarged neck lymph node (especially in patients with an anamnesis of head or neck malignancies) or thyroid nodule. In those cases, US-guided FNAB is feasible (Abraham 2007).

11.3 Parathyroid Cancer

Parathyroid cancer is a rare abnormality observed in 1–2% of all cases of primary HPT. Differential diagnosis of adenoma is difficult. The diagnosis is made in the majority of cases during a pathomorphological examination.

According to Kinoshita (1985) malignant tumors show the highest echodensity of all parathyroid lesions. This makes them similar to the colloid nodules of the thyroid gland. Parathyroid cancer usually exhibits a roundish or oval shape, irregular indistinct margins, and an absence of an echogenic capsule (Fig. 11.9). Extremely high levels of blood PTH and calcium are also characteristic. One indirect feature is large lesion size (the mass can reach 15–200 g). The metastatic lymph nodes of the neck can serve as an additional sign of parathyroid cancer in the absence of malignancies in the other organs of the head, neck, and mediastinum. Alternatively, they can easily mask the abnormal parathyroid, which appears to have a similar echostructure on US.

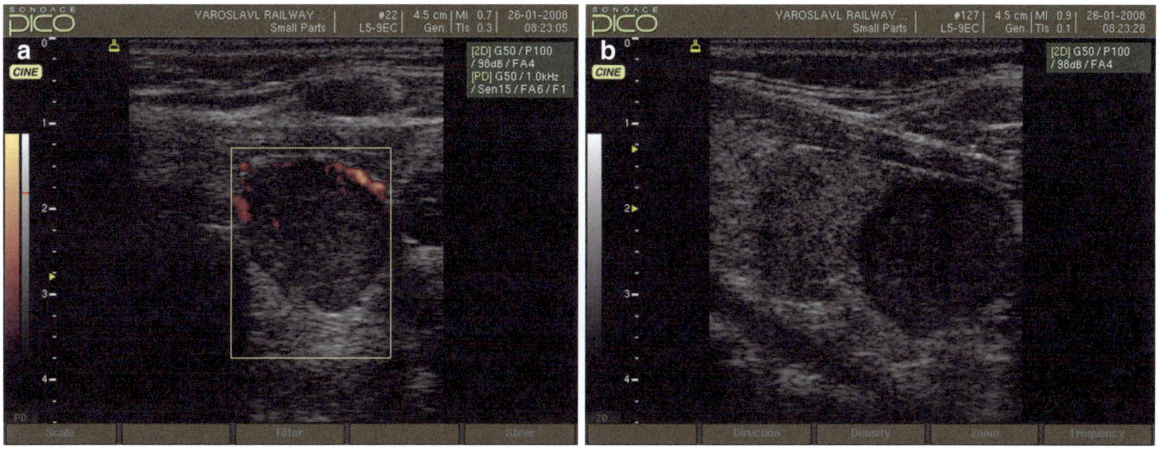

Fig. 11.9 (**a**, **b**) Parathyroid cancer. Grayscale and PDI

The size of the parathyroid tumor is important for accurate sonography in patients with primary HPT. Special difficulties arise in detecting small parathyroid tumors. According to Moca (2000), parathyroid lesions less than 500 mg in mass are not detected sonographically. Thus, US is not efficient for tumors less than 10 mm in size. It is also of little value for retrotracheal, retroesophageal, mediastinal, and other atypical locations of parathyroid lesions. Scintigraphy with MIBI, CT, or MRI are preferable in such cases.

11.4 Parathyroid Hyperplasia

Parathyroid hyperplasia is characterized by the symmetric or asymmetric enlargement of two or more glands. Hyperplasia of one parathyroid gland is only seldom observed. The most frequent cause of parathyroid hyperplasia is a secondary (renal) HPT due to chronic program hemodialysis in patients with chronic renal failure. This results from hyperphosphatemia and hypocalcemia.

Both parathyroid hyperplasia and parathyroid adenoma are associated with an increased weight of parathyrocytes and a significant decrease in adipocytes. Parathyroid hyperplasia may be classified into diffuse, nodular, and mixed types (Lomonte et al. 2005). The sonographic features of the different types of parathyroid hyperplasia are quite subjective. Common morphological changes in adenoma and hyperplasia of the parathyroid gland exclude the possibility of their differentiation by means of sonography (Fig. 11.4).

The differential diagnosis of parathyroid hyperplasia and adenoma is difficult, and not only for ultrasound specialists. Most often they cannot be distinguished visually during surgery either. The final conclusion is drawn based only on morphological examination.

The differential diagnosis of diffuse and nodular types of parathyroid hyperplasia in secondary HPT is a challenge for an ultrasound specialist (Fig. 11.10). In most cases, the areas of nodular hyperplasia in parathyroid tissue are small and are difficult to spot with US.

11.5 Parathyroid Cyst

True parathyroid cysts are observed quite rarely (Solbiati et al. 1993; Mitkov et al. 2006). Most of these cysts are found by chance during a scheduled neck US. Parathyroid cysts are mainly of the nonfunctioning type. True functioning parathyroid cysts that result in primary HPT appear to be extremely rare (Sugimoto 1997). Nonfunctioning cysts are always located in the inferior parathyroid glands. The location of a functioning cyst is less predictable; they can be detected in the range from the angle of the mandible to the mediastinum (Pinney and Daly 1999).

Parathyroid cysts appear as anechoic lesions of roundish or oval shape with regular accurate margins located at the sites of parathyroid glands. The capsule is thin, echogenic, or sometimes not visualized by standard sonography (Fig. 11.11). CDI, PDI, and 3DPD observe only the peripheral blood pattern around the cyst. Sometimes it is possible to identify the afferent artery.

Parathyroid cysts should be differentiated from fluid nodules and true cysts of the thyroid gland, median and lateral neck cysts, and metastases of well-differentiated thyroid cancer into neck lymph nodes.

Parathyroid cysts do not demonstrate any specific US features. Therefore, US-guided FNAB should be utilized to assess the PTH level and the parathyrocytes in the aspirate (Birnbaum and Van Herle 1989). In

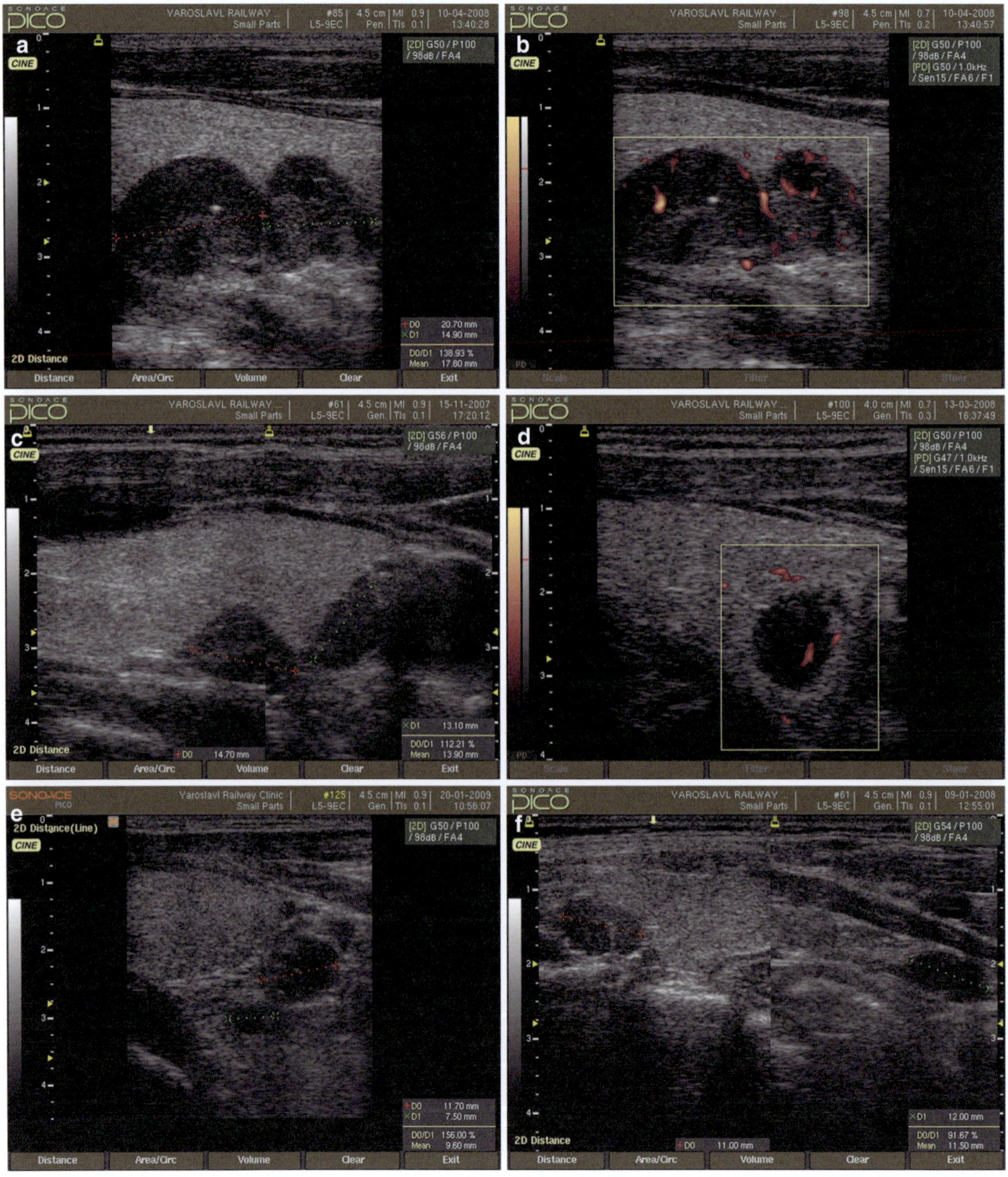

Fig. 11.10 (**a–h**) Parathyroid hyperplasia. Grayscale, PDI, and macroscopic view

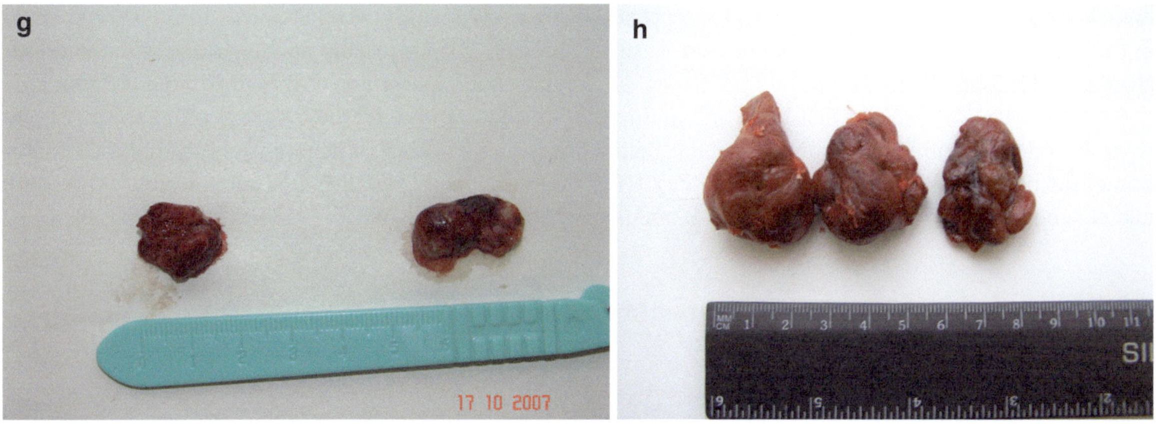

Fig. 11.10 (continued)

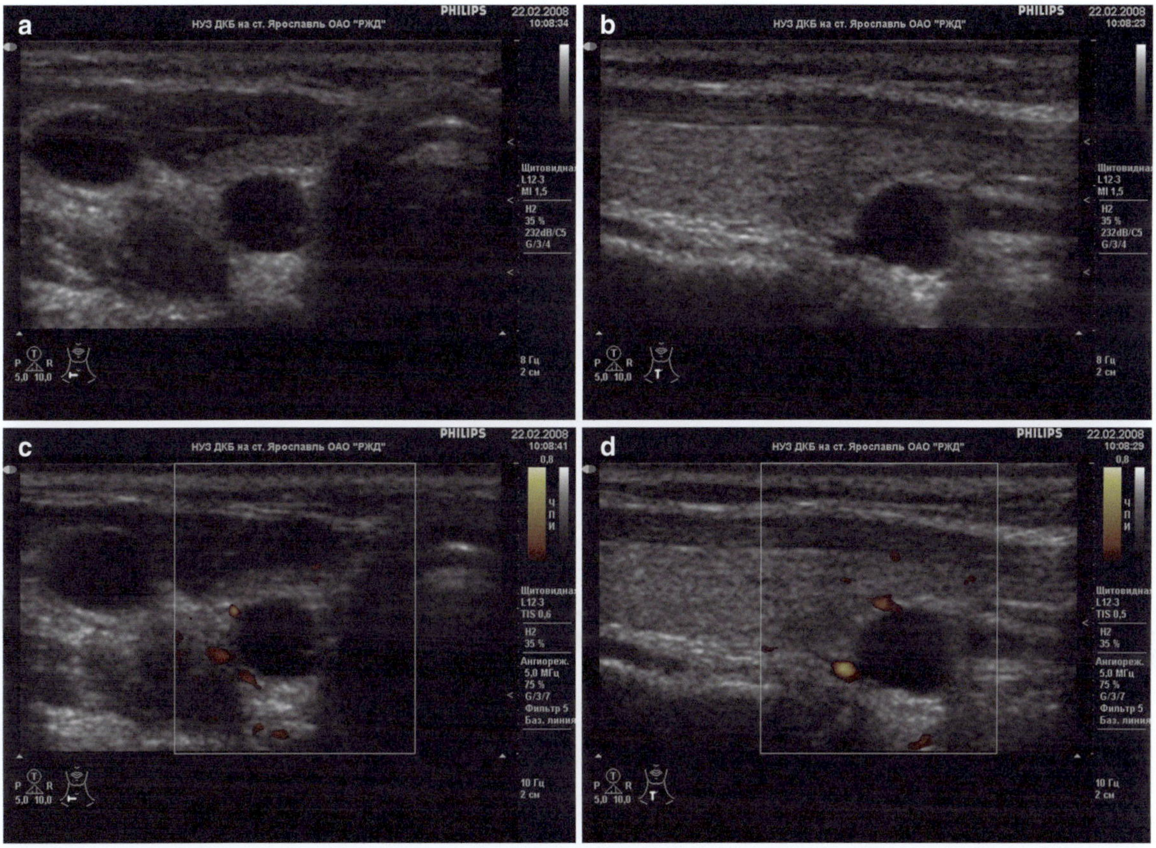

Fig. 11.11 (**a–d**) Parathyroid cyst with high PTH level. Grayscale and PDI

cases with functioning cystic lesions, scintigraphy with ^{99m}Tc-sestamibi can supply additional data. However, some authors report that scintigraphy with ^{99m}Tc-sestamibi is not capable of depicting functionally active parathyroid cysts (Ak 2007).

Despite research that demonstrates the capacity of sonography to localize abnormal parathyroids, most publications provide reasonable objections to the "routine" visualization of parathyroid glands with different visualizing modalities, including US. One argument is that even the best methods of visualization yield exact results in less than 80% of cases. The methods are also insufficiently reliable for multiple lesions.

It is important to consider that large and multiple thyroid nodules significantly complicate the detection of the parathyroids in patients with primary HPT and concomitant thyroid pathology. Thyroid nodules often mask parathyroid abnormalities Asymptomatic primary HPT is usually not diagnosed with multinodular goiter. Despite FNAB being "the gold standard" for nodular goiters, the cytology often appears to be misinterpreted as follicular thyroid neoplasia in samples obtained from the parathyroid lesion (Weymouth 2003).

The example of US report in abnormal parathyroid

First name, middle initial, last name:
Age:
Date:
The number of case history:
US scanner:
The thyroid gland is typically located with regular well-defined margins and homogeneous isoechoic structure. The capsule is uniform and continuous on all extent. Cystic and solid lesions are not detected.

The depth of the **isthmus** - 2 mm					
Right lobe			**Left lobe**		
Depth	15	mm	Depth	14	mm
Width	16	mm	Width	15	mm
Length	51	mm	Length	47	mm
Volume	6.1	cm^3	Volume	4.9	cm^3

The total volume 11 cm^3 does not exceed the upper limit for the endemic region and the WHO recommendations.
The vascular pattern of the parenchyma of the gland is normal and symmetric in CDI, PDI, and 3D reconstruction of vascular structures.
The topographic relation of the thyroid gland with the muscles and neck organs is typical.
An oval shaped hypoechoic lesion of 1.2x1.4x2.3 cm in size with accurate regular margins, homogeneous structure, and decreased intranodular vascular pattern is located adjacent to the back surface of the inferior segment of the left thyroid lobe. The capsule of the thyroid gland is unchanged. No lesions are detected in the orthotopic sites of other parathyroid glands.
The lymph nodes in the neck and supraclavicular areas are not enlarged.
CONCLUSION: Normal thyroid. A neck lesion (the image may correspond to the adenoma of the left inferior parathyroid gland).
US specialist:

12 Ultrasound Diagnostics of Neck Masses

A neck mass is an abnormal change in the volume and/or structure of organs or tissues of the neck. Neck masses usually arise due to a thyroid pathology (nodular goiter, tumors, etc.). Other neck lesions are much rarer.

Most of the neck masses observed can be classified as follows:

1. Primary tumors
   - Tumors of the neck organs (the thyroid, salivary glands, ENT organs, parathyroids, and others)
   - Extra-organ neck tumors
2. Lymphadenopathies
   - Reactive
   - Metastatic
   - Lymphoproliferative
3. Congenital anomalies
   - Neck cysts (midline and lateral)
   - Thyroid ectopia
   - Teratoma
   - Cysts of the thyroid and salivary glands
4. Vascular abnormalities
   - Aneurysm
   - Hemangioma
   - Lymphangioma
5. Inflammatory processes
   - Thyroiditis
   - Sialolithiasis
   - Sialadenitis

Extra-organ primary tumors account for 1.25% of all human neoplasms. According to Kamardin and Romanchishen (1991), neck tumors of mesenchymal origin constitute 52.4% of all extra-organ primary tumors, cysts 34.9%, and tumors of neuroectodermal origin 12.7%. Extra-organ tumors arising from soft tissues of the neck comprise a small but highly polymorphous group of lesions.

Extra-organ neck tumors can be grouped as follows:

1. Tumors of mesenchymal derivatives
   - Fat tissue tumors (lipoma and liposarcoma)
   - Fibrous (fibroma, desmoid, and fibrosarcoma)
   - Vascular (lymphangioma, hemangioma, and angiosarcoma)
   - Muscular (rhabdomyosarcoma and leiomyosarcoma)
   - Rare tumors (chondrosarcoma, synovioma, mesenchymoma, and others)
2. Dysembryonic tumors
   - Branchial cyst (or branchial cancer)
   - Thyroglossal neck cyst (or cyst cancer)
   - Rare tumors (chordoma, teratoma, and others)
3. Tumors of neuroectodermal origin
   - Paraganglioma (carotid, vagal, atypical)
   - Neurinoma and ganglioneuroma
   - Meningioma
4. Lymphadenopathy (metastatic, inflammatory, and hemoblastoses)

More than 70 tumor types with different morphological structures can arise in the soft tissues of the neck. Sarcomas, especially rare types, account for up to 30% of all soft-tissue tumors and less than 1% of all malignant neoplasms (King et al. 1997; Agapov et al. 1998; Fink et al. 2002). Their incidence peaks at the age of 20–40 years, and afflict more women than men (ratio of 2:1). The majority of soft-tissue tumors show benign character with slow growth and cause only cosmetic discomfort. Asymptomatic development, noninvasive, nonaggressive growth, and (rarely) the compression of

V.P. Kharchenko et al., *Ultrasound Diagnostics of Thyroid Diseases*,
DOI: 10.1007/978-3-642-12387-0_12, © Springer-Verlag Berlin Heidelberg 2010

adjacent structures complicate early clinical diagnosis. Additionally, the great diversity of pathological processes within the neck makes differential diagnosis difficult.

Diagnostic methods that are utilized to diagnose neck masses, can be classed as either visualizing (US, CT, radionuclide scan, MRI, PET, etc.), morphological (cytological and histological examination), or auxiliary (serological, laboratory, etc.).

In most cases, US aids in achieving an exact diagnosis or, at least, in determining the relation of the lesion to one or another neck organ, as well as its size, structure, margins, and vascularity. Morphological examination is necessary in cases with suspected Hodgkin's disease, malignancy of any neck site, or conglomeratic lesions. If the neck lesion is large, extends to sonographically inaccessible sites, or contacts with octal structures, CT is recommended. MRI is feasible for detailed assessment of soft tissues and blood vessels in particular. Large, benign, extra-organ tumors with fluid collections and large neck cysts are subjected to diagnostic US-guided FNAB with full fluid aspiration. Chest X-ray, abdominal US, scintigraphy of bones, and other methods are performed to rule out remote metastases in cases of malignant neoplasm.

Extra-organ neck tumors are sonographically characterized according to their locations in the following anatomical neck regions:

- Submental triangle
- Submandibular triangle
- Hyoid area
- Carotid triangle (the area of CCA bifurcation)
- Sternocleidomastoid area
- Lateral neck triangle
- Back surface of the neck

Various sites of neck masses are shown in Fig. 12.1. Neck lesions are most often located superficially and are normally easily accessible to confident US visualization.

Some neck masses that are often defined by neck US are described below.

Neck lesions that contain fluid are cysts. These are grouped into median and lateral types.

A *median cyst* (thyroglossal cyst) of the neck is an embryonic dysplasia resulting from a failure to obliterate the thyroglossal duct. It can occur anywhere from the base of the tongue to the thyroid gland, but is usually located under the deep cervical fascia between the hyoid bone and the upper edge of the thyroid cartilage, and sometimes in the submandibular triangle. It is midline or just off the midline and necessarily connected to the hyoid bone. It is represented by a painless fluid structure of flattened or roundish shape that moves up and down upon swallowing. It exhibits a thin regular capsule and homogeneous anechoic fluid contents. A certain amount of suspension may be detected. It may grow slowly. Up to half of all thyroglossal cysts are not diagnosed until adulthood. The size of the cyst can change periodically if the connection with the oral cavity through the thyroglossal duct is preserved. If the cyst is infected, the inflammation manifests as pain at swallowing and a painful midline infiltrate. Sonographically, this corresponds to the dilation of the cyst with an increase in suspension. The margins appear indistinct and thickened. Thin septa may arise within the cyst. The empyema of the cyst often results in the destruction of the capsule and overlaying soft tissues with the formation of a fistula.

Lateral cysts of the neck are a consequence of congenital developmental defects arising from branchial arches, clefts, and pouches. Lateral cysts may be divided according to their origin into lymphogenous

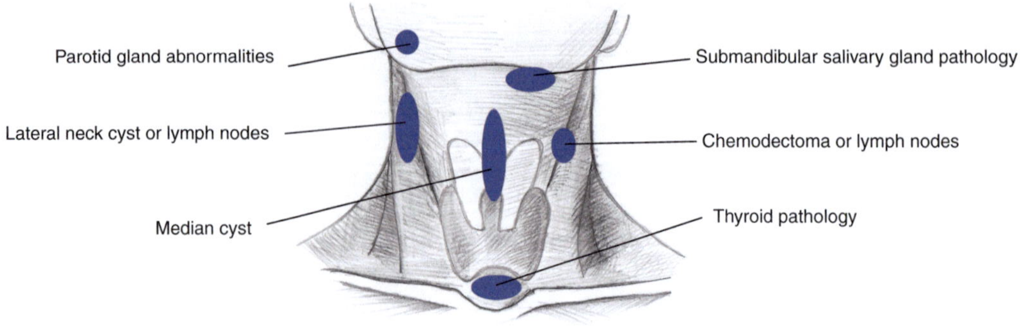

Fig. 12.1 Characteristic sites of some neck masses (Petrov et al. 2001)

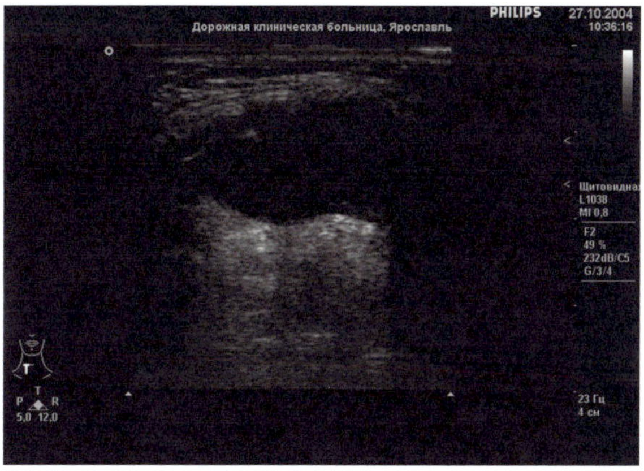

Fig. 12.2 Midline neck cyst. Grayscale sonography

(inflammatory and dysembryogenic) and branchial. Upper lateral cysts are located at the level of the mandible angle and are usually of inflammatory origin. Inferior lateral cysts are located in supraclavicular areas and are dysembryogenic (Karmazanovsky et al. 2005). Second branchial cleft cysts are most common. They are found in the upper neck along the anterior border of the sternocleidomastoid at the level of carotid bifurcation, more often on the left side. Grignon et al. (1998) consider that cyst position ahead of the sternocleidomastoid muscle at the level of the angle of the mandible is the basic feature for differential diagnosis. The cyst is, as a rule, unilateral. Bilateral cysts still occur in 2% of cases. They may develop branchial cancer, which is morphologically represented by either squamous cell carcinoma or adenocarcinoma. The incidence of this disease is higher in people over 50 years of age and is equal in men and women. Unless infected, these cysts can exist in a dormant state for a long time. Infected cysts may result in fistulas.

Lateral and median cysts are sonographically defined among the neck muscles without an organ-specific location. They demonstrate an image that is characteristic of cystic lesions (Figs. 12.2 and 12.3): roundish or oval shape; regular, well-defined margins; anechoic, homogeneous structure, sometimes with suspension, echogenic inclusions or solid component; posterior echo enhancement; avascularity in CDI, PDI, and 3DPD; limited mobility; elasticity with compression. The capsule of the cyst in usually easily identified as the echogenic linear avascular margin of the thickness up to 1–2 mm (depending on whether the cyst is infected). Inflammation leads to cyst dilation with much suspension, clots, and changes in the capsule. The capsule of the cyst becomes thicker or

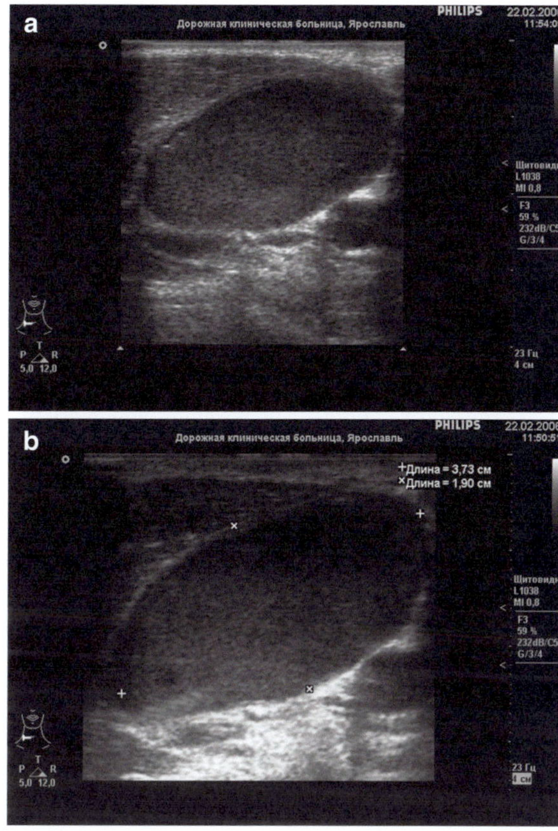

Fig. 12.3 (**a**, **b**) Lateral neck cyst. Grayscale sonography

thinner (and sometimes cannot be differentiated). Edema and infiltration of the surrounding tissues may accompany the inflammation in some cases. This is sonographically observed as a decrease or increase in echodensity, protruding heterogeneity, and a blurring of the differentiation of the structure. Lymph node enlargement associated with inflammation may occur.

Neuroectodermal tumors of the neck are represented by *paragangliomas* (chemodectomas, glomus tumors). These form part of the extra-adrenal neuroendocrine system. There are two main location-specific types of neck paraganglioma: carotid and vagal paragangliomas. Carotid paragangliomas—also called carotid body glomus tumors—are the most common of the head and neck paragangliomas. They occur at the bifurcation of the CCA and arise from the tissue of the normal carotid body. Vagal paragangliomas are the least common of the head and neck paragangliomas. Paragangliomas are more often observed in women 40–45 years old. They usually appear as solitary lesions, although multiple lesions at multiple sites may be seen in 3–5% of cases. The vast majority of glomus tumors are benign and slow to grow. In rare cases they may become active and secrete catecholamines, which can lead to clinical manifestations similar to pheochromocytoma.

Carotid paragangliomas are found at the site of CCA bifurcation and are tightly connected to the vessels. The tumor is sonographically represented by a large lesion (up to 10 cm) of oval or roundish shape, iso- or hypoechoic homogeneous structure, with accurate regular contours (Fig. 12.4). It shows very limited mobility and appears dense upon compression by the US probe. Because it is part of the neuroendocrine system, this tumor is highly vascularized. A large amount of arterial and venous vessels is rather characteristic. Zhurenkova (2002) reported a high intensity of vascularity of paragangliomas with a prevalence of arterial blood flow of the collateral type with PW Doppler interrogation. CDI and PDI are also necessary in such patients to assess both the anatomical course and hemodynamic changes in proximal and distal parts of the carotid artery. In cases of malignant tumor, metastases in regional lymph nodes are possible.

US permits the differentiation of *malignant pathology of the larynx*. Laryngeal cancer is the most common malignancy of the larynx (50–60%), and one that mainly affects men 40–70 years old. Larynx sarcomas are most often represented by rhabdomyosarcomas, liposarcomas, fibrosarcomas, and angiosarcomas. Carcinosarcomas are rare. Malignant tumors of the larynx show different clinical signs that complicate the differential diagnosis.

They exhibit sonographic features similar to cancers of other neck organs (e.g., the thyroid or salivary glands), and are characterized by lesions in the projections of median structures of the neck with the following features (Fig. 12.5): decreased echodensity, irregular shape, indistinct contours, heterogeneous structure often with echogenic inclusions, immobility, incompressibility, painlessness, and frequent enlargement of regional lymph nodes. Large carcinomas are characterized by disorganized hypervascular patterns in CDI, PDI, and 3DPD. Hypo- and avascularity are seen less often. CT of the larynx is always needed in order to assess the lesion more precisely.

Hodgkin's lymphoma is a type of malignancy originating from lymphocytes. It affects cervical lymph nodes in 60–70% of cases. It commonly arises in combination with abnormal axillary, mediastinal, inguinal, retroperitoneal, or other groups of lymph nodes. The disease is more often observed in males and exhibits two peaks in incidence: at 20–30 years and over 60 years of age.

During the initial stage of the disease, the lymph nodes show the following US picture: enlarged size of 1–3 cm; roundish, oval, or irregular shape; regular or irregular accurate margins; decreased echodensity; frequent heterogeneity of echostructure (Fig. 12.6). CDI, PDI, and 3DPD reveal various types of vascularity. Hypovascularization or hypervascularization with a hypertrophic hilar blood flow pattern is observed. Compression with the US probe demonstrates low mobility, a dense body, and painlessness. Further development of the disease is characterized by conglomerations of lymph nodes of various sizes and densities. The natural course of the disease is characterized by spontaneous remissions and flares. As the disease progresses, new groups of lymph nodes become affected and the disease generalizes. Abnormal lymphatic nodes

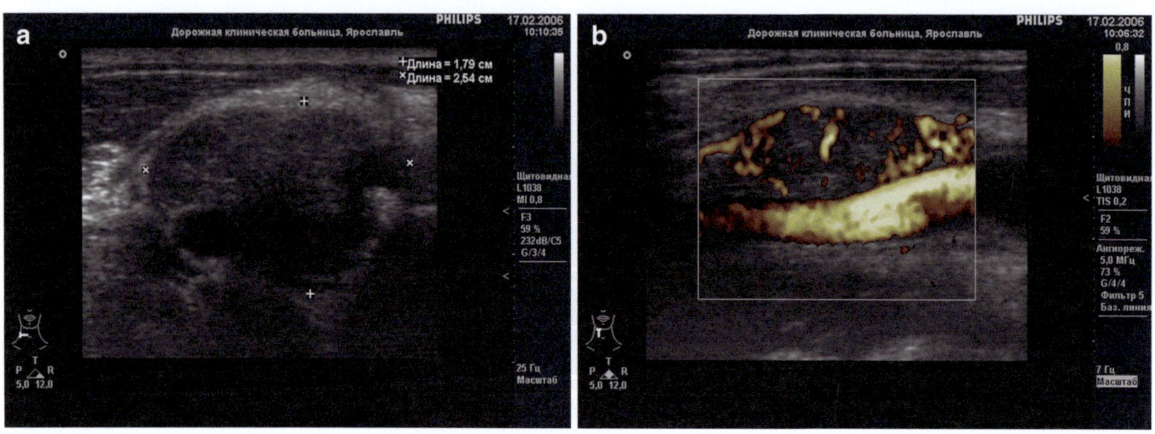

Fig. 12.4 (**a**, **b**) Carotid paraganglioma. Grayscale and PDI

in Hodgkin's disease are differentiated from metastases of thyroid cancer (see Chap. 8) or malignant tumors of other head and neck organs (Fig. 12.7).

Sialadenitis is inflammation of a salivary gland, which may result in the appearance of a neck lesion. Causes range from simple infection to autoimmune etiologies. It is often a consequence of bacterial infection ascending from the oral cavity. It usually arises due to an obstructing stone or gland hyposecretion in people of 50–60 years of age and/or those with immune

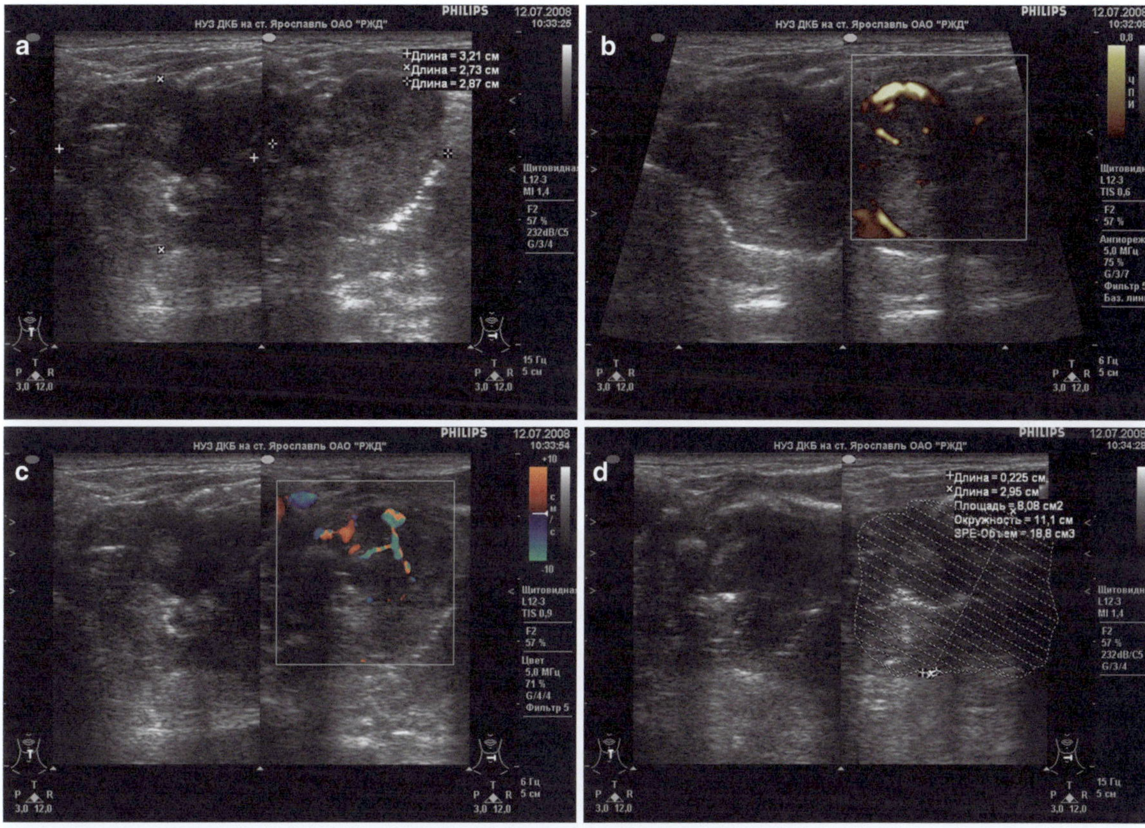

Fig. 12.5 (**a–c**) Laryngeal cancer. (**a**) Grayscale sonography. (**b**) CDI and (**c**) PDI

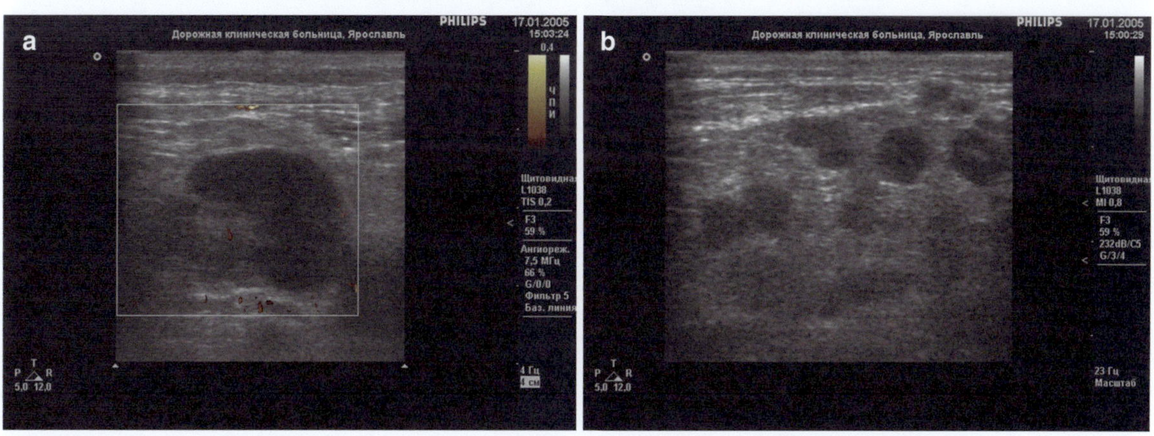

Fig. 12.6 (**a–d**) Enlarged neck lymph nodes in Hodgkin's disease. (**b**) Grayscale. (**c**) CDI and (**a, d**) PDI

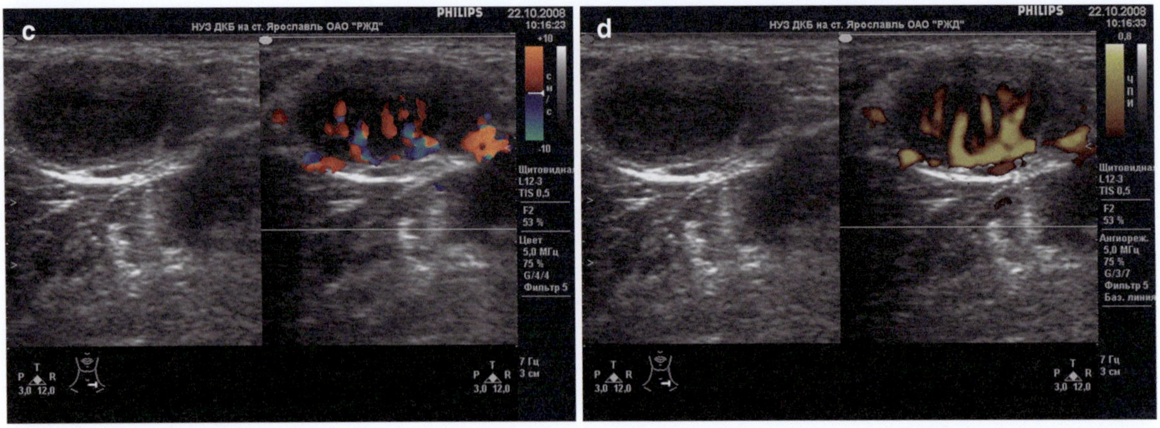

Fig. 12.6 (continued)

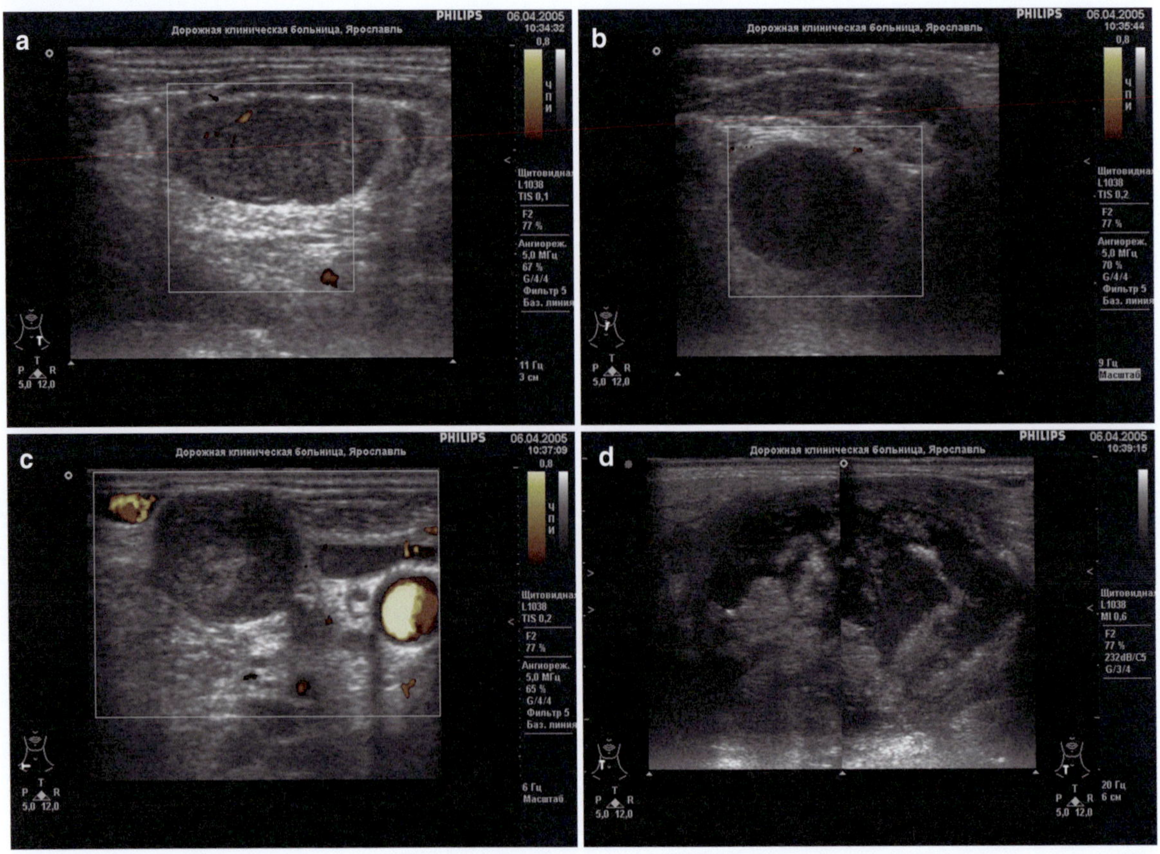

Fig. 12.7 (**a–d**) Metastases of tongue cancer in neck lymph nodes. (**d**) Grayscale. (**a–c**) PDI regimen

deficiency conditions. Inflammatory infiltrates of salivary glands are normally differentiated from tumors.

According to US, salivary glands with inflammation appear enlarged, hypoechoic, and heterogeneous. They may show indistinct contours, irregular borders, and irregular vascularity with hypervascular and hypovascular areas in CDI, PDI, and 3DPD (Fig. 12.8). They are also significantly painful, fixed, dense with compression, and accompanied by inflammatory changes in adjacent soft tissue. Dilated hypo- or

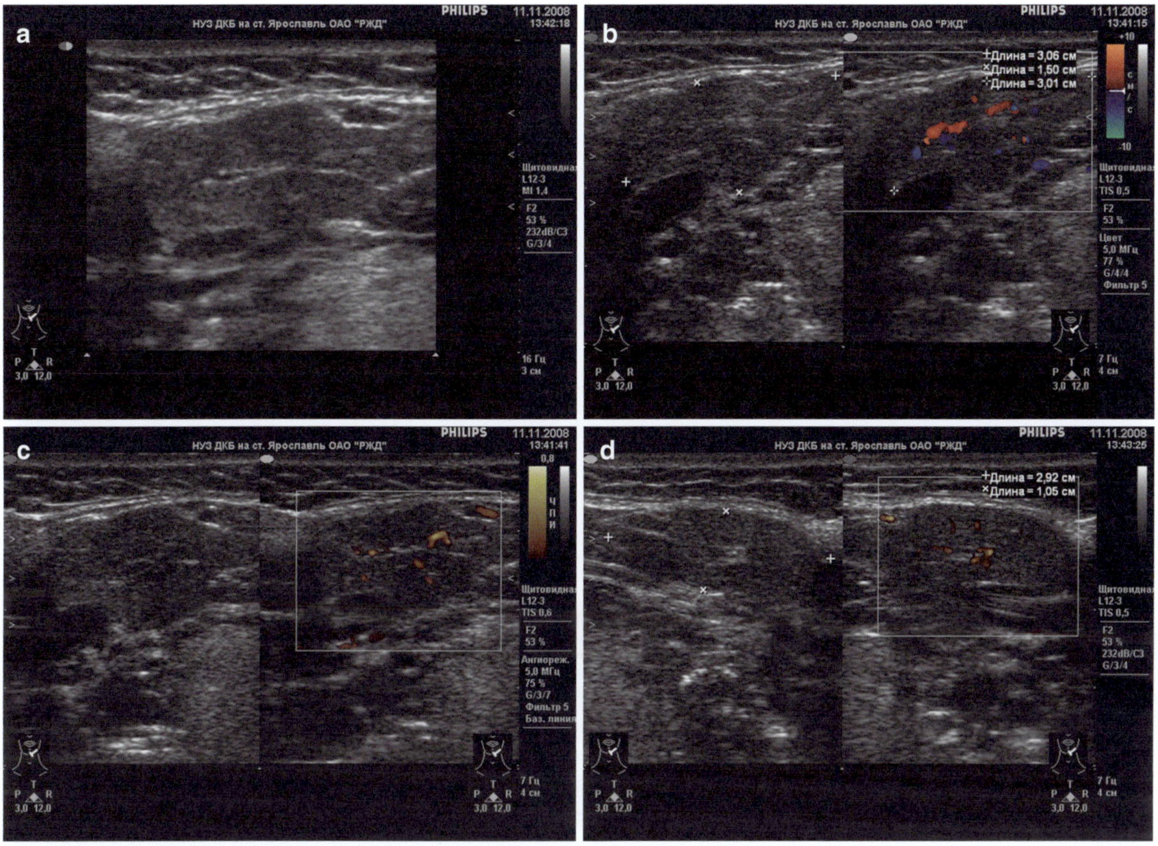

Fig. 12.8 (**a–d**) Acute sialadenitis. (**a**) Grayscale sonogram, (**b**) CDI and (**c, d**) PDI

anechoic salivary ducts are often defined. Acute inflammation may result in an abscess, which exhibits a different sonographic picture depending on the stage. It is most often visualized as a hypo- or anechoic lesion of roundish or irregular shape and heterogeneous structure. The central compartments often contain various amounts of fluid due to tissue destruction. CDI, PDI, and 3DPD reveal a short period of hypervascularization of the solid component during the initial stages with a subsequent decrease in vascularity up to total avascularity. The presence of a capsule depends on the age of the abscess, since it takes time for it to form. US permits the visualization and precise localization of salivary gland stones, irrespective of the degree of mineralization.

Cervical esophageal diverticulum is a rare diagnostic finding with US (Fig. 12.9). Esophageal diverticulum is a diversely shaped evagination of the esophageal wall that is connected with the esophageal lumen. True and false types of diverticula can be distinguished. The walls of the first type contain all of the layers of the normal esophageal wall. The walls of the latter type consist of the mucosa that outpouches through the defect in the muscular layer. Esophageal diverticulum may have a congenital or acquired origin. The latter develop due to the following mechanisms: pulsion (appears with an increase in pressure within the esophagus resulting from a disturbance to its motility or distal stenosis), traction (arises as a result of adhesion between the esophageal wall and the surrounding structures due to an inflammatory process, etc.), and pulsion-traction (mixed). Diverticula may exist in any part of the esophagus and be solitary or multiple.

Esophageal diverticulum is sonographically visualized as a roundish isoechoic or hypoechoic lesion of regular shape with accurate margins and a length of 0.5 to 2–3 cm that is avascular in CDI, PDI, and 3DPD. It contains heterogeneous, mostly hyperechoic, inclusions in the central part that are similar to those of a microcalcification or an arc-shaped calcification, and

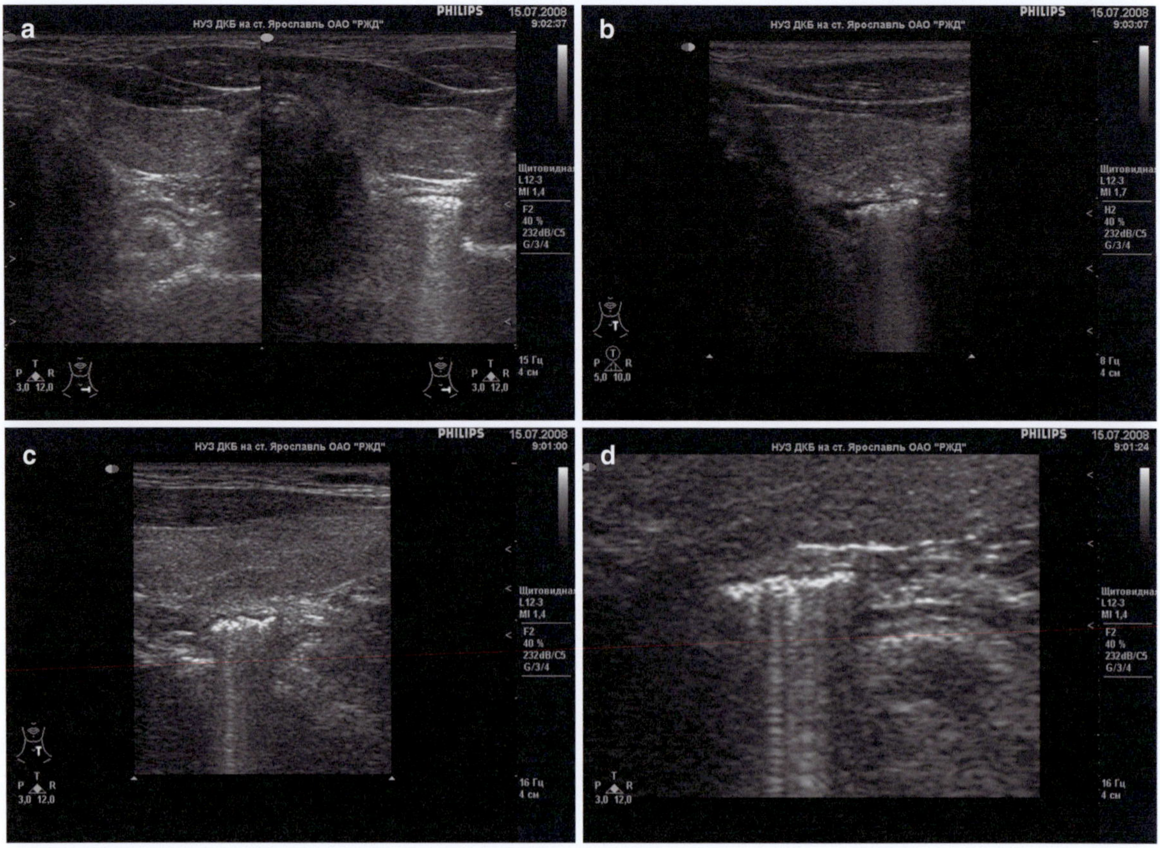

Fig. 12.9 (**a–d**) Cervical esophageal diverticulum. Grayscale sonography

which move and change shape upon swallowing. The lesion may change in size and content depending on the patient's head or body position. The esophageal wall is most often differentiated as a hypoechoic boundary structure up to 2 mm thick that surrounds the lesion. The echodensity and echostructure of the wall may differ from homogeneous and hypoechoic to heterogeneous and mostly hyperechoic depending on the morphological stricture and the type of diverticulum. Careful examination can reveal its connection with the adjacent esophageal wall. Esophageal diverticula can easily be misdiagnosed as thyroid nodules, since they often occur on the posterior portion of the thyroid gland, especially on the left side. Turning the patient's head maximally results in the esophagus changing position. It is normally located close to the dorsal part of the left thyroid lobe. Upon turning the head to the left, the esophagus moves to the right and appears adjacent to the right thyroid lobe. The diverticulum, if not fixed, may change position. Swallowing also helps to distinguish the diverticulum from a thyroid nodule.

The location and spread of *inflammatory processes* in the soft tissues of the neck are defined by the complexity of the anatomy of the neck, with tender fat separated by multiple fascias, muscles, neck internals, and other structures. Sisley (2005) defines the following sonographic stages of inflammation: edema, infiltrate, preabscess, and hypo-, and anechoic abscesses. All of these stages represent the transition of serous inflammation to purulent, resulting in an abscess. They have certain features and can be defined sonographically. Neck inflammation may lead to phlegmons and abscesses at different locations, which imply a high risk of descent into the mediastinum, sepsis, purulent blood vessel destruction with bleeding, development of venous thrombosis, thrombosinusitis, and brain abscess.

US allows the type of inflammation and its stage of development to be specified. The site, volume, structure, margins, relation to blood vessels and surrounding organs should be outlined to follow-up the infiltrate during treatment. Purulent inflammation can be identified precisely, and pus collections can be located to assist the surgery. In the case of osteomyelitis it is sometimes possible to detect marginal destruction, cortical sequesters, and subperiosteal abscesses.

US is a valuable modality among the group of diagnostic visualization procedures for neck lesions. It has a number of advantages. The main ones are undoubtedly availability, harmlessness, high diagnostic value, accuracy in localizing neck structures, easy follow-up, and real-time guidance for minimally invasive modalities.

13 Fine-Needle Aspiration Biopsy

Percutaneous puncture biopsy is now an obligatory modality in thyroid diseases. It can utilize fine needles with inner diameters of up to 1 mm or thick needles with diameters of over 1 mm. In some cases, thyroid biopsy is performed using special needles: trepan biopsy. Boey et al. (1986) and Carson et al. (1996) have demonstrated that this method leads to unreliable results for thyroid cancer due to the difficulties involved in obtaining a specimen at the border between the pathological and normal tissue. Alternatively, Pinsky et al. (1999) have reported that trepan biopsy led to an accurate diagnosis in 86.8% of patients with thyroid lesions.

Fine-needle aspiration biopsy (FNAB) is now the most popular procedure. A number of authors regard it as the main screening method for diagnosing thyroid diseases, and the only preoperative modality for directly assessing morphological tissue changes (Paches et al. 1995; Burch 1995; Alexandrov 1996). Cytological examination permits the differentiation of thyroid diseases in their early stages, when clinical implications are absent.

The indications for US-guided FNAB are as follows:

- Nodules of various sizes and echostructures, in order to specify morphological structure (especially in the first nodules detected, cases that exhibit fast growth, malignant features, significant changes in echostructure, vascularization or other US or clinical features over a short period of time, i.e., 6–12 months)
- Multichamber and complex cysts (especially with a hypervascular solid component)
- Nodules of ectopic or aberrant thyroid
- Substernal goiter
- Recurrent goiter
- Contradictory data from US or other diagnostic methods with clinical implications
- Metastatic neck lymph nodes of unknown origin
- Cytological verification prior to minimally invasive modalities or surgery

Many authors consider that all thyroid nodules should be necessarily biopsied. Palpable nodules are biopsied more often. Nonpalpable nodules that are smaller than 1 cm tend to be followed up. They should be biopsied if malignant US features are present or there is a family history of medullary carcinoma. Sonography permits the detection and biopsy of small, deeply located, nonpalpable lesions at least 3–4 mm in size. In cases with multiple lesions, the question of whether to biopsy each nodule is controversial. Nodules that are over 3.5–4 cm in size should be biopsied at several sites.

Contraindications for FNAB are as follows (Trofimova 1999):

- Severe coagulation system disorders
- Diseases associated with abnormalities of the vascular wall when the risk of the procedure exceeds its diagnostic value
- Flat refusal of the patient to undergo the procedure
- Acute psychiatric disorders

Thyroid puncture may be carried out using the following methods:

1. "Blind" puncture. This is performed without instrumental guidance. The nodule is detected with palpation.
2. With preliminary US marking. This implies that the nodule site has been previously specified by US and that its projection onto the skin of the neck has been indicated.
3. US-guided biopsy. The guidance ensures precise placement of the needle tip within the lesion.

V.P. Kharchenko et al., *Ultrasound Diagnostics of Thyroid Diseases*,
DOI: 10.1007/978-3-642-12387-0_13,

Kratochwil first introduced US guidance for puncture into the medical record in 1969. The utilization of sonography to determine the site for biopsy significantly increases the diagnostic value of thyroid biopsy (Bogin et al. 1990; Takashima et al. 1994; Alexandrov 1996; Gritzmann 2007).

US guidance for FNAB of thyroid lesions confers the following advantages:

- Fast real-time management
- Precise targeting when obtaining the specimen
- It is harmless to the patient and the staff; there is no ionizing radiation involved
- High resolution (although this depends significantly on the quality of the scanner)

The disadvantages of US guidance for thyroid biopsy are as follows:

- Dependence on the class of equipment used
- High dependence on the experience and skill of the operator
- Dependence of the quality of visualization on the individual patient's features (density of tissues, site of the nodule, position and somatic status of the patient, etc.)

The productivity of FNAB is significantly influenced by the skills of the personnel performing the biopsy, the accuracy of needle introduction, the amount of material obtained, the use of the correct smear technique, and the skill of the cytologist. The rate of uninformative biopsies of nodular goiter performed at specialized centers is less than 5–10%. According to Lee et al. (1993), using the method of repeated puncture reduces the rate of uninformative biopsies further, to 4%, increases the accuracy of cytological examination up to 91%, and allows the histological type of the tumor to be defined in 71% of cases. Takashima et al. (1994) report that FNAB without guidance shows a higher incidence of diagnostic mistakes than cases with US guidance (19.5% vs. 0.04%, respectively). According to Alexandrov et al. (1996), the sensitivity of US-guided FNAB is 80.3%, that of FNAB with US marking is 72.1%, and that of "blind" FNAB is 68.5%; the incidence rates for uninformative samples are 0.2%, 4.2%, and 17%, respectively.

US-guided FNAB can be performed by the following techniques:

1. Freehand biopsy is often utilized by specialists with confident puncture skills, especially for large lesions or in the absence of a puncture adapter to mount on the US probe. The advantages of this technique are a high degree of freedom to manipulate the needle and a high level of needle visualization.
2. Utilizing a puncture probe allows the the needle course to be determined prior to the puncture. However, the needle is often poorly visualized during the procedure, course correction is limited, and special needles are required.
3. Mounting a puncture adapter on the US probe allows precise needle course determination and good visualization of the needle, but limits the needle's mobility due to its rigid construction. The number of biopsies is limited by the package of sterile instruments.

US guidance of FNAB of thyroid nodules is performed with linear 7.5–15 MHz probes. A team of two specialists (the sonographer and surgeon/endocrinologist) is preferable (Fig. 13.1).

Special preparation of the patient for the procedure is not required. The patient is positioned supine with a cushion under the shoulders and the head hyperextended. Local anesthesia is usually not necessary, since the pain of injection is comparable to that of biopsy. Additionally, the administration of anesthetic can lead to deterioration in the US visualization of the target region and change the quality of the smear. The US probe is positioned on the neck in the most convenient way. The path of the needle to the target lesion is determined. The probe is covered and prepped with an antiseptic. The skin of the neck is carefully cleaned with an antiseptic; a sterile coupling gel is utilized.

The biopsy is carried out under aseptic conditions with a disposable 5–10 mL syringe and a 21G needle,

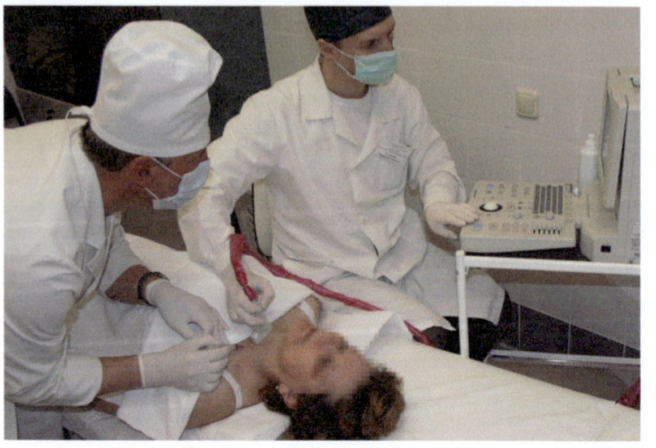

Fig. 13.1 FNAB. Freehand technique

and generally takes only a few minutes to perform. The motion of the needle in the lesion is registered on the screen of the US scanner. The needle may be introduced from the lateral side of the US probe or directly over the nodule (midway along the probe's length). This corresponds to an echogenic point in a transverse scan or an echogenic line in a longitudinal scan, which changes position in accordance with the motion of the needle (Fig. 13.2).

The needle is introduced into the target lesion. Samples for cytological examination are aspirated from at least three areas within the lesion. When the nodule has heterogeneous echostructure, the samples should be obtained from the most suspicious areas in the center and periphery of the lesion. The solid component of the cyst must also be biopsied.

The material obtained is spread across a glass slide, smeared (Fig. 13.3), and delivered to a cytological laboratory for analysis. The site of puncture is compressed with a sterile dressing for 15 min to prevent hemorrhage.

The sensitivity of FNAB for thyroid cancer is 70–98%, its specificity is 70–100%, its accuracy is 87–92%, its rate of false-positive results is up to 20%, and its rate of false-negative results is 2–15% (Burch 1995; Alexandrov 1996). Valdina (1996) reports that cytological and histological conclusions match in 78.2–83% of cases. According to Shulutko et al. (2004), the sensitivities of FNAB for thyroid goiter, adenoma, and carcinoma are about 87.1, 92.9, and 69.7%, respectively.

Giuffrida et al. (1995) suggested that FNAB could be used to specify the origins of enlarged neck lymph nodes (true-positive results were obtained in 96%, true-negative in 99% of cases). The most reliable FNAB data are obtained for lymph nodes larger than 1.5 cm in size (Nakhjavari et al. 1997).

The incidence of complications depends on how experienced the experts who carry out the biopsy are, the concurrence of their actions, how closely the correct technique is followed during the procedure, the equipment utilized, and other aspects. According to different

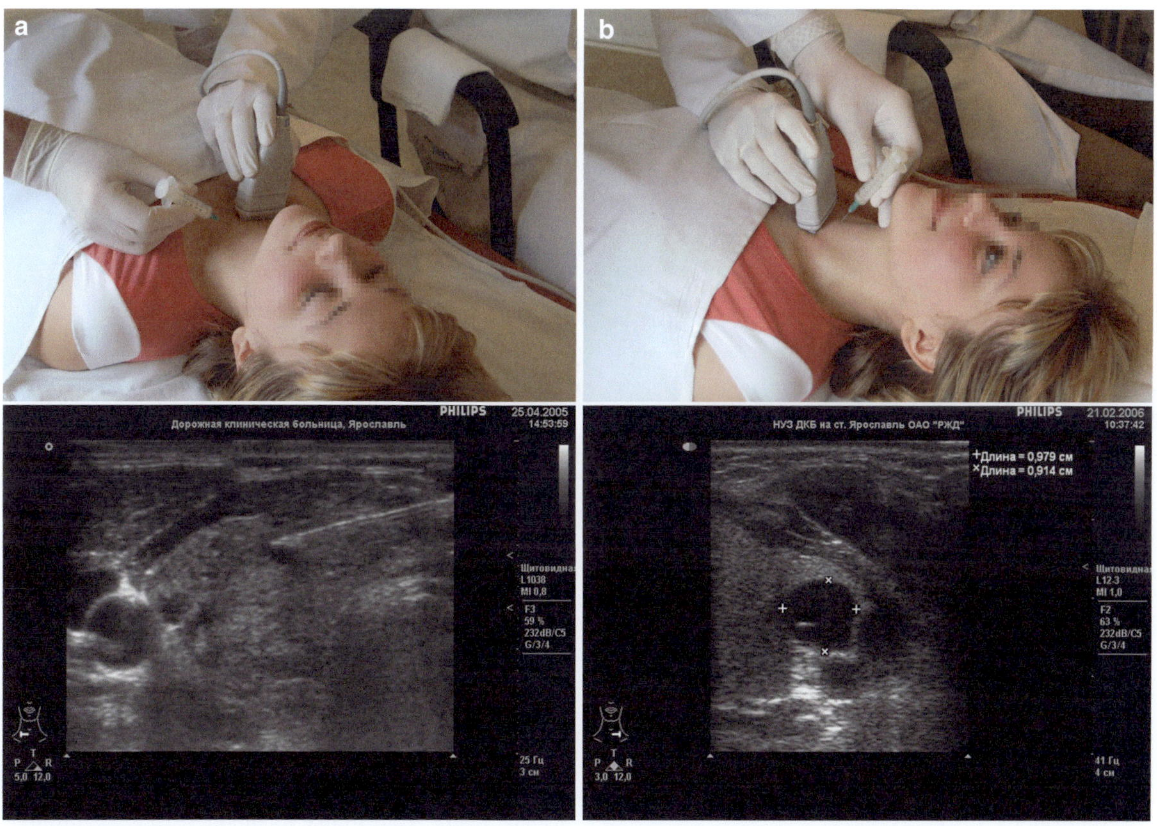

Fig. 13.2 (**a**, **b**) FNAB. Needle visualization

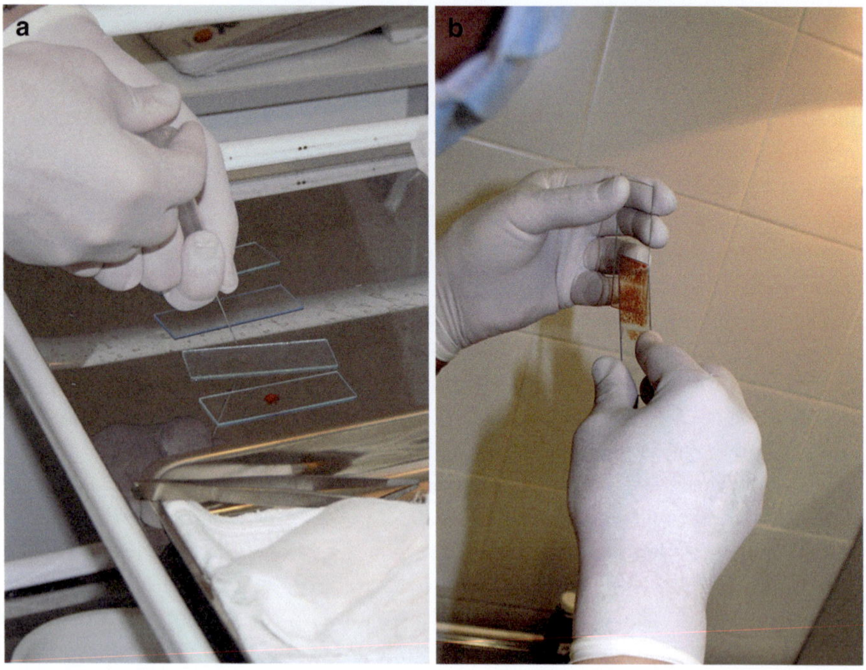

Fig. 13.3 (**a**, **b**) FNAB. The obtained sample on the glass slide

Table 13.1 Side-effects and complications of FNAB

Side-effects and complications	References	Incidence	Own data ($n=760$)
Cervical pain	Trofimova et al. (1999)	18 of 32	7%
Dysphonia	–	–	0.65%
Hemorrhage into the nodule or cyst	–	–	0.65%
Puncture of large nervous trunks	Bubnov et al. (2002)	Registered	0.5%
Hemorrhage from subcutaneous veins, subcutaneous hematomas	Trofimova et al. (1999)	14 of 32	0.25%
Large vessel injury with hematomas	Angelini et al. (1996) Pashchevsky (2004)	Registered 4 of 2010	Not registered
Puncture of the trachea	Bubnov et al. (2002)	Registered	Not registered
Puncture of the esophagus	Sun et al. (2002)	Registered	Not registered
Subendothelial carotid hematoma	Anastasilakis et al. (2008)	Registered	0.05%
Tumor implantation along the puncture channel	Weisinger (1993)	Registered	Not registered

authors, complications can develop in 1–12% of patients (Brom Ferral et al. 1993; Alexandrov et al. 1996–2005; Privalov et al. 2001) (Table 13.1).

Side-effects and complications may be divided into local (pain, local inflammation, paresis or paralysis of the recurrent nerve, etc.) and general (discomfort, fever, hormonal disorders, etc.).

The early occurrence of pain at the site of puncture may be a consequence of local tissue damage or hematoma. Its intensity depends on the severity of the damage.

Local hemorrhagic complications, such as subcapsular, interfascial, intermuscular or subcutaneous hematomas, result from injury to blood vessels at different

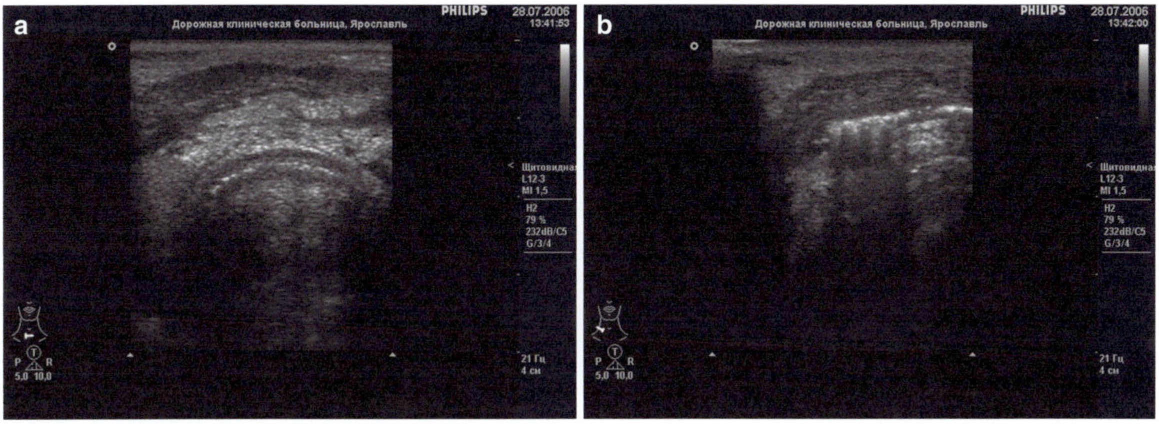

Fig. 13.4 (**a**, **b**) FNAB complication. Interfascial hematoma

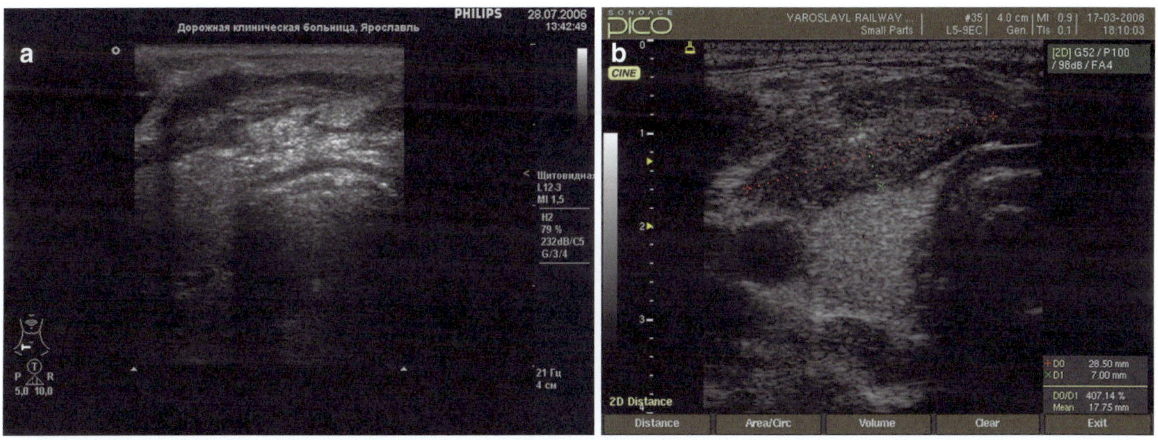

Fig. 13.5 (**a**, **b**) FNAB complication. Interfascial and subcapsular hematomas

locations, including subcutaneous veins (Figs. 13.4 and 13.5). They may also arise with hypervascular lesion puncture, and with some diffuse thyroid diseases associated with thyroid parenchyma hypervascularity (AITD or Graves' disease).

Subcapsular hematoma is accompanied by the enlargement of the thyroid lobe and is sonographically represented by a hypoechoic avascular area under the thyroid capsule with irregular margins. It does not change shape with compression. The patient sustains increasing pain in the region of puncture. The hematoma, as a rule, disappears within a period of 2–5 days.

Interfascial and intermuscular hematomas may be detected as relatively homogeneous hypoechoic structures that cover the anterior and lateral thyroid surfaces, spreading along interfascial spaces. The shape of such a hematoma changes with compression. The enlargement of the hematoma can be seen as an increase in its thickness between the surface of the thyroid and the neck muscles. These hematomas are normally a relatively small size, expand downwards, and do not enlarge after the puncture is ceased. Nevertheless, the occurrence of a hematoma demands an US follow-up and certain measures to prevent its enlargement. Interfascial hematomas are sometimes accompanied by a bruise in the suprasternal fossa or on the anterior surface of the neck within 2–3 days of the procedure. This quickly resolves and is sonographically unidentifiable after a few more (5–7) days.

In some cases, usually in nodules with prevalent fluid components and cysts, the hemorrhage can affect not the surrounding tissues but the cystic lumen (Fig. 13.6). After aspirating the contents, the cystic lumen is filled to primary volume with blood, and in some cases enlargement is possible. US reveals heterogeneous masses with hypoechoic and echogenic inclusions within the nodule. The heterogeneity increases for a few days and the echostructure shows a cellular pattern with echogenic structures of various shapes along the inner surface. CDI and PDI demonstrate the avascularity of the lesion. Such a hemorrhage may develop full or partial lysis with sonographic features of a cyst or organization resulting in a heterogeneous hypoechoic nodule with echogenic inclusions and calcifications. These nodules can later be penetrated by blood vessels, so the nodule vascularity may correspond to a true thyroid nodule.

The puncture of large venous or arterial vessels may occur if the path of the needle passes close to these structures. A blood vessel is evidently punctured if the syringe is filled with blood at aspiration. US images the needle as an echogenic point or a line within the vessel lumen. Injuries to large arteries, including the carotids, can lead to a hematoma in the vascular wall with stenosis. This is sonographically observed as a hypoechoic crescent-shaped lesion with eccentric wall thickening and protrusion of endothelium into the lumen. Hematomas outside of arteries are rare (Fig. 13.7). Injuries to large veins are also seldom accompanied by hematomas, although they increase the risk of thrombosis (Fig. 13.8).

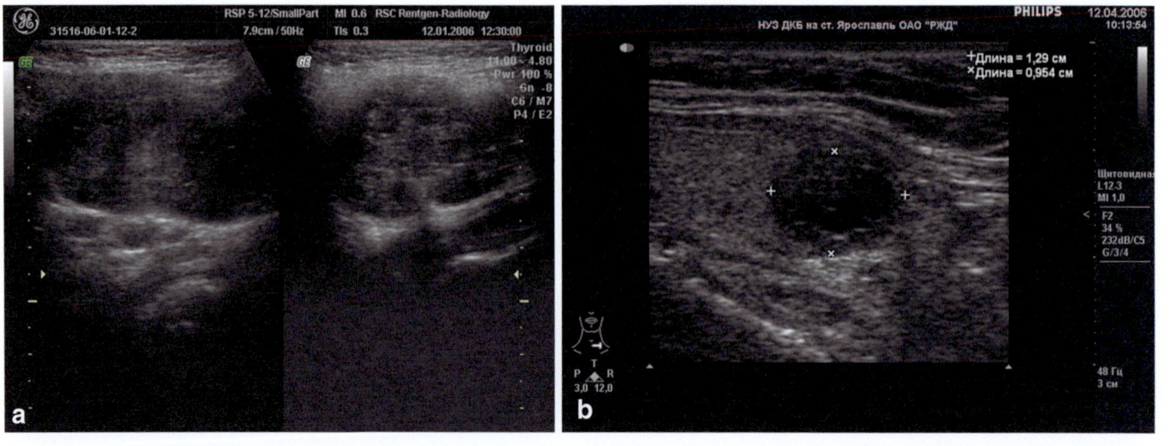

Fig. 13.6 (**a**, **b**) FNAB complication. Hemorrhage into cystic lumen

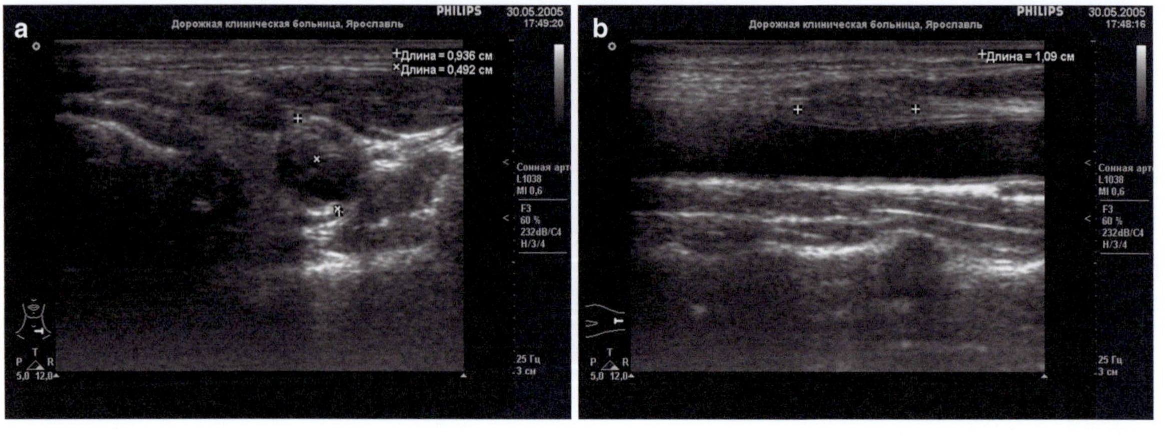

Fig. 13.7 (**a**, **b**) FNAB complication. Hematoma within CCA wall

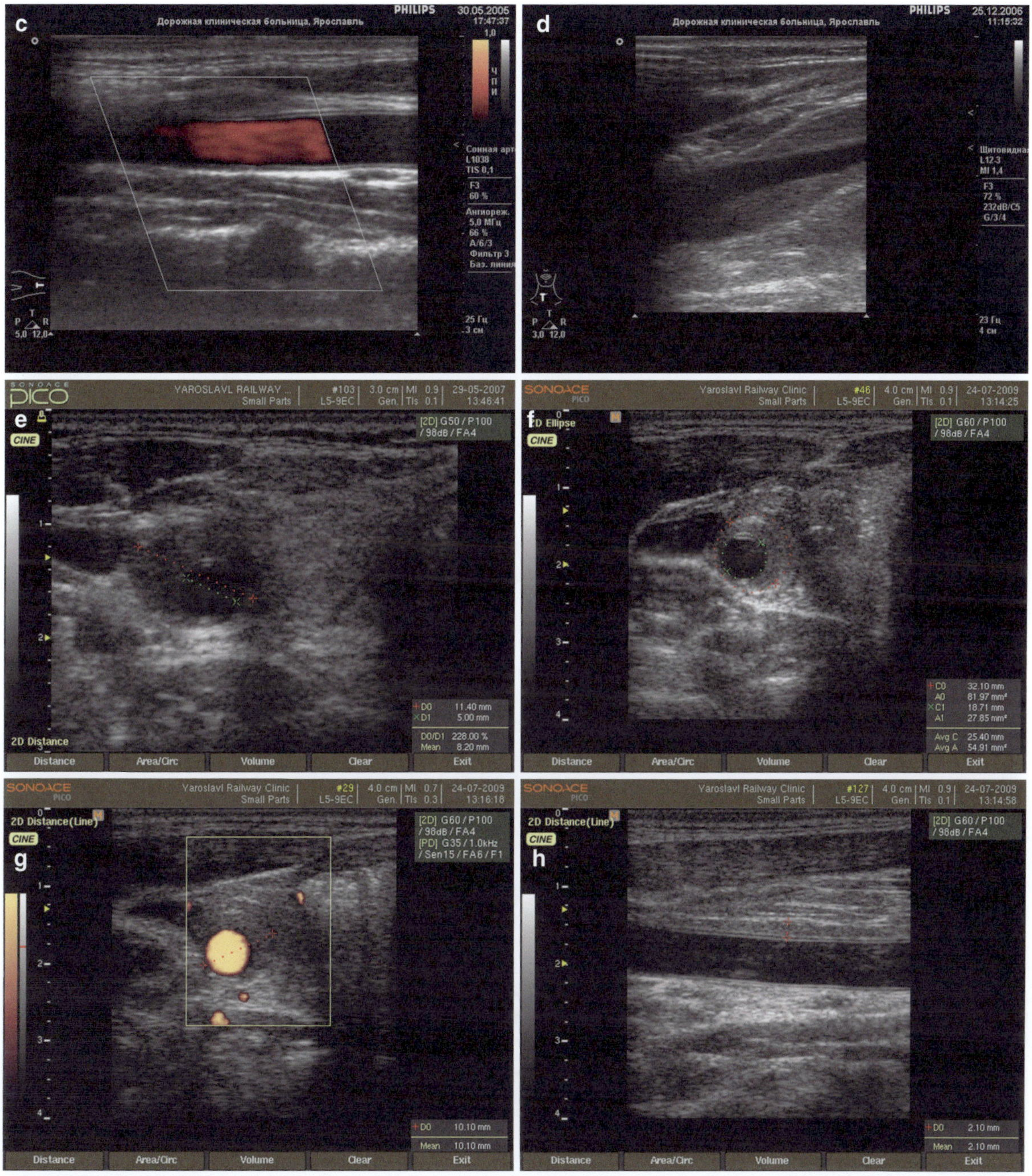

Fig. 13.7 (continued)

A rare complication of FNAB is the puncture of large nerves, including the elements of the cervical plexus. Such a nerve injury is followed by severe pain in the corresponding half of the neck, shoulder joint, or the upper extremity. Damage to the superior or inferior (recurrent) laryngeal nerves results into corresponding neurologic symptoms, such as hoarse voice (recurrent nerve), fast fatigue during loud speech, and choking, especially with liquids (superior laryngeal nerve).

Paratracheal nodule puncture may be complicated by the puncture of the trachea in cases with inaccurate US visualization of the needle tip. This causes an

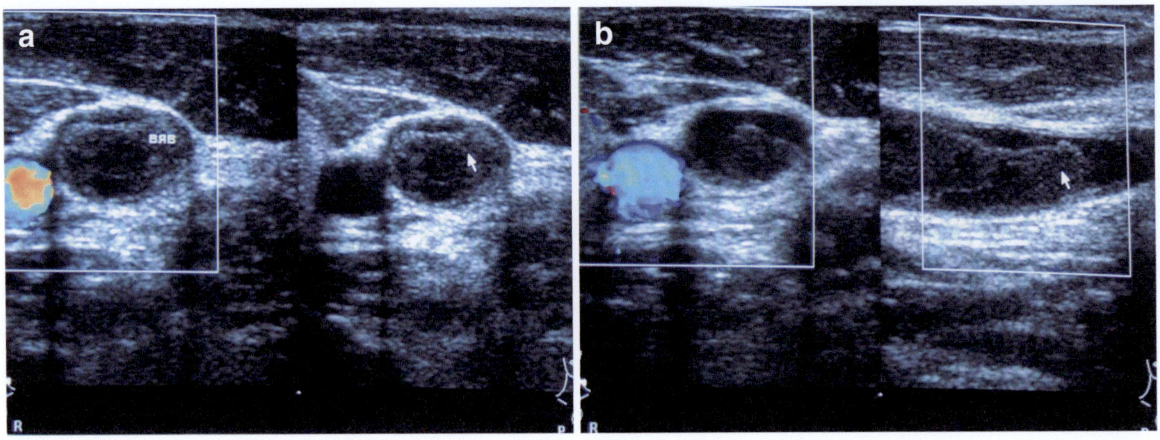

Fig. 13.8 (**a**, **b**) FNAB complication. Left internal jugular vein thrombosis

instant dry, hoarse cough for 1–5 min. Insignificant subcutaneous emphysema is sometimes possible. This does not require any special therapy.

The probability of puncture of the esophagus largely depends on the experience of the US specialist. A roundish (oval) lesion seen in the dorsal aspect of the left thyroid lobe with a transverse scan can be misinterpreted as a nodule. Therefore, such a lesion should be considered with special care; assessment in several planes is necessary.

Complications resulting from improper asepsis (inflammatory infiltrates, abscesses) are quite rare.

After FNAB, the patient does not normally require US follow-up.

The efficacy of cytological diagnosis is defined by the skills of four experts: the surgeon performing the FNAB; the US specialist, who provides accurate visualization; the laboratorian staining the smears; and the pathologist.

The example of US report of FNAB of a thyroid lesion:

First name, middle initial, last name:
Age:
Date:
In aseptic conditions fine needle aspiration biopsy of the 2.9x3.1x3.2 cm (volume 14.4cm^3) heterogeneous avascular nodule with fluid collections in the inferior compartment of the right lobe of the thyroid gland was performed under US guidance with a 21G needle and free hand technique.
Visualization during the procedure was satisfactory.
The received sample from 3 nodule areas (central, posterior, and anterior) is sent to the cytology department.
The patient tolerated the procedure satisfactory, somatic status without changes. Compression with aseptic bandage was applied to the puncture site for 10 minutes.
The surgeon (endocrinologist):
The US specialist:

14 Diagnostic Algorithms in Thyroid Pathology

New diagnostic modalities and the individual advantages of each method of radiology lead to the problem of selecting which to use in diagnostic algorithms. The methods chosen should not repeat each other, and they should supply all of the required data. Modern complex diagnostics does not imply the obligatory use of all accessible methods. For each individual case, the specialist defines the sequence of diagnostic procedures that permits the maximum useful information to be obtained with the minimum effort and expense.

We use the diagnostic algorithms shown in Figs. 14.1 and 14.2 in our daily work to define the thyroid pathology.

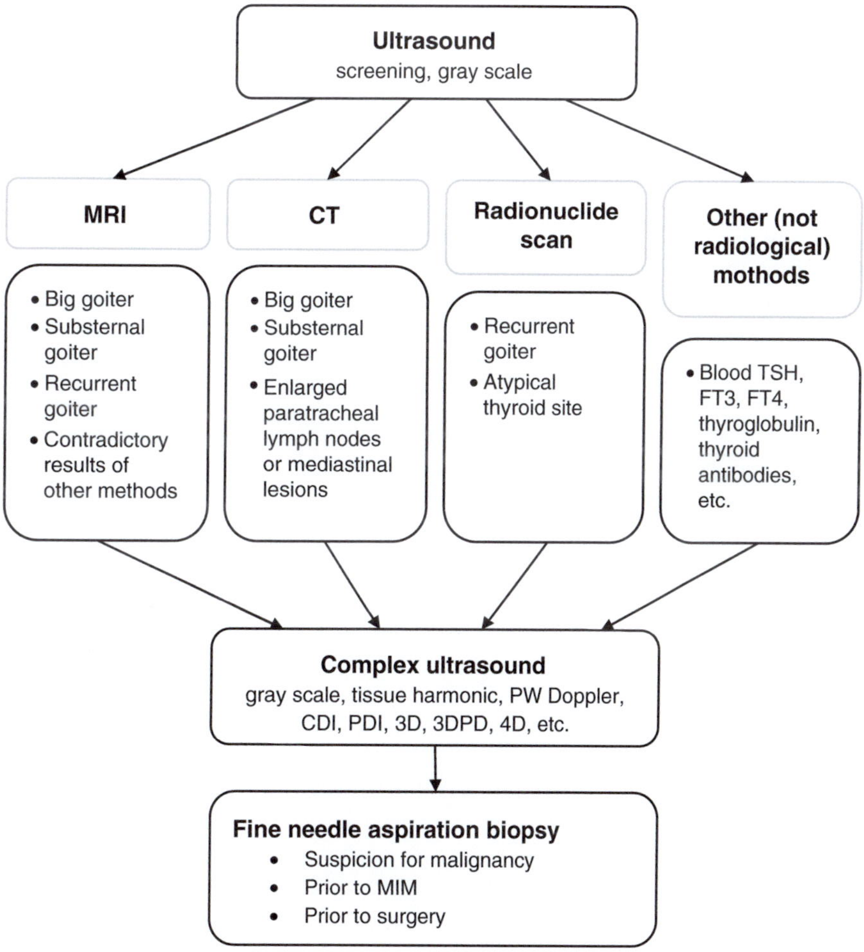

Fig. 14.1 Radiological methods for diagnosing thyroid pathologies

V.P. Kharchenko et al., *Ultrasound Diagnostics of Thyroid Diseases*,
DOI: 10.1007/978-3-642-12387-0_14, © Springer-Verlag Berlin Heidelberg 2010

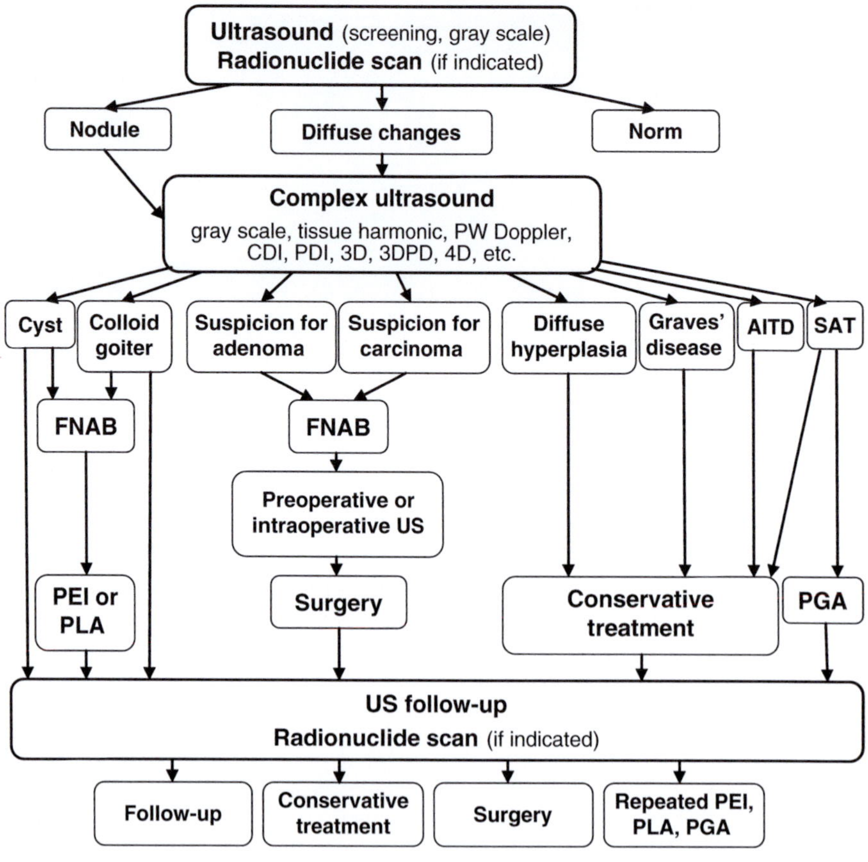

Fig. 14.2 Algorithm of the use of radiological methods and interventions in thyroid diseases

A wide range of diagnostic procedures for the pathology of the thyroid gland are now available. US has a specific role in modern diagnostics. The diagnostic value of sonography is constantly increasing due to rapid advances in the equipment used and new diagnostic options. US guidance is of undoubted importance for MIM in thyroid lesions. The complex application of US in most cases permits the correct diagnosis to be made and the appropriate treatment to be administered.

Applications of US are blossoming due to the rapid development that this field is undergoing, the prospect of new discoveries, and the gradual perfection of current US equipment. The full potential of US is not yet known, but it is clear that it can still make a significant contribution to improving the diagnostic value of medical visualization.

15 Ultrasound Aspects of Minimally Invasive Procedures on the Thyroid Gland

Interventional ultrasound is still a young discipline, yet rapid advances mean that it has already acquired an important position within various fields of medicine, including surgical endocrinology. It has considerably expanded the possibilities of radiological methods with respect to both diagnosis and treatment. Ultrasound assistance is an essential component of minimally invasive procedures (MIPs) on the thyroid gland. It provides important preliminary information, enables estimation of the procedure course, is predictive of early and late complications, and permits subsequent follow-up. Having said that, it must also be acknowledged that many aspects of the use of MIPs in the treatment of thyroid diseases (including the role of ultrasound) will require further study if general acceptance by radiologists, surgeons, and endocrinologists is to be achieved.

The use of MIPs in the treatment of thyroid diseases is advantageous because such procedures cause minimal damage to surrounding tissue, avoid the need for local or general anesthesia, reduce the frequency and severity of side-effects and complications (thus shortening hospital stay), reduce the cost of treatment, and facilitate rehabilitation. Often there is no alternative to MIPs, as they can be performed in seriously ill patients who represent an extremely high operative risk.

The primary aims of using ultrasound during MIPs on the thyroid are as follows:

Before the MIP:

- Enable preliminary conclusions about the lesion structure and vascularization, its localization, and the state of adjacent tissue and organs
- Permit selection of the appropriate MIP for that particular patient, with this decision being reached in cooperation with the endocrine surgeon (or endocrinologist)
- Define the optimal needle path to a focal lesion
- Assess the probability and nature of potential side-effects and complications during and after the MIP

During the MIP:

- Guide the introduction of the needle into the nodule (the lesion locus) in accordance with the previously chosen optimal path
- Visualize and confirm the needle end positioning (and the optical fiber tip in the case of percutaneous laser ablation) within the target structure (the region of interest)
- Continuously monitor the condition of the structures surrounding the target region
- Permit dynamic supervision of the procedure, with registration of efficiency criteria
- Define side-effects and complications

After the MIP:

- Assess the procedure efficiency in the target region
- Assess the condition of surrounding organs and tissues
- Reveal early (up to 30 min) and delayed (3–4 weeks) complications
- Analyze the nodule echostructure and vascularity in the early (3–4 weeks) and later (more than one month) post-MIP periods, and define changes in US characteristics

US guidance for MIPs is much more effective than guidance by other radiology methods. It is comparatively cheap, widely available, safe for the patient and personnel, and works in real time. The use of CDI and PDI allows characterization of lesion vascularization and easy differentiation of pathological liquid collections from vascular structures, thereby preventing serious complications.

V.P. Kharchenko et al., *Ultrasound Diagnostics of Thyroid Diseases*,
DOI: 10.1007/978-3-642-12387-0_15, © Springer-Verlag Berlin Heidelberg 2010

Sonographically guided MIPs are much better tolerated by patients, are accompanied by fewer complications, and can be easily repeated if necessary.

15.1 US-Guided Percutaneous Glucocorticoid Administration

One method of treating subacute thyroiditis (granulomatous, nonsuppurative, de Quervain's) is percutaneous glucocorticoid administration (PGA) into the thyroid gland under US guidance (e.g., Depo Medrol (methylprednisolone acetate), injectable suspension, in three strengths: 20, 40, or 80 mg/mL).

PGA can be used when the traditional treatment of SAT is contraindicated, in order to achieve a reduction in the dose of peroral glucocorticoid during the stage of clinical recovery. As monotherapy, it can be used in patients with slight thyroid enlargement and an ESR no greater than 25 mm/h.

PGA is preceded by standard clinical examination with obligatory thyroid US. The latter is carried out by a qualified expert using high-quality equipment to define how acute the process is, the predominant location, and the possibility of and need for the PGA procedure.

The PGA procedure is carried out in the surgical dressing room or a specially equipped room with an US scanner. The patient lies on his back with a bolster under the shoulders and with the head thrown back (standard position for thyroid US and MIPs). Special preparation of the patient and general or local anesthesia are not required. After positioning the US probe in the most convenient way, the site of injection and needle path are outlined (Fig. 15.1).

The puncture is carried out in aseptic conditions with a disposable 5–10 mL syringe and a standard needle for intramuscular injections (22–21G × 1.1/2"). The needle motion in the lesion can be observed on the screen of the US scanner, and the introduction of the needle can easily be corrected (in terms of path and depth) if necessary. The principal conditions for successful PGA are confident definition of the target region, accuracy of needle introduction, reliable visualization of the needle throughout the procedure, and correct choice of preparation quantity to be administered. The drug is injected into those regions which have the greatest density and morbidity at palpation, and the maximum decrease in echodensity and blood flow on color Doppler or power Doppler imaging.

The criterion for the accuracy of needle end positioning in the target locus is the appearance of a hyperechoic point in the region of maximum decrease in echodensity at cross-section scanning or a hyperechoic line at longitudinal scanning, which changes position in accordance with the needle motion (Fig. 15.2).

As the injection starts, multiple small echogenic signals appear around the needle tip. Those signals form a heterogeneous area of increased echodensity with blurred irregular margins (Fig. 15.3). The thyroid capsule limits their diffusion, so some amount of the introduced drug can be registered under the capsule, thus increasing its thickness and echodensity. When the drug is injected completely the needle is withdrawn.

It is recommended that the site of puncture should be compressed with a sterile dressing within 10–15 min after the procedure to prevent hemorrhage.

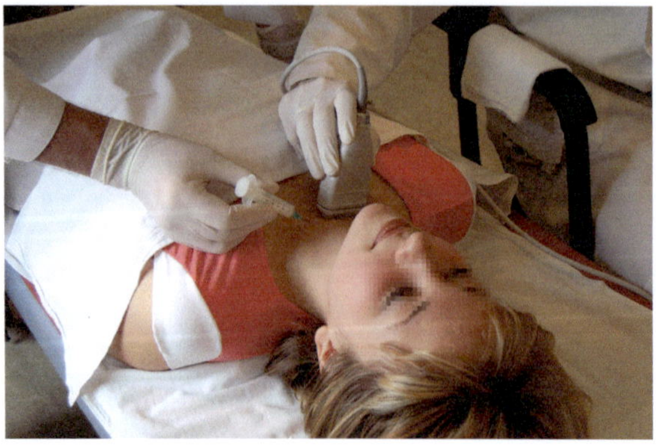

Fig. 15.1 PGA procedure

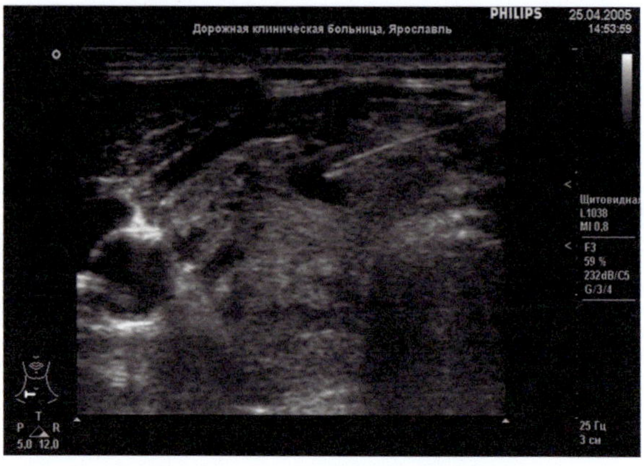

Fig. 15.2 PGA. The needle end in the target region

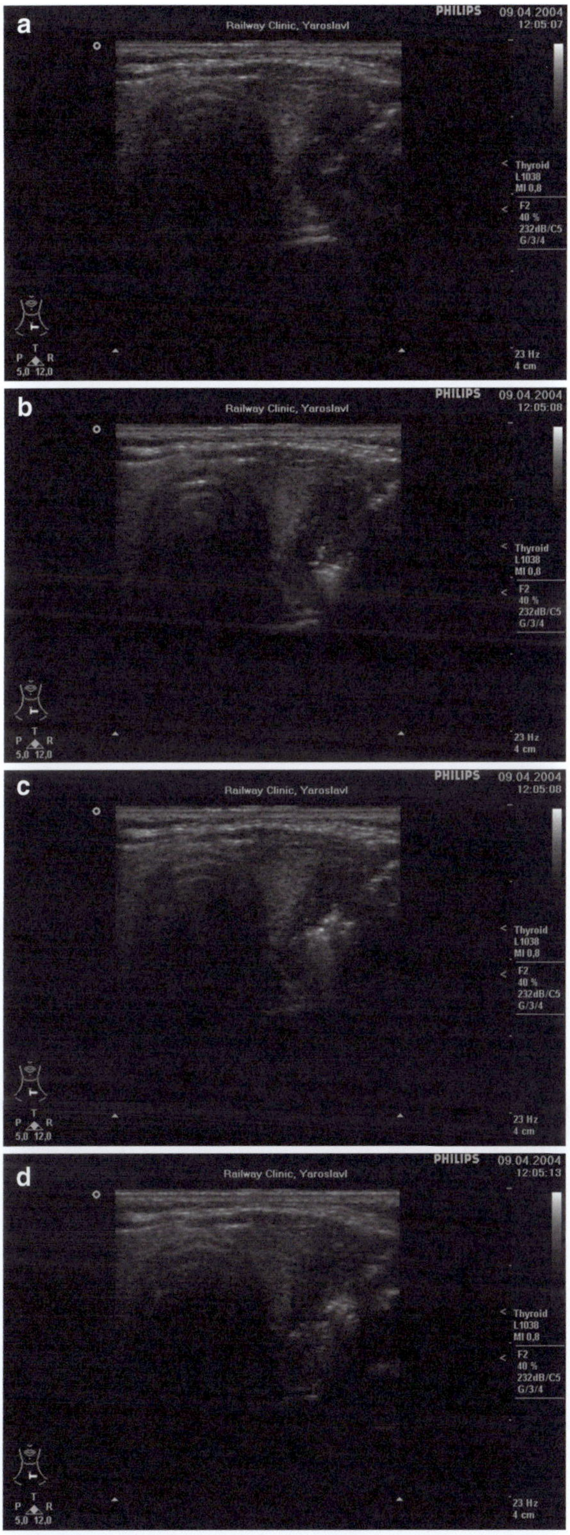

Fig. 15.3 (**a–d**) PGA. Drug introduction

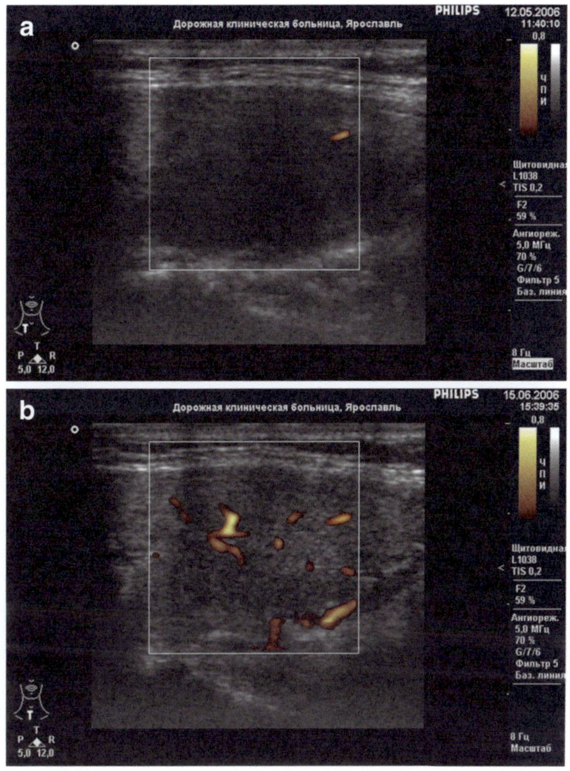

Fig. 15.4 (**a–b**) Change in echostructure and vascularity of SAT locus one month after PGA

US criteria for positive dynamics of SAT after PGA are as follows (Fig. 15.4):

- Reduction in thyroid volume
- Reduction in the size of hypoechoic lesions, their fragmentation, and an increase in echodensity
- Restoration of grainy structure
- Change in margins from indistinct and irregular to well defined and regular
- Recovery of vascularity within the lesion to the normal pattern
- Reduction of cervical lymphadenitis

PGA may be repeated in 1–3 days. There can be up to 5–6 procedures performed sequentially if necessary. More than 5–6 injections are worrisome for the risk of fibrous changes in the thyroid lobe.

Improvement is sonographically observed in 63% of cases after PGA (Fig. 15.5). No change or a

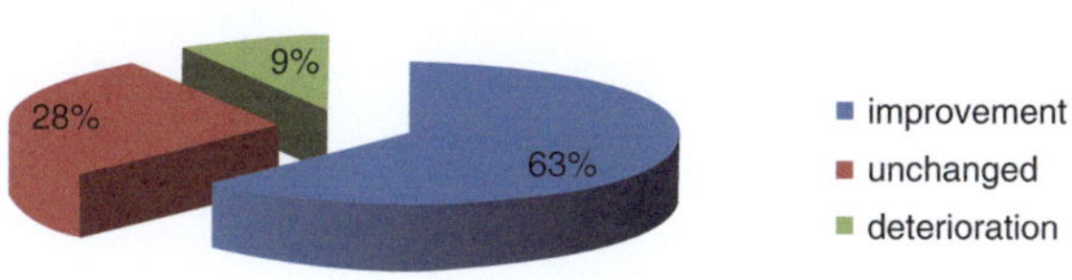

Fig. 15.5 Efficacy of PGA in subacute thyroiditis

Example of US report at PGA:

First name, middle initial, last name:
Age:
Date:
In aseptic conditions under US guidance with free hand method a 21G needle was introduced into the 19x18x15 mm homogenous avascular hypoechoic locus with irregular shape, indistinct margins, dense, moderately painful at compression in the inferior segment of the right lobe of the thyroid gland (proved subacute thyroiditis). 1 ml of "Depo Medrol" suspension for injections (40mg/ml) was introduced into the locus. Visualization during the procedure was satisfactory. The patient tolerated the procedure satisfactory, somatic condition without changes. Aseptic bandage was applied to the puncture site with compression within 10 minutes. The next visit is recommended in 3 days.
The surgeon (endocrinologist):
The US specialist:

deterioration of the US image after six sessions of PGA are detected in 28% and 9%, respectively.

15.2 Percutaneous Ethanol Injections

Percutaneous ethanol injections (PEI) in thyroid nodules are now widely utilized (Monzani et al. 1994; Barsukov 2000; Martino and Bogassi et al. 2000; Seliverstov 2003; Alexandrov et al. 2005).

US-guided PEI has several advantages:

- High efficacy
- Minimal damage of the thyroid gland and surrounding structures of the neck
- Low risk of complications
- Technical simplicity and use for outpatients
- Good tolerance by patients of any age

Indications for PEI are as follows:

- Solitary thin-walled thyroid cysts larger than 10 mm
- Cystic nodules big nodules with compression of neck organs in elderly and seriously ill patients in order to reduce the lesion volume
- Recurrence of euthyroid nodular goiter in cases with postoperative complications
- Autonomous nodules and toxic adenomas
- In some cases where the nodules cause a cosmetic defect

Contraindications for PEI are as follows:

- Epilepsy, mental instability of the patient
- Coagulopathies
- Hodgkin's disease
- Acute respiratory diseases
- SAT
- High blood pressure (160–180 mmHg and higher)

PEI is most effective in predominantly fluid nodules smaller than 10 mm and larger than 30 mm (Fig. 15.6). Use of PEI is limited in multichamber cysts, multiple small cysts, or isoechoic nodules larger than 30 mm. The method cannot be recommended in 10–30 mm isoechoic nodules and nodules with calcification and fibrosis. It is thought that ethanol should only be introduced into the nodules with a distinct capsule (halo). Otherwise alcohol can escape out of the nodule and damage intact surrounding thyroid tissue. Special attention should be paid when PEI is performed in the nodules located in the dorsal compartments of the thyroid lobes, considering the neighboring location of nerves, vascular structures, trachea, and esophagus (Fig. 15.7).

A qualified thyroid US on a high-quality scanner and a US-guided FNAB should be performed to exclude malignancy prior to PEI. An US scanner with CDI and PDI modes, equipped with 7.5–12 MHz linear transducer, is used for PEI and follow-up. Special preparation of the patient is not required. The patient is supine with a bolster under the shoulders and the head thrown back (Fig. 15.8).

Depending on the nodule site in one of the lobes of the thyroid gland, the patient's head might be turned to the opposite side. Use of local anesthesia is usually not required, so the patient can take an active part in the procedure and his/her sensations can supply additional information about ethanol diffusion. Moreover, local anesthesia can deteriorate the visualization quality due to superficial microbubbles of gas in the target lesion. The patient is asked to remain still, not to talk, and not to swallow.

US-guided PEI is performed in the following stages:

- The nodule puncture
- Fluid aspiration
  - Genuine cysts: full aspiration.

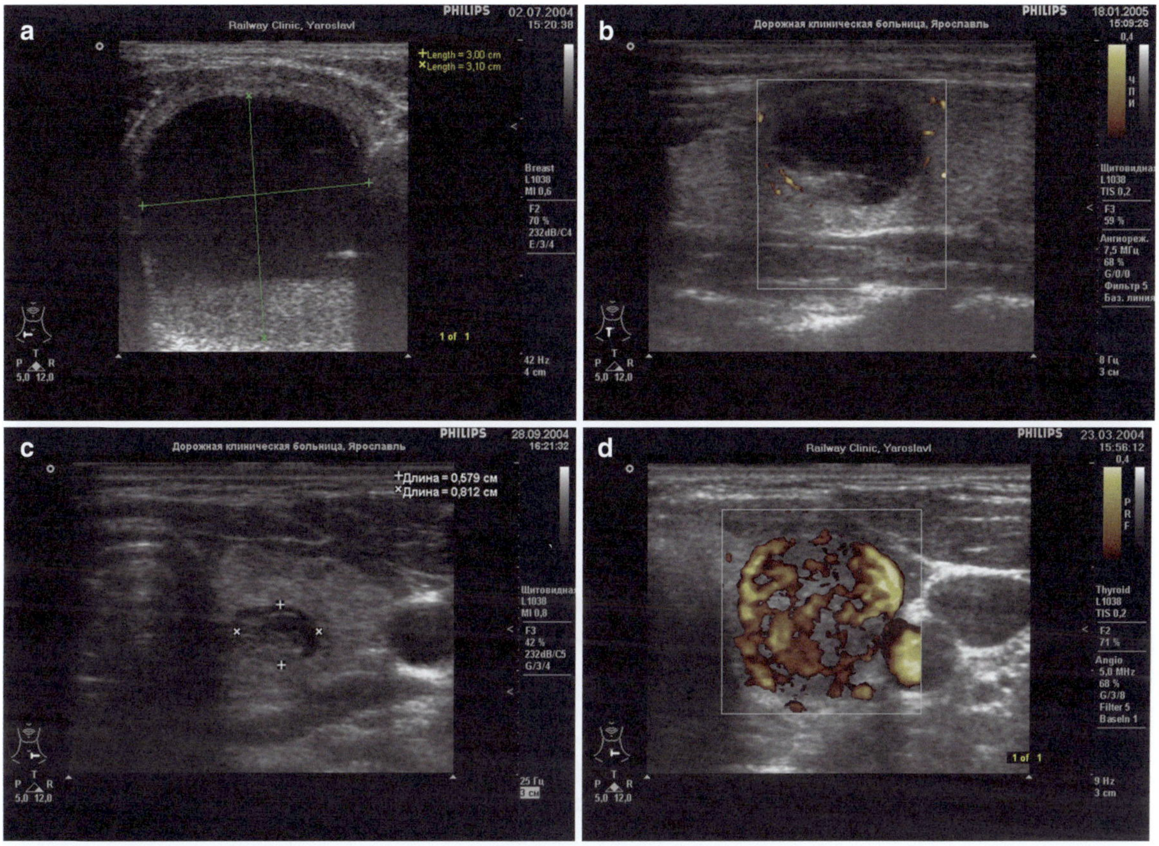

Fig. 15.6 Nodules subjected to PEI. (**a**) Genuine solitary (thin-walled) cysts; (**b**) cystic nodules with predominance of fluid collections; (**c**) recurrent euthyroid nodular goiter; (**d**) toxic adenoma

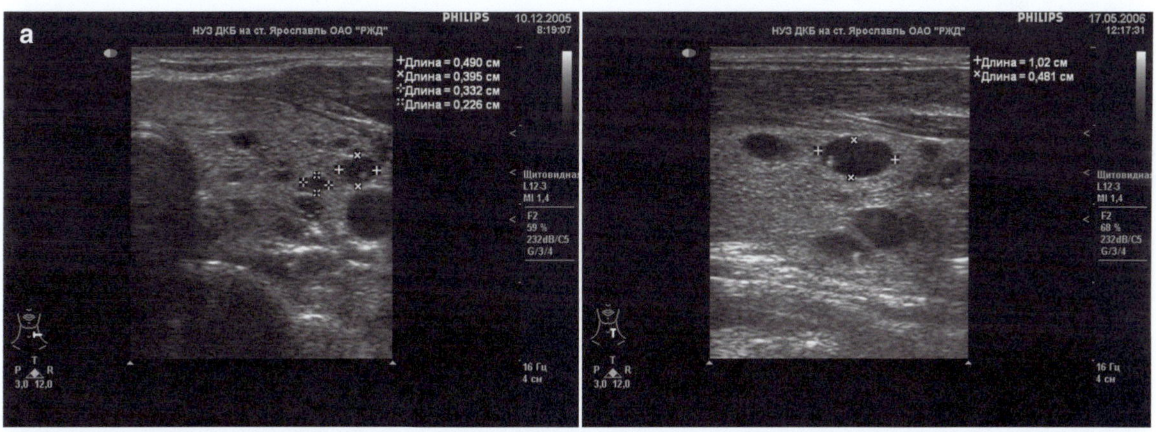

Fig. 15.7 (**a–e**) Nodules not subjected to PEI. (**a**) Multiple small cysts; (**b**) multichamber cystic lesions; (**c**) isoechoic nodules larger than 30 mm; (**d**) paravasal location of the nodule; (**e**) subcapsular location of the nodule

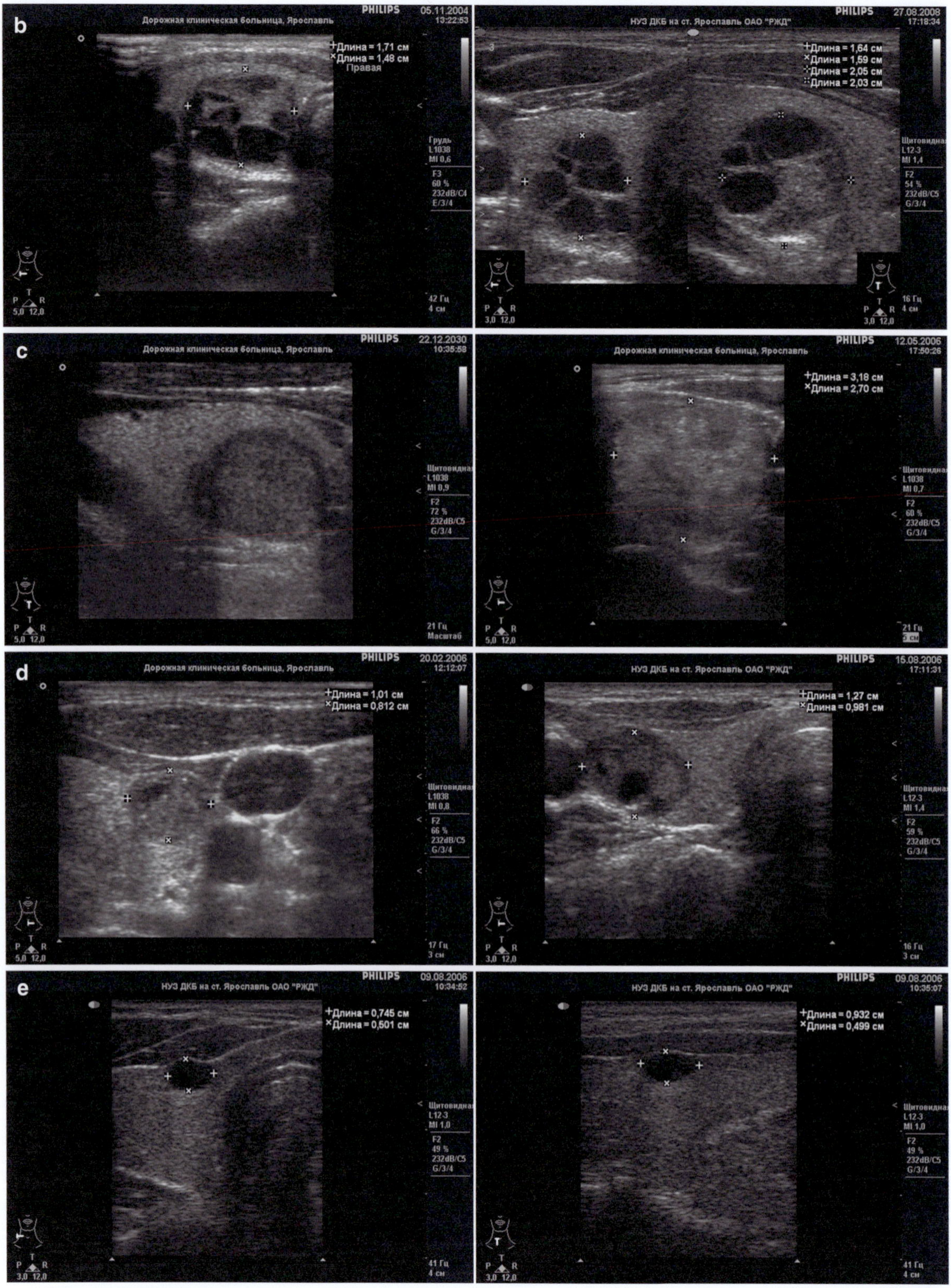

Fig. 15.7 (continued)

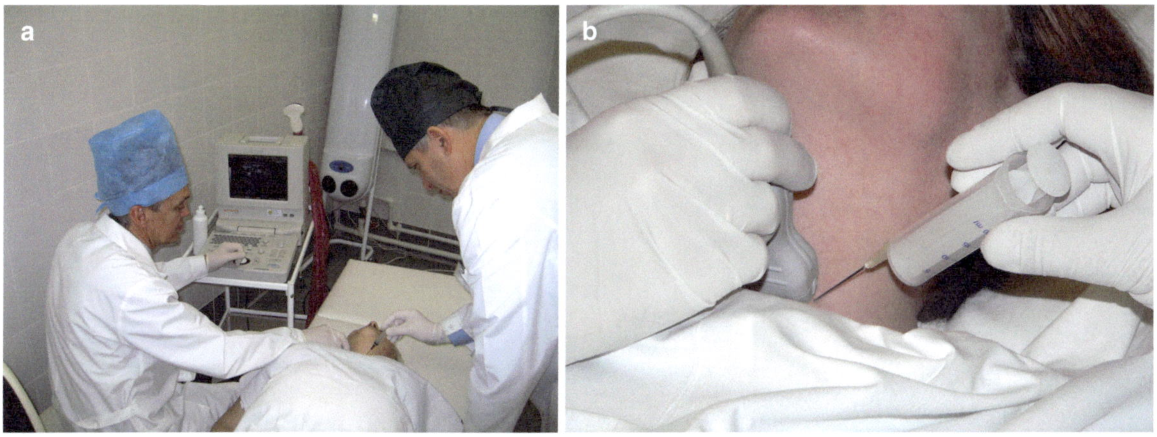

Fig. 15.8 (**a**, **b**) PEI. Position of the patient and medical staff

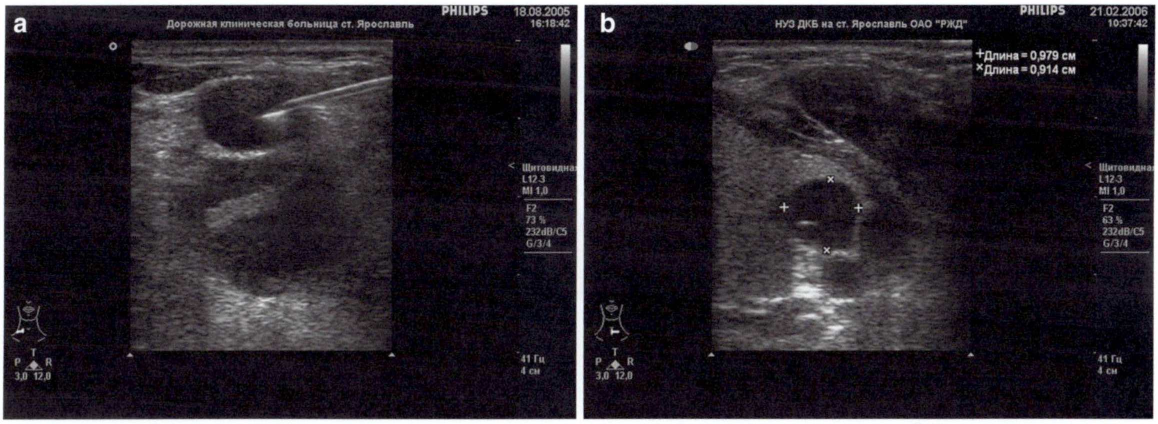

Fig. 15.9 (**a**, **b**) PEI. Needle end in a cyst

- – Complex cysts: fluid evacuation from all chambers, one after another.
- – Isoechoic nodules: attempt at aspiration fails. The needle is fixed in the location of increased vascularity.
- Assessment of the aspirate, determining the amount of ethanol to be introduced
- Ethanol injection
- Exposure
- Reaspiration
- Follow-up

After the US survey, the site of puncture and the needle course are outlined. The probe is covered and prepped with an antiseptic. The neck skin is carefully cleansed with an antiseptic; sterile coupling gel is utilized. The puncture is carried out under aseptic conditions with a disposable 3–5 mL syringe and a 22–21G needle. The needle motion in the nodule is observed on the screen of the US scanner. Depending on the US probe orientation, this corresponds with a hyperechoic point or a hyperechoic line, which changes its position in accordance with the needle motion (Fig. 15.9). The needle path can easily be corrected if necessary.

The fluid is aspirated completely from the cystic nodules. In some cases this leads to the disappearance of the nodule on the screen (Fig. 15.10). In solid nodules, the needle is targeted to the area with maximum vascularity.

The volume and the character of the obtained fluid are estimated after the aspiration. The ethanol volume to be introduced into the nodule is determined individually, depending on nodule size and echostructure.

Ninety-six percent ethanol is normally used. The volume of ethanol to be injected is usually up to 50–70% of the aspirated fluid. The injection is observed ultrasonically. Slow alcohol injection leads to the enlargement of the corresponding cyst. Its cavity is filled with turbulently moving signals with various

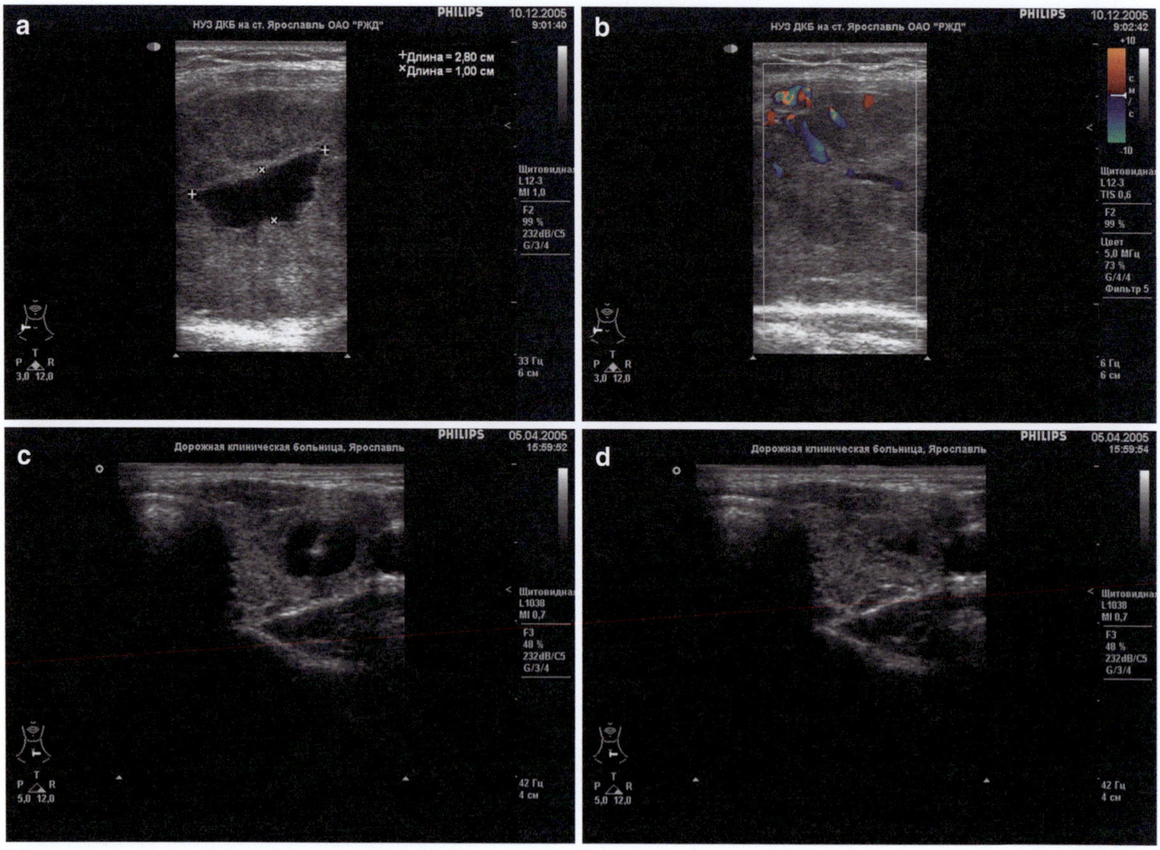

Fig. 15.10 (**a–d**) PEI. Aspiration of cystic nodule

echodensities (Fig. 15.11). The hyperechoic particles (air bubbles, turbulent fluid motion with suspension and coagulated albuminous units) quickly change the echodensity of the lesion. Intranodular ethanol injection does not markedly affect the echodensity and echostructure of surrounding tissue. In cases with solid nodules, CDI and PDI register a quick vascularity decrease with completely avascular regions corresponding to blood stasis, local small vessel thrombosis, and coagulative necrosis.

As a rule, ethanol exposure in cystic nodules should last for at least 30 s, although some authors recommend longer exposure, from a few minutes to 24 h. After that, the ethanol is reaspirated. Reaspiration of ethanol from the cystic nodules normally does not present any difficulty, but it is usually impossible to reaspirate ethanol from solid nodules. After reaspiration the needle is withdrawn. The place of puncture is compressed with a sterile dressing for 15 min.

The US follow-up after the procedure should define the size, echostructure, margins, and vascularization of the nodule, and the state of the surrounding structures (Table 15.1). It makes sense to perform US in 10–15 min, and 3, 6, 12 months after PEI.

US criteria for PEI efficacy in nodular goiter are as follows:

- Reduction in nodule size
- Change in its echostructure
- Irregular blurred margins
- A decrease in vascularity in CDI and PDI in solid nodules

Zubeev and Konovalov (2004) define five outcomes of treatment of thyroid cysts by PEI:

- Cyst enlargement
- Without significant changes (±5% of initial volume)
- Reduction in volume by 6–30%
- Reduction in volume by 31–75%
- Full cyst regression to a scar

According to Pashchevsky (2004), successful PEI in thyroid nodules is characterized by a reduction in nodule size of 2–3 times with replacement by connective tissue within six months.

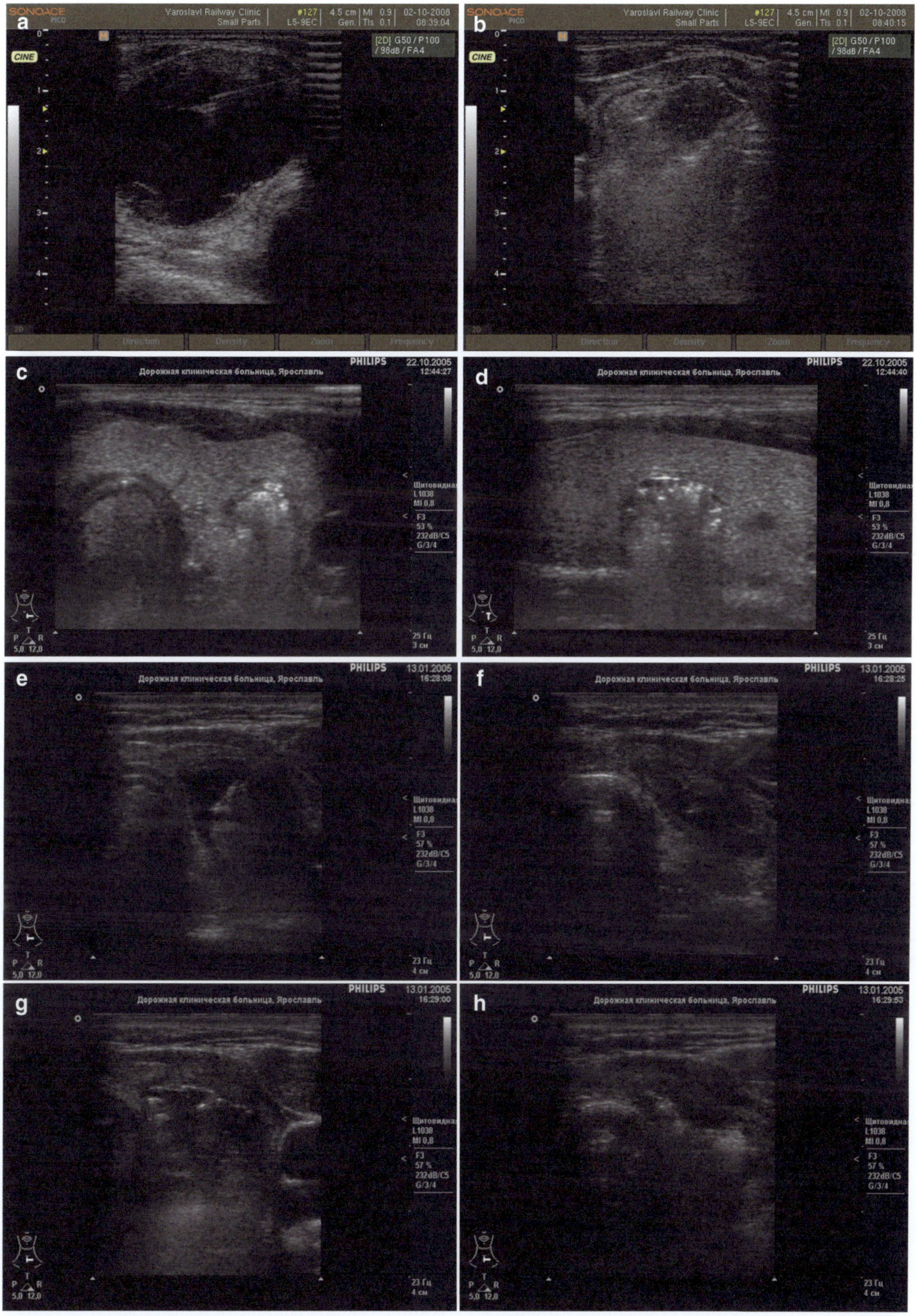

Fig. 15.11 (**a–h**) PEI. Fluid aspiration, ethanol injection, and reaspiration

Table 15.1 Changes in US features of lesions after PEI ($n = 145$), M ± sd%

US features	Before PEI	After 1 month	After 6 months	After 12 months	Reliability of differences			
					p_{0-1}	p_{0-6}	p_{0-12}	p_{1-12}
Average maximum lesion size (mm)	26.36 ± 1.8							
Character of changes in the dimensions:								
Unchanged	–	84.2 ± 3.0	77.3 ± 3.5	68.3 ± 3.9				
Reduction	–	10.3 ± 2.5	10.3 ± 2.5	11.0 ± 2.6				
Enlargement	–	4.8 ± 1.8	8.3 ± 2.3	11.0 ± 2.6				+
Scar	–	0.7 ± 0.7	4.1 ± 1.6	9.65 ± 2.5				+
								+
Shape:								
Oval	67 ± 3.9	57.2 ± 4.1	55.2 ± 4.1	53.7 ± 4.1		+	+	
Spherical	24.1 ± 3.6	20 ± 3.3	17.9 ± 3.2	24.8 ± 3.6				
Irregular	8.9 ± 2.4	22.8 ± 3.5	26.9 ± 3.7	21.5 ± 3.4	+	+	+	
Margins:								
Smooth	91.7 ± 2.3	6.9 ± 2.1	30.3 ± 3.8	48.2 ± 4.1	+	+	+	+
Rough	8.3 ± 2.3	93.1 ± 2.1	69.7 ± 3.8	51.8 ± 4.1	+	+	+	+
Contours:								
Well defined	97.9 ± 1.2	6.2 ± 2.0	28.2 ± 3.7	77.2 ± 3.5	+	+	+	+
Indistinct (or locally indistinct)	2.1 ± 1.2	93.8 ± 2.0	71.2 ± 3.7	22.8 ± 3.5	+	+	+	+
Echodensity:								
Hyper-	6.2 ± 2.0	0.7 ± 0.7	4.1 ± 1.6	10.3 ± 2.5				+
Iso-	9.0 ± 2.4	4.8 ± 1.8	4.1 ± 1.6	4.1 ± 1.6				
Hypo-	31.0 ± 3.8	24.1 ± 3.6	31.0 ± 3.8	35.2 ± 4.0				+
An-	51.7 ± 4.1	70.4 ± 3.8	60.8 ± 4.1	50.4 ± 4.2	+			+
Echostructure:								
Homogeneous	37.9 ± 4.0	17.9 ± 3.2	17.9 ± 3.2	15.2 ± 3.0	+			
Heterogeneous	62.1 ± 4.0	82.1 ± 3.2	82.1 ± 3.2	84.8 ± 3.0				
Calcifications:								
Present	–	–	–	2.9 ± 1.4			+	+
Absent	100	100	100	97.1 ± 1.4			+	+
Fluid collections:								
Present	95.9 ± 1.6	95.9 ± 1.6	95.9 ± 1.6	90.4 ± 2.4			+	+
Absent	4.1 ± 1.6	4.1 ± 1.6	4.1 ± 1.6	9.6 ± 2.4			+	+
Vascularity:								
Hypervascular (including solid component)	10.3 ± 2.5	2.1 ± 1.2	4.1 ± 1.6	5.5 ± 1.9	+	+		
Hypovascular (including solid component)	30.4 ± 3.8	11.7 ± 2.7	15.2 ± 3.0	17.2 ± 3.2	+	+	+	
Avascular	59. ± 4.1	86.2 ± 2.9	80.7 ± 3.3	77.3 ± 3.5	+	+	+	+

+, differences significant at $p < 0.05$

The results of recurrent euthyroid nodular goiter treatment are assessed as follows:

- Positive effect: disappearance of the nodule or its reduction by 50% or more of the initial volume
- Satisfactory effect: reduction by 25–50% of the initial volume
- Unsatisfactory effect: reduction by less than 25% of the initial volume

PEI allows 6.9% of benign thyroid nodules to be cured completely, and achieves a positive result (a reduction in nodule volume by 50% or more) in 80.1% of cases (Fig. 15.12).

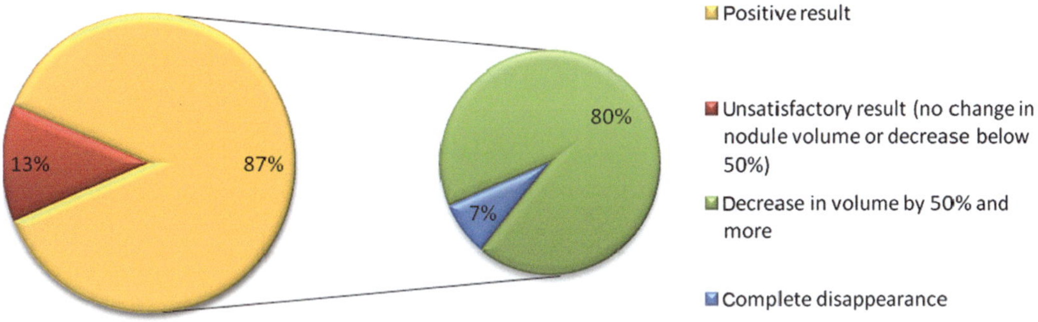

Fig. 15.12 Efficacy of PEI in benign thyroid nodules

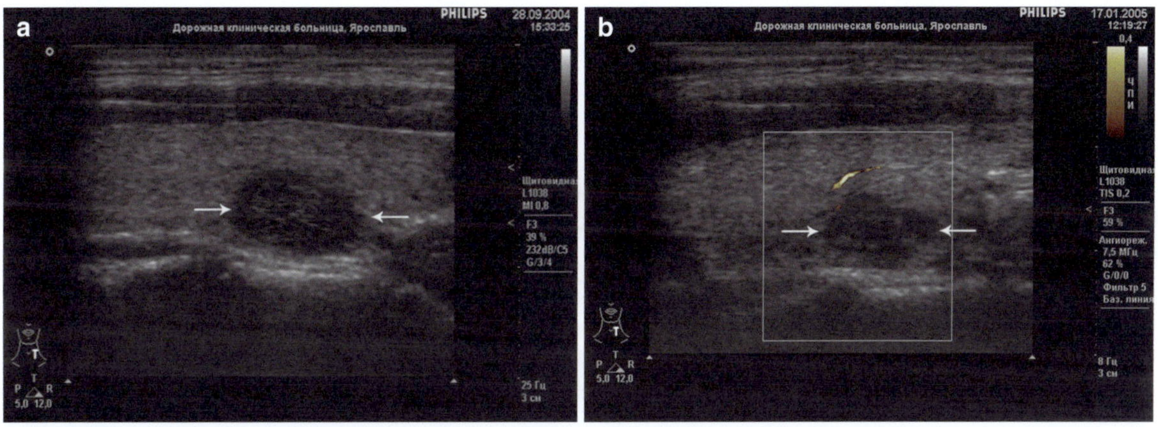

Fig. 15.13 (**a**, **b**) Status after PEI. Change in nodule margins

Post-PEI changes in the size of a nodule may vary from fast regression to progressive enlargement. The outcome mainly depends on the local inflammatory reaction and nodule vascularity. It can be expected that the more pronounced the changes that occur immediately post-PEI, the faster the subsequent dynamics.

Indistinct contours usually reflect a tissue inflammatory process. One to two months after PEI, the nodules are usually hypoechoic with indistinct irregular margins (Fig. 15.13). These signs predict subsequent nodule involution.

Positive dynamics at three months after PEI were observed in 81.6% of cases when the volume of the original nodule was less than 1 mL, in 95.5% when the volume was 1–3 mL, and in 80.9% when the volume was more than 3 mL. Uryvchikov (2004) demonstrated that PEI was efficacious in 88.6% of patients; among them, it was efficacious in 91.3% with nodules smaller than 10 mm and 83.3% with nodules larger than 10 mm. Chu et al. (2003) considered PEI to be effective in cases where the cyst disappeared or its volume reduced to less than 0.5 mL. Treatment was considered unsuccessful if the effect was not achieved with five injections. Antonelli (1994) and Alberti (1994) note that the positive effect of MIP should only be discussed if in cases with complete absence of the lesion (cyst or nodule) or a reduction in its volume by more than 50% within twelve months of the procedure (Fig. 15.14).

Three months after US-guided PEI, the average volume of cystic nodules was 28.7%, isoechoic nodules 58%, and hypoechoic nodules 43%, in comparison with the initial data (Fig. 15.15). Small calcified foci may be detected within the nodules within three years of PEI.

The application of CDI and PDI provides extra opportunities to define the efficacy of PEI in solid nodules. Vascularity changes in all cases of successful treatment. It may either precede or accompany the reduction in nodule size. Soon after PEI (3–7 days after), the regions of aseptic necrosis within the nodule are seen as avascular foci, and the surviving tissue as foci with a preserved blood supply. During the first three months, the vascularity reduces in 64.8% of patients (Fig. 15.16).

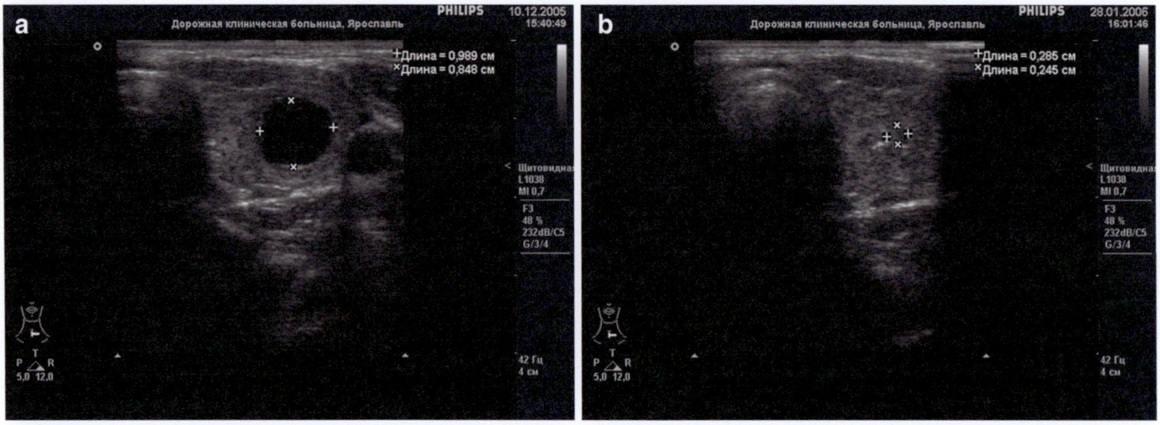

Fig. 15.14 (**a**, **b**) Status after PEI. Change in nodule size

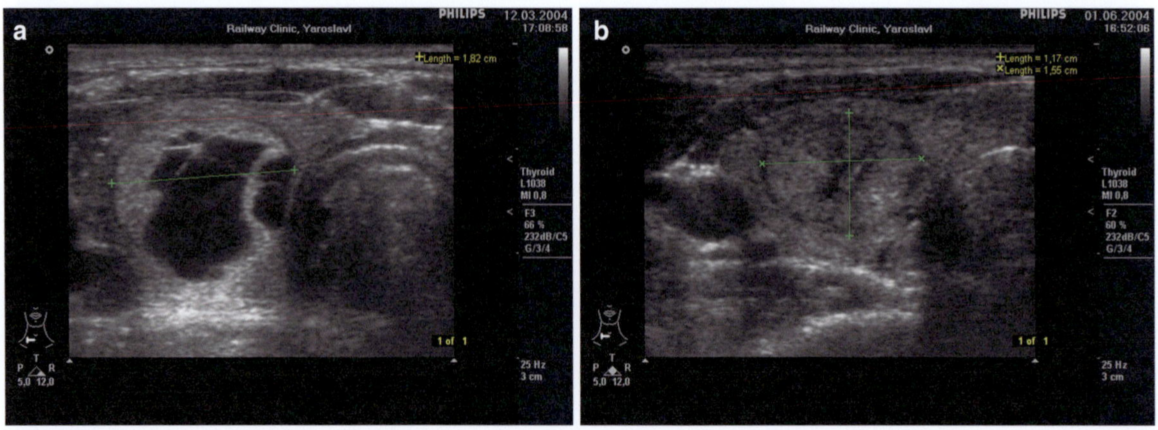

Fig. 15.15 (**a**, **b**) Status after PEI. Change in nodule echodensity

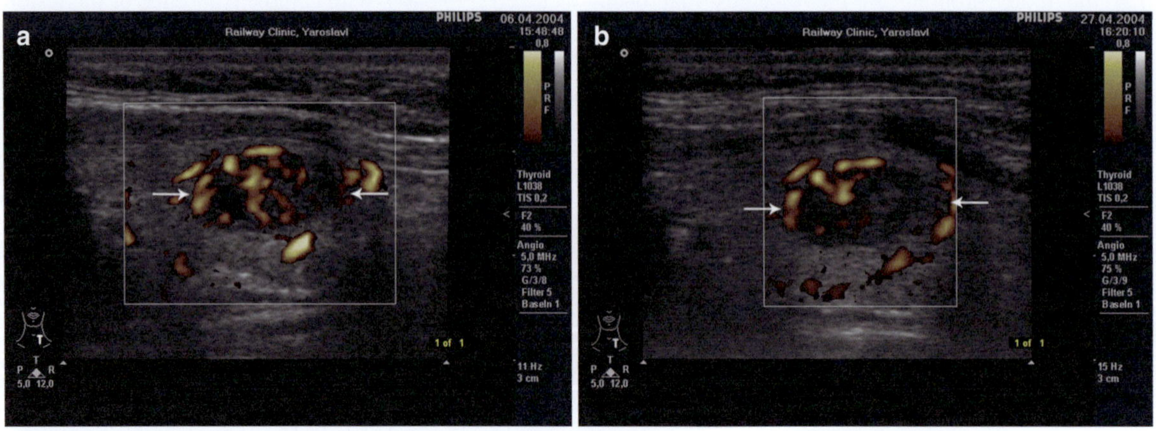

Fig. 15.16 (**a**, **b**) Status after PEI. Change in nodule vascularization

The change in vascularity of the nodule after PEI depends on its initial vascular pattern:

1. In avascular nodules, CDI and PDI are of no benefit. The desired positive effect is obtained through fluid aspiration, suppression of luminal secretion, and destruction of wall tissue. PEI is monitored by the quantity of introduced ethanol and perinodular blood flow depression.
2. In hypovascular nodules, it is difficult to assess the development of stasis and local necrosis in the thyroid nodule during the first few minutes. A reduction in perinodular and intranodular vascularity within 1–2 weeks after PEI predicts fast nodule involution.
3. CDI and PDI are of maximum benefit in cases of intranodular and perinodular patterns of hypervascularity and a nodule size of 10–20 mm. Within 3–10 min of ethanol injection avascular areas appear within the nodule. Such areas morphologically correspond to coagulative necrosis and local small-vessel thrombosis. They are observed not only within the nodule but also around it due to perinodular vessel thrombosis. These changes are also registered by pulse Doppler as a decrease in the velocity of blood flow. Since ethanol infiltrates the nodule in an unpredictable manner, blood supply may remain preserved in some areas of the nodule. In such cases, immediate ethanol reinstillation is avoided. Instead, it is preferable to delay any subsequent procedure, which may not necessarily be a PEI. On day 3–7 post-PEI, aseptic necrosis develops within the avascular foci. Meanwhile, the surviving nodule tissue is visualized as the foci of the preserved blood supply. During the resorption of the necrotic tissue, the former foci shrink and the latter foci take their place. Lack of a decrease in nodule vascularity on CDI and PDI within 1–2 weeks suggests inefficiency of nodule treatment. In such cases the nodule size remains unchanged. Therefore, it is necessary to consider that a decrease in vascularity is an early and almost an absolute feature that defines successful treatment of hypervascular nodules. Detection of significant vascularization after ethanol injection predicts treatment inefficiency and is a probable (though not absolute) feature of the viability of the nodule.

Side-effects and complications of PEI usually result from faulty procedure technique, such as inconsistency in the actions of the personnel, insufficient experience of an operator, inappropriate needle course, inaccurate US visualization, improper indications for the procedure, contraindications not taken into account, excessive alcohol volume, etc.

The most frequent side-effects of PEI are front neck discomfort, cervical pain, low-grade fever, and local edema (Table 15.2). The cervical pain usually lasts for 2–3 h. The pain most often appears in cases where the US registers ethanol flowing out of the nodule, under the thyroid capsule, and out of its margins. It is difficult to predict the patient's pain reaction.

Several complications (ethanol injection in the hypodermic fat, muscles, and healthy thyroid tissue) are a consequence of inadequate US guidance (Fig. 15.17). In cases with injection into hypodermic fat, ethanol can induce local hyperemia, infiltrate, necrosis, or abscess formation. Forcing excessive ethanol into the nodule can lead to the overflow and diffusion of alcohol through the nodule margins, resulting in damage to the surrounding tissues. Ethanol can also expand along the puncture canal both during injection and after the needle has been withdrawn. This can result in the development of intra- and extrathyroidal fibrosis. The risk of extrathyroidal fibrosis is particularly high in PEI of the subcapsular nodules. It also leads to the necrosis of normal thyroid tissue. In the case of the outpouring of 3–7 mL of 96% ethanol into the paranodular tissue, total necrosis of the thyroid lobe may be induced with a subsequent significant reduction in lobe size.

PEI into the nodules located in the dorsal compartment of the inferior segment of the left lobe should be performed with extra caution. In cases of ethanol misadministration or injection of an excessive volume, recurrent nerve alcoholization with vocal chord paresis and transient dysphonia may appear (Zingrillo 1998). This complication can also develop due to recurrent nerve compression due to an increase of nodule volume after the injection (Martino and Bogassi 2000).

PEI demands careful planning, definition of indications and contraindications, calculation of ethanol volume, and careful performance of the procedure. US helps to guide the procedure and to assess its effect. The most strongly expressed changes in the nodules occur within the first 1–6 months after intranodular ethanol administration.

Table 15.2 Side-effects and complications of PEI

Side-effect or complication	References	Rate
Cervical pain	Antonelli (1994)	Present
	Monzani et al. (1994)	Present
	Grineva et al. (2000)	100%
	Sikharulidze (2001)	73.6%
	Dossing et al. (2002)	1 case
	Hegedüset et al. (2003)	90%
	Marchenko (2003)	96%
	Seliverstov and Yarovoy (2004)	Present
	Zubeev et al. (2004)	Present
	Sung et al. (2008)	Present
	Tarantino et al. (2008)	21.3%
	Kanotra et al. (2008)	24 of 40
	Own data (n=360)	68.3%
Hypodermic alcohol injection with infiltrates, hematomas, local edema	Seliverstov et al. (1999)	0.4%
	Grineva et al. (2000)	2 of 14
	Sikharulidze (2001)	1 case
	Dossing et al. (2002)	4%
	Hegedüs et al. (2003)	Present
	Barsukov (2003)	Present
	Zubeev et al. (2004)	1 case
	Own data (n=360)	6.4%
Local hyperemia	Garg (2000)	Present
	Own data (n=360)	4.7%
Fever	Monzani et al. (1994)	3%
	Martino (2002)	2–8%
	Dossing et al. (2002)	1 case
	Marchenko (2003)	1.3%
	Barsukov (2003)	Present
	Own data (n=360)	3.6%
Dysphonia, vocal chord paresis or paralysis	Zingrillo (1998)	Present
	Martino et al. (2000)	Present
	Dossing et al. (2002)	1 case
	Hegedus et al. (2003)	5%
	Lee and Ahn (2005)	0.7%
	Tarantino et al. (2008)	2.4%
	Own data (n=360)	3.33%
Blockage of large nervous trunks (paresis of recurrent or laryngeal nerve)	Bubnov et al. (1997)	2 cases
	Seliverstov and Yarovoy (1999)	0.4%
	Sikharulidze (2001)	3.5%
	Hegedüs et al. (2003)	0–3%
	Marchenko (2003)	1.8%
	Barsukov (2004)	3 of 702
	Own data (n=360)	1.11%
Intra- or extrathyroidal fibrosis	Martino (2000)	Present
	Own data (n=360)	1.11%
Tracheitis	Sikharulidze (2001)	1 case
	Own data (n=360)	0.27%

Table 15.2 (continued)

Side-effect or complication	References	Rate
Necrosis of thyroid tissue, lobe atrophy	Ilyin (2002) Marchenko (2003) Barsukov (2004) Own data ($n=360$)	Registered 0.9 % Registered Not registered
Hemorrhage into the cyst	Seliverstov and Yarovoy (1999) Own data ($n=360$)	0.2% 0.27%
Thrombosis of the jugular vein	Angelini et al. (1996) Hegedüs et al. (2003) Own data ($n=360$)	Registered 1 case Not registered
Aseptic thyroiditis	Barsukov (2004) Own data ($n=360$)	5 of 702 Not registered
Horner syndrome	Bubnov et al. (1997) Own data ($n=360$)	Registered Not registered
Transitory hyperthyroidism, increase in blood thyroglobulin	Monzani (1994) Own data ($n=360$)	Registered Not registered
Hypothyrosis	Monzani et al. (1997) Own data ($n=360$)	0.9% Not registered
Granuloma at the position of the nodule	Rajatanavin (1994) Own data ($n=360$)	Registered Not registered
Acute respiratory insufficiency	Iacconi et al. (1996) Own data ($n=360$)	Registered Not registered
Paroxysms of sinus tachycardia	Zieleznik (1997) Own data ($n=360$)	Registered Not registered

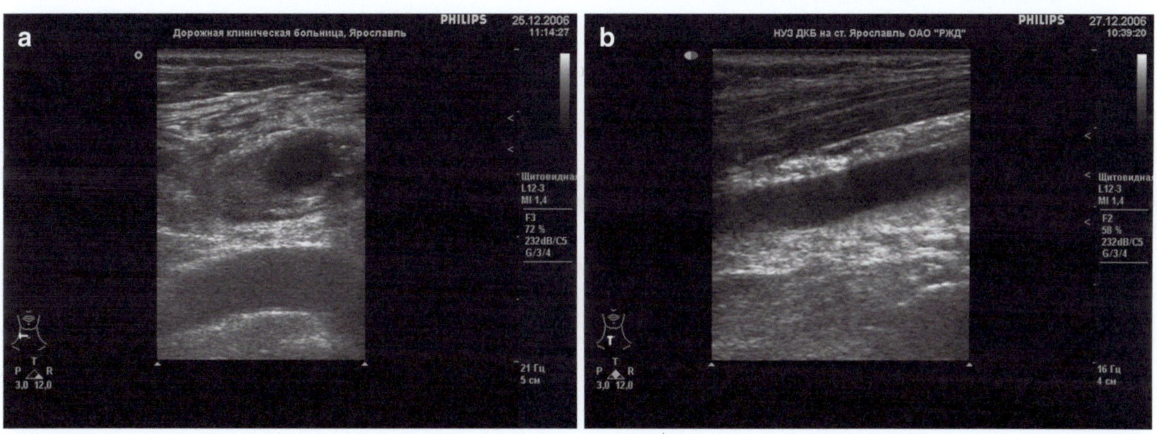

Fig. 15.17 (**a–f**) PEI complications. Alcohol outflow in thyroid parenchyma surrounding the nodule and beyond the thyroid margins

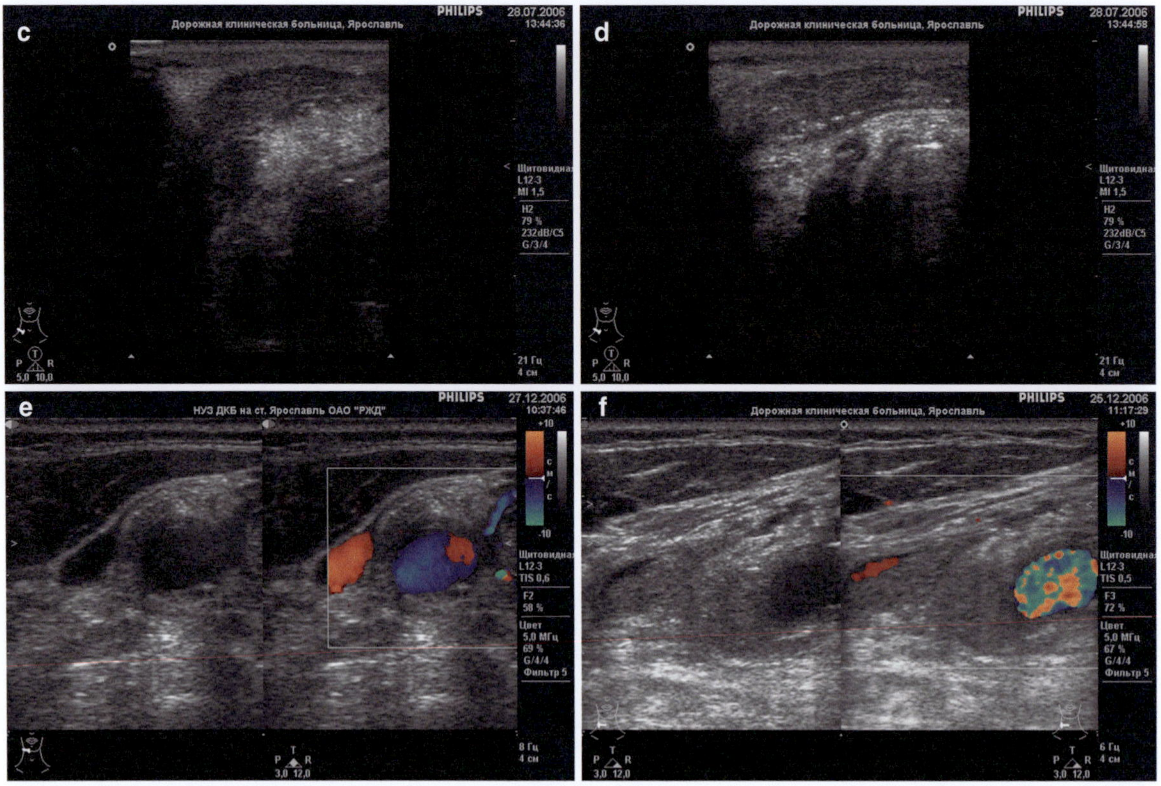

Fig. 15.17 (continued)

Example of US report at PEI:

First name, middle initial, last name:
Age:
Date:

In aseptic conditions under US guidance with free hand method a 22G needle was introduced into the 14x16x22 mm (volume 2.4cm3) anechoic avascular (in CDI and PDI) nodule with minor solid component in the upper segment of the left lobe of the thyroid gland. 2.1 ml of light yellow transparent fluid was aspirated. 1 ml of 96% ethanol was introduced into the nodule. Exposition within 30 seconds, complete reaspiration.

Visualization during the procedure was satisfactory. The patient tolerated the procedure well, somatic status without changes. Compression with aseptic bandage was applied to the puncture site for 15 minutes. The next visit is recommended in 3 months.

The surgeon (endocrinologist):
The US specialist:

Example of US report in 3 months after PEI:

First name, middle initial, last name:
Age:
Date:

3 months after PEI of the 14x16x22 mm (volume 2.4cm^3) anechoic avascular (in CDI and PDI) nodule with minor solid component in the upper segment of the left lobe of the thyroid gland. Nodule size has decreased to 3*3*6 mm (volume 0.03 cm^3). The nodule is predominantly hypoechoic with hyperechoic central part, with indistinct margins, avascular. The next visit is recommended in 3 months.

The surgeon (endocrinologist):
The US specialist:

15.3 Percutaneous Laser Ablation

Percutaneous laser ablation (PLA) of thyroid lesions now has many supporters. It is the alternative to the conservative management of patients with nodular goiter. Since medical laser equipment has become widely available, this procedure, initially only performed in a research setting, has been introduced into daily clinical practice (Revel-Muroz 1999; Seliverstov 2001; Dossing et al. 2002; Pacella 2004; Alexandrov et al. 2005).

Indications for thyroid PLA are as follows:

- Benign solid or predominantly solid nodules
  - Benign solitary nodules with unchanged surrounding tissue or combined with diffuse thyroid enlargement without any change in its echostructure and echodensity
  - Nodules of up to 20 mm in size
- Postoperative recurrent goiter
- Patient declines surgery or surgery cannot be performed due to serious comorbidities.

US guidance ensures correct PLA performance, guarantees its safety, and determines the efficacy.

PLA is preceded by a standard clinical examination with thyroid US. The latter is carried out by a qualified expert using high-quality equipment. Prior US-guided FNAB is mandatory in order to exclude a malignancy. Immediately prior to PLA, the dimensions of the nodule, its echostructure, blood supply, and its site (depth, lobe, segment, and relation to thyroid capsule, trachea, vascular bundle, and esophagus) are assessed with high-resolution US.

The efficacy of PLA is mainly determined by nodule size, structure, and vascularity (Figs. 15.18 and 15.19).

The most convenient position for the US probe for PLA guidance and the optimal needle course should be chosen. The participation of two experts, a surgeon and an US specialist is a reasonable approach to improve the quality of PLA (Fig. 15.20). The surgeon introduces the needle into the nodule, positions it correctly, defines the regimen of laser irradiation, and establishes and moves an optical fiber. The sonographer guides the

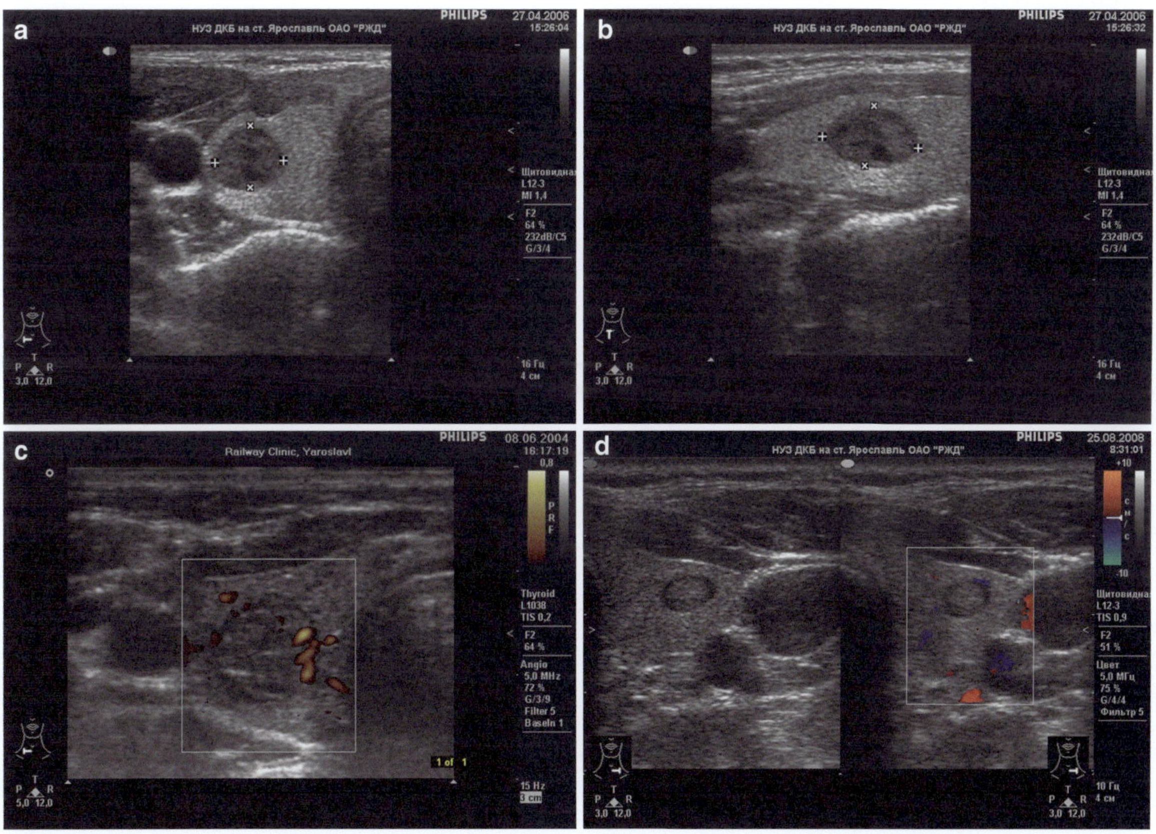

Fig. 15.18 (**a–c**) Nodules subjected to PLA

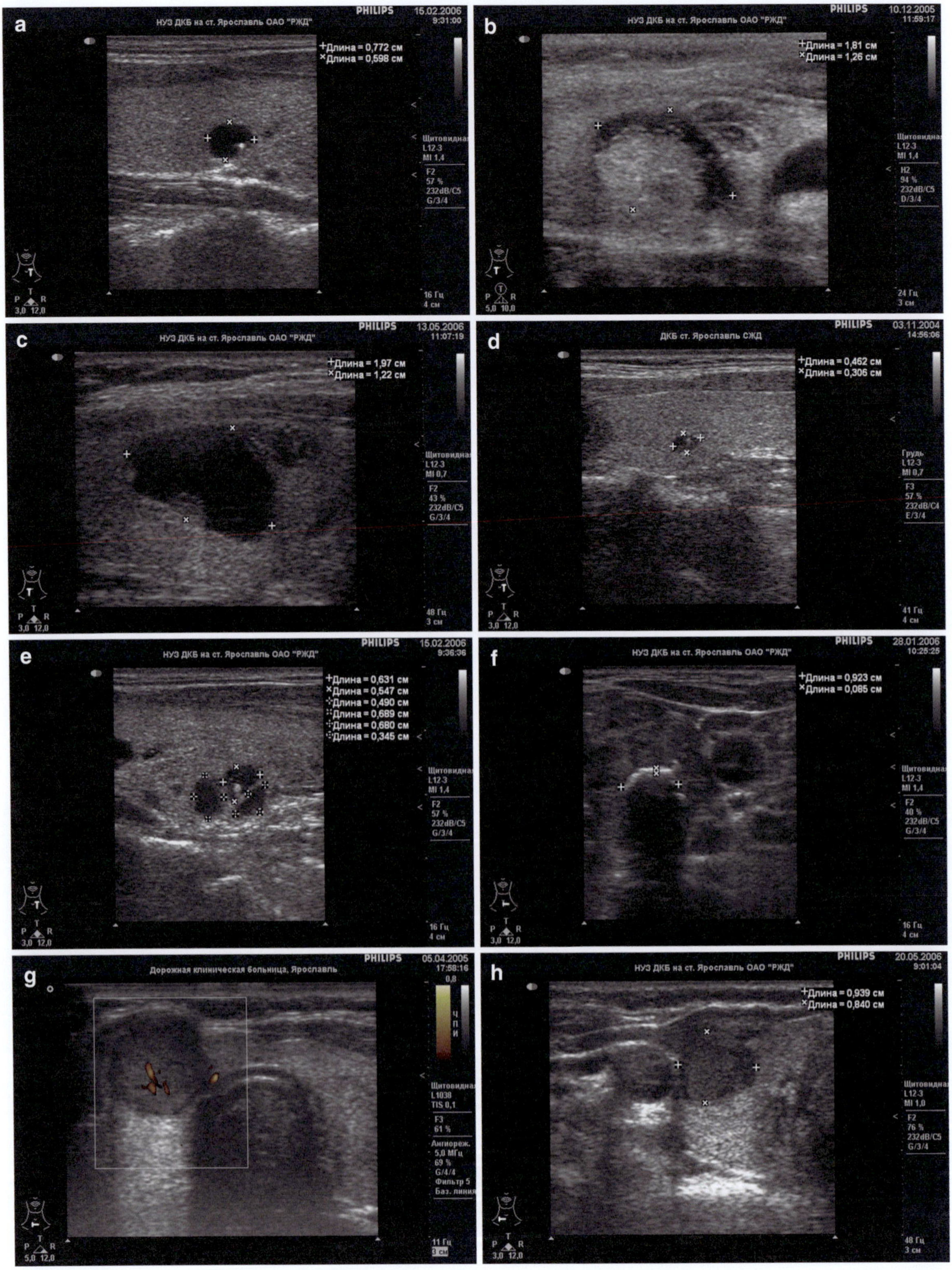

Fig. 15.19 Nodules not subjected to PLA. (**a**) Cysts; (**b**) complex solid nodules with large fluid collections; (**c**) complex cysts with solid component; (**d**) nodules smaller than 0.5 cm or larger than 3 cm in size; (**e**) multiple nodules; (**f**) nodules with calcifications; (**g**) subcapsular location; (**h**) paravasal location

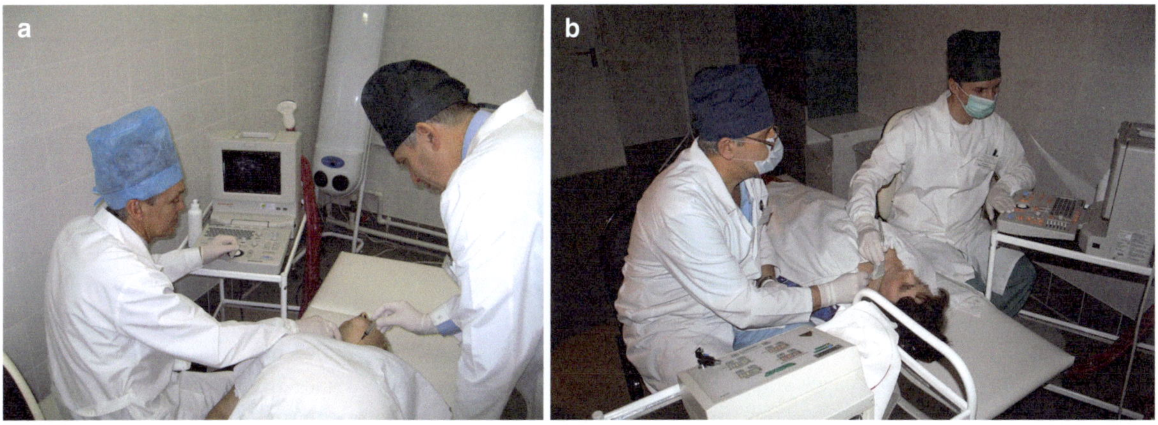

Fig. 15.20 (**a**, **b**) PLA. The position of the patient and medical staff

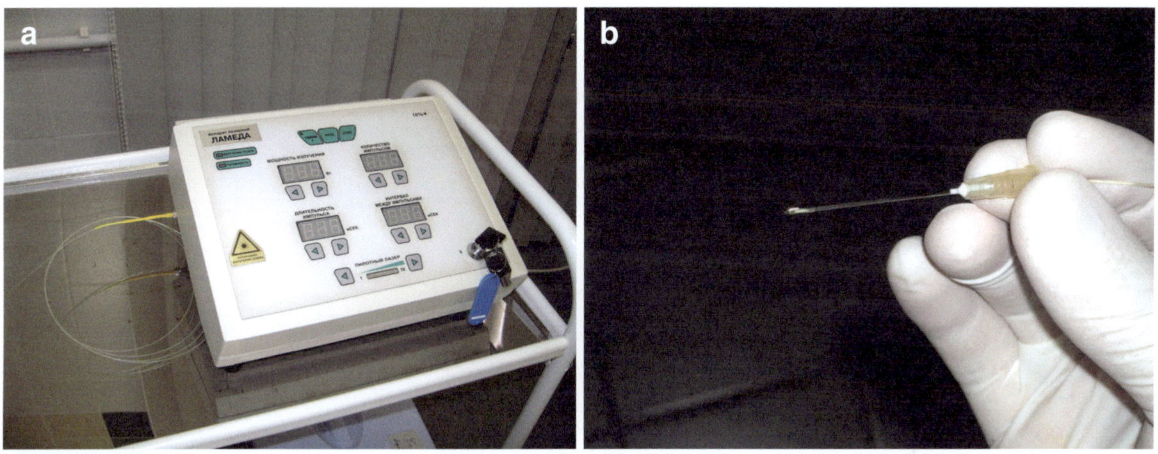

Fig. 15.21 (**a**, **b**) Medical diode laser and the optical fiber in the needle

introduction of the needle, defines the necessary duration of the procedure, and follows up the lesion after PLA.

PLA of thyroid nodules is carried out in the surgical dressing room or a specially equipped room with an US scanner. The latter should have a linear 7.5–12 MHz probe, and CDI and PDI modes. An infrared medical laser can be used for the procedure. A disposable sterile 19-gauge (1.1 mm) needle capable of conducting a 0.4 mm optical fiber (the diameter of the inner quartz fiber without its plastic covering) is utilized (Fig. 15.21).

During the procedure the patient is supine. A bolster is positioned under the patient's shoulders with the head thrown back for convenient access to the thyroid gland. The patient's head may be turned to the opposite side for convenience. Anesthesia is not usually used; this allows the patient to report on the occurrence of pain and thus to prevent several complications.

US-guided PLA has the following stages:

1. Puncture of the nodule and needle positioning
2. Introduction of the optical fiber and visualization of its tip within the nodule
3. Laser irradiation and vaporization of the lesion
4. Stopping the delivery of laser radiation upon the appearance of signs of complete nodule "processing" in the US image, complications, or a deterioration of the state of the patient
5. Withdrawal of the needle together with the optical fiber
6. Follow-up

After treating the neck skin with antiseptic, the US-guided puncture of the nodule is carried out in accordance with a freehand technique used for FNAB.

The access should be convenient for the surgeon, and should allow wide maneuverability and the possibility of adjusting the angle of the needle, as well as constant US guidance at every position of the needle. The path of the needle should be chosen carefully in order to avoid any vital structures both along its course and below the needle (Figs. 15.22 and 15.23).

US effects observed at PLA are an important part of the procedure. These include phenomena induced by the laser and artifacts associated with it (Table 15.3). The phenomena can be divided into two groups: main (which are seen in 100% of cases where PLA is performed correctly, supply important information, and must be taken into consideration) and additional (which do not provide significant additional information and do not influence the procedure). US artifacts give false information and complicate the procedure. Artifacts can appear different upon grayscale and color-flow Doppler imaging, and largely depend on the settings of the ultrasound equipment.

Important changes in the nodule and surrounding thyroid tissue form the basis of PLA and are main US phenomena. The first stage of PLA is puncture of the lesion. Depending on the US probe position, the needle is visualized either at its full length as a moving hyperechoic line or as a hyperechoic point. Its end position should be accurately defined. The direction and depth can be corrected during its introduction. Laser ablation is only carried out under the condition of confident visualization of the needle tip in the nodule. After the needle is precisely positioned, a sterile optical fiber is administered through the needle lumen until it comes into contact with nodule tissue. The introduction of the optical fiber is visualized as a moving linear hyperechoic structure inside the needle lumen. The optical fiber tip protruding from the needle into the nodule

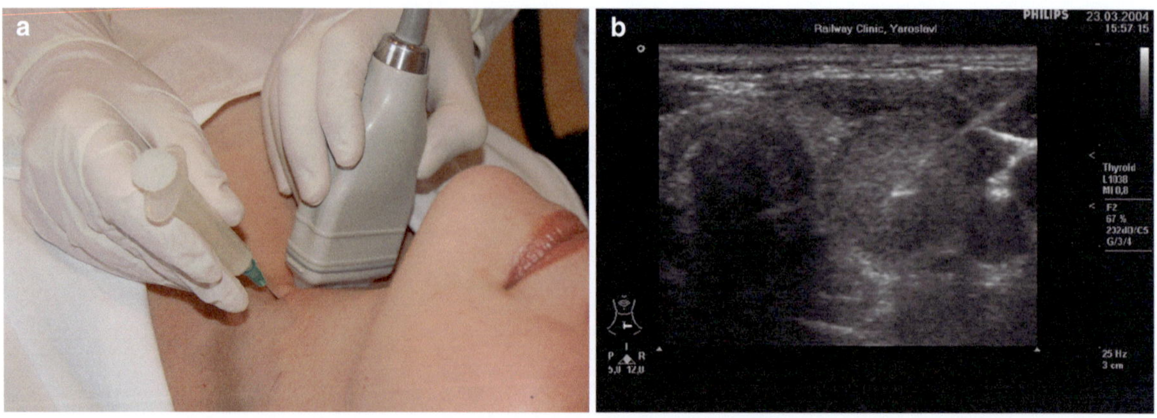

Fig. 15.22 PLA. (**a**) Needle administration by the lateral side of an US probe. (**b**) Visualization of the needle end

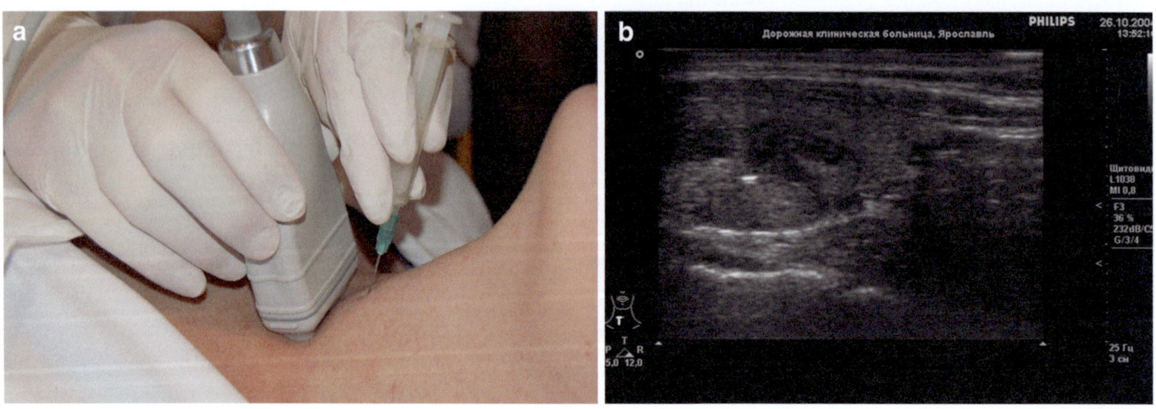

Fig. 15.23 PLA. (**a**) Needle administration directly over the nodule. (**b**) Visualization of the needle end

takes the form of a point or a line that is comparable in its echodensity to the needle, and which moves along its axis (Fig. 15.24).

Table 15.3 US effects linked to the influence of a laser

Effect	Rate, % (n=852)
Main phenomena:	
Visualization of the needle and optical fiber	100
Visualization of hyperechoic vaporization zone and the phenomenon of nodule contrasting	100
Staining of the vaporization zone in CDI and PDI modes	100
Additional phenomena:	
Contrasting of the nodule capsule	60.0
Microbubble motion in the needle lumen	91.9
Microbubble motion in blood vessels	65.0
Contrasting of the walls of blood vessels	21.1
Contrasting of fascias and septa	40.0
Contrasting of thyroid capsule and its visual thickening	36.0
Artifacts:	
Artifact of multiple "false needles"	9.97
"Fan" artifact at the needle tip	5.0
Atypical posterior acoustic shadowing after vaporization zone and expanding gas	80.0
Doppler staining of the acoustic shadow	44.95
Doppler staining of the needle	11.97

It is necessary to push the optical fiber tip 3–7 mm out of the needle to achieve reliable contact with tissue and avoid heating the needle. In cases with large nodules, several optical fibers can be introduced simultaneously (Spiezia et al. 2003; Pacella et al. 2004). At the start of laser irradiation, the US picture typically remains unchanged (depending on the laser irradiation power) for several seconds. Then a heterogeneous dynamic hyperechoic area begins to surround the optical fiber tip. This has an irregular shape, indistinct margins, and atypical posterior acoustic shadowing. This zone characterizes vaporization (the evaporation of tissue and intercellular fluid; Fig. 15.25).

The vaporization zone gradually enlarges during the procedure and serves as a rough reference for subsequent necrosis. A delay in the appearance of this zone may be due to the morphological features of the nodule, but much more often results from the dislocation of the optical fiber tip. The tip can be dislocated into the needle lumen, in which case the patient reports sharp pain due as the metal part of the needle overheats. Alternatively, it can be pushed deeply into the location of the "blind" zone, for example near the trachea, with subsequent complications.

As the PLA session proceeds further, microbubbles of gas in the form of small hyperechoic particles with reverberation appear within the nodule. They expand irregularly within the hyperechoic vaporization zone and centrifugally within the nodule. Their motion depends on the morphological structure and density of the nodule. Microbubbles also move in nodule vessels and are accumulated under its capsule. This results in the US phenomenon of the contrasting of the nodule capsule due to

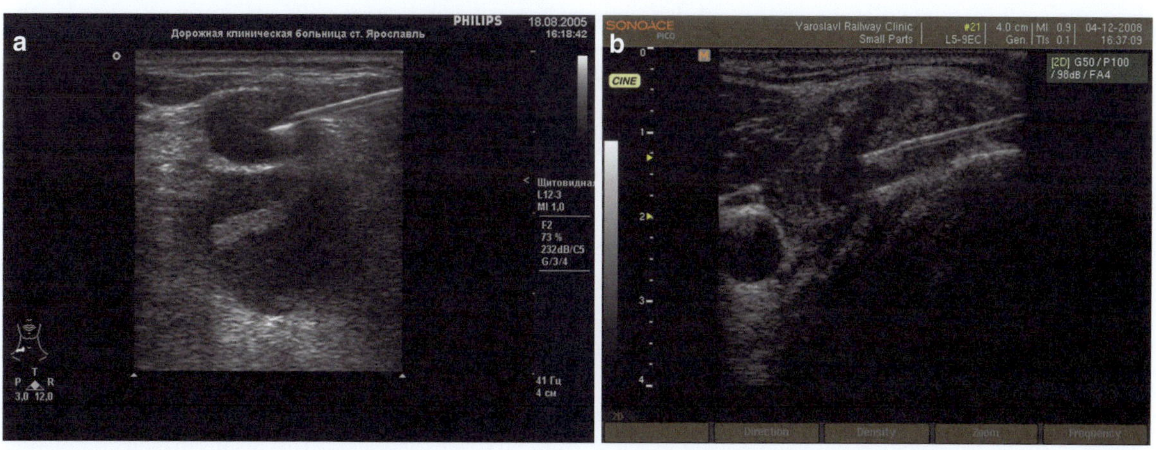

Fig. 15.24 (**a**, **b**) PLA. The phenomenon of visualization of the needle and the optical fiber

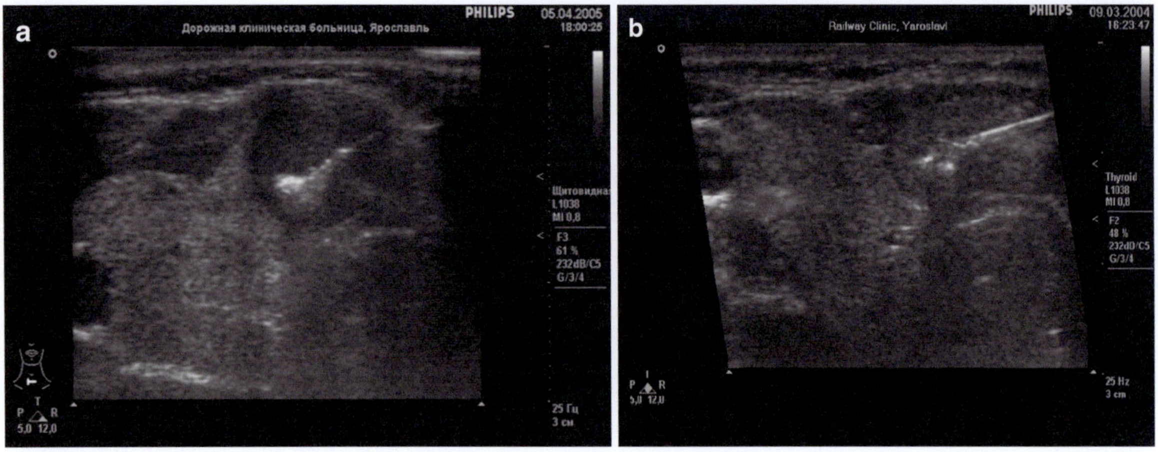

Fig. 15.25 (**a–b**) PLA. The phenomenon of visualization of the hyperechoic vaporization zone

the increase in its echodensity with visual thickening. The growth of the vaporization zone and the contrasting of the nodule capsule merge and lead to the phenomenon of nodule contrasting (Fig. 15.26). Its echodensity significantly increases and the nodule becomes clearly delimited from its surrounding thyroid tissue.

CDI and PDI reveal intensive staining of the hyperechoic vaporization zone during laser irradiation (Fig. 15.27).

The intensity of staining is so high that most of the scanning range appears colored. In this case, it is necessary to correct the color-flow Doppler sensitivity until the size of the stained range is less than 1–1.5 cm. This allows this phenomenon to be utilized to specify the location of the optical fiber tip during the procedure. The stained area is roundish and dynamic with short "beams" corresponding to centrifugal diffusion of gas. The visualization quality progressively deteriorates during the procedure. This is a consequence of the merging of the echodensity of the zone of laser influence and the needle with the optical fiber, as well as the accumulation of gas in the thyroid gland and surrounding neck tissue along with corresponding artifacts. The appearance of the phenomenon of the Doppler staining of the vaporization zone does not depend on the quality of grayscale visualization. Thus, CDI or PDI may assist in verifying the exact position of the optical fiber tip.

The introduction of the laser beam into live tissue results in tissue vaporization with subsequent evacuation of the vapors. This process constitutes the essence of the additional phenomena observed in PLA. The isolated phenomenon of nodule contrasting is observed after 15–30 s. Then the vapor diffuses from the nodule into the bloodstream. The diffusion of the vapors results in contrasting and visual thickening of the blood vessels and connective tissue septa. This is observed as an US phenomenon (Figs. 15.28 and 15.29).

The movement of fine hyperechoic particles one after another, forming "paths" and "clumps," sometimes with reverberation, can be seen in the blood vessel lumens. Their velocities depend on the laser irradiation power and the intensity of vaporization. The phenomenon of the contrasting of fine vessel walls results in their clear US visualization in thyroid tissue in the form of parallel linear hyperechoic structures and the manifestation of the vessels that were not visualized prior to PLA. Contrasted fine vessel walls are clearly visualized in the ultrasound image as parallel linear hyperechoic structures within the thyroid tissue, which are not discernible prior to PLA.

Gas accumulates under the thyroid capsule in large amounts. The echodensity of the capsule and its visual thickness both increase. The capsule becomes distinctly apparent as it contrasts against the thyroid tissue and surrounding muscles (Fig. 15.30). Intense laser irradiation leads to the movement of the steam outside the gland. Continued intense laser irradiation leads to gas bubbles spreading outside the gland. The gas bubbles move through blood vessels and along the interfascial spaces and septa. This results in their contrasting and visual thickening.

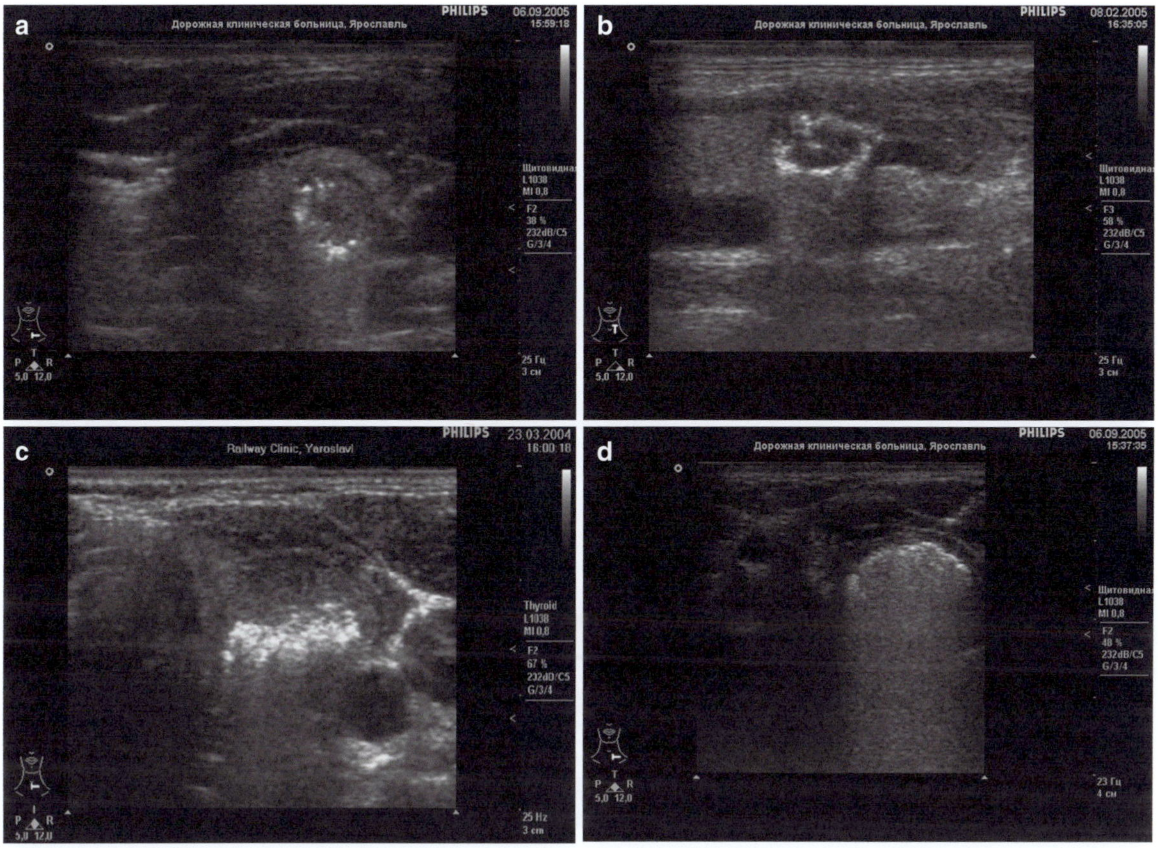

Fig. 15.26 (**a–d**) PLA. The phenomena of the contrasting of the nodule capsule and the contrasting of the nodule

Gas can be evacuated from the vaporization zone by large veins, which are sonographically observed as "streams" of hyperechoic bubbles in their lumen. The movements of the bubbles may be also registered in the needle lumen and along the puncture path (Fig. 15.31).

A "plateau" effect within the hyperechoic vaporization zone is reached in 300–400 s after the initiation of laser treatment. The area becomes stable without further enlargement. The maximum volume of tissue damage in this area is thus reached. The efficacy of further laser irradiation significantly decreases. The procedure should be terminated at this point. Alternatively, the optical fiber may be moved to a different area within the target lesion. Seliverstov et al. (2004) recommends changing the location of the optical fiber tip within the nodule 60–90 s from the beginning of the procedure, especially in the case of large nodules. Thus, the optical fiber tip may be initially positioned deep within the lesion and subsequently shifted by 5–7 mm to a more superficial location for the ablation of additional nodule volume. Initiating the PLA procedure within the posterior portion of the nodule reduces interference and minimizes the difficulties related to vaporization artifacts. In this fashion, the superficial portion of the nodule remains accessible to sonographic visualization. This allows the consistent ablation of the whole nodule volume by moving the optical fiber during the procedure. Various areas of the nodule may be influenced more precisely by individual laser ablation regimens. PLA proceeds until the nodule is completely replaced with the heterogeneous hyperechoic zone.

Acoustic artifacts that accompany PLA can deteriorate visualization, induce alterations in data, and complicate the procedure.

Artifacts can appear while the needle is being positioned. As the needle approximates the perpendicular to the probe's surface, its visualization inevitably deteriorates. When the positioning angle is decreased and the needle runs close to parallel to the probe surface, reflection artifacts naturally appear. The true needle is

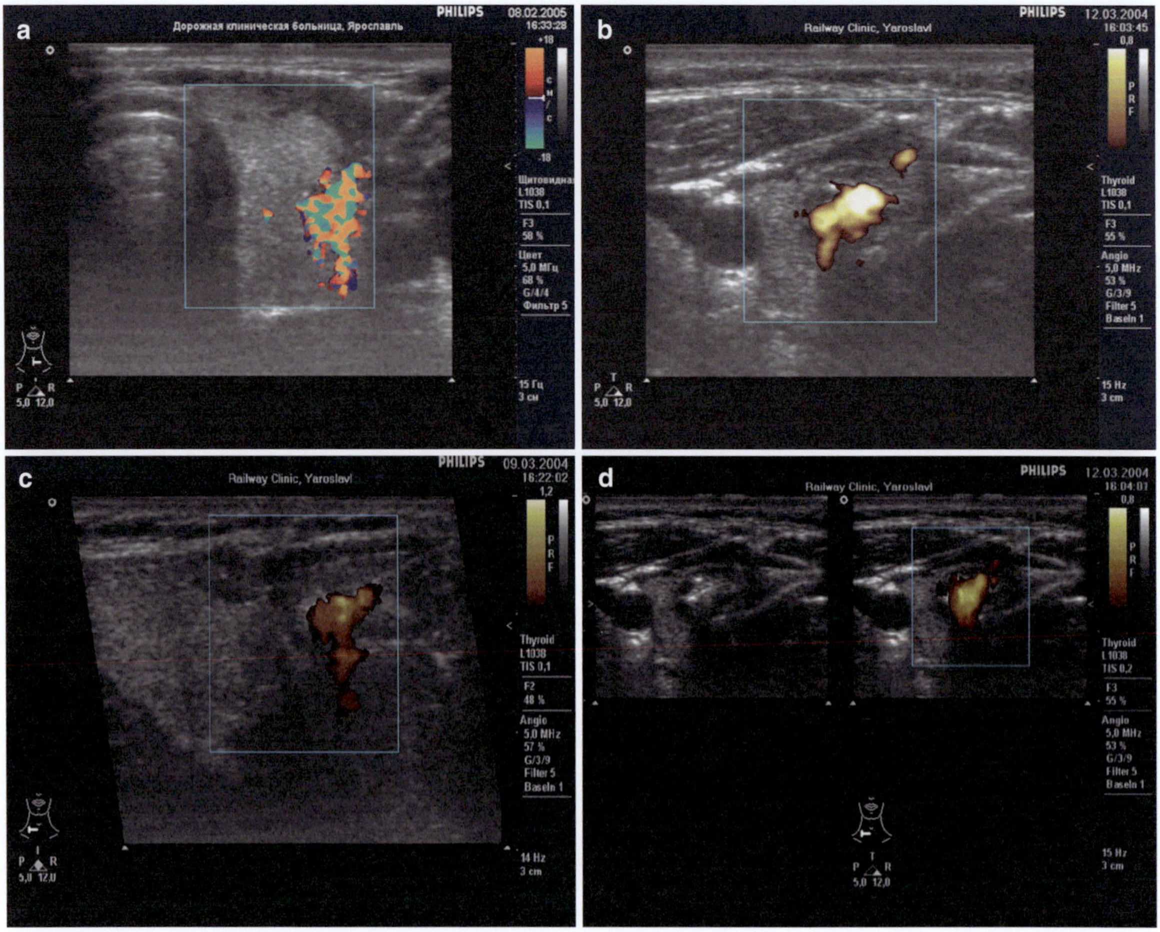

Fig. 15.27 (a–d) PLA. The phenomenon of vaporization zone staining in CDI and PDI

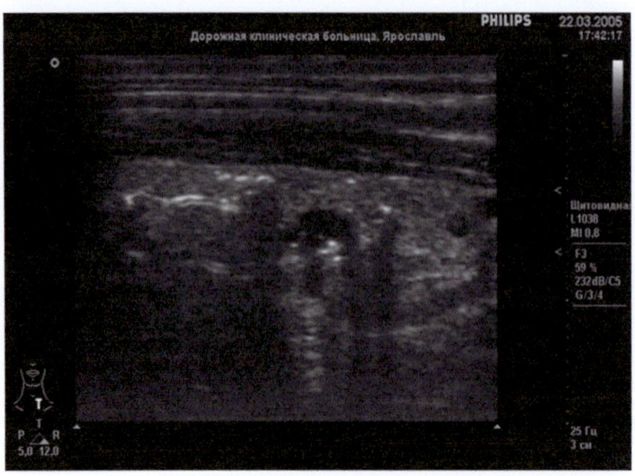

Fig. 15.28 PLA. The phenomenon of microbubble motion in blood vessels and the contrasting of vessel walls

thus accompanied by additional "false needles" of lower echodensity (Fig. 15.32).

A "fan" artifact dispersing from the needle end in the form of a fading tail may occasionally be observed (Fig. 15.33). This is due to the orientation of the cut plane of the needle end against the scanning plane. Such artifacts give false information and can lead to undesirable iatrogenic damage.

When doubts exist regarding the true position of the needle it is advisable to tilt either the needle or the US probe. The true needle image does not change, but the artifacts usually attenuate or disappear.

During the fast reciprocal movement of the optical fiber in the tissue during laser irradiation, there is insufficient time for the abovementioned spherical hyperechoic vaporization zone to form. Therefore, US

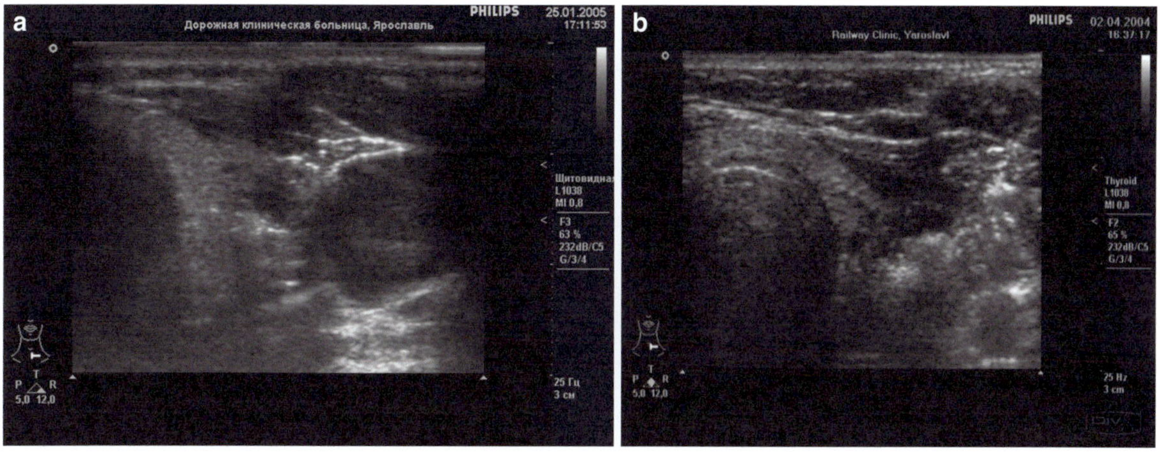

Fig. 15.29 (**a**, **b**) PLA. The phenomenon of the contrasting of fascias and connective tissue septa

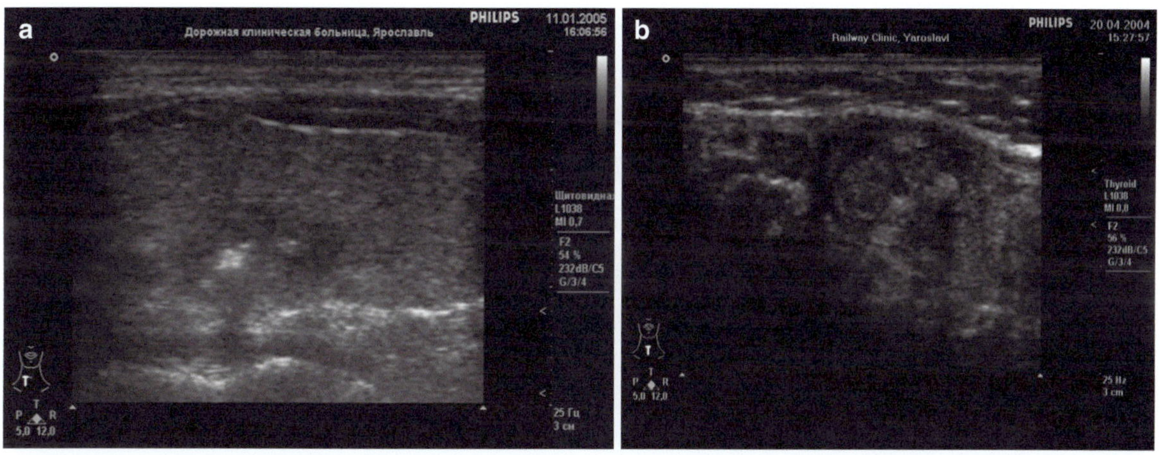

Fig. 15.30 (**a**, **b**) PLA. The phenomenon of the contrasting of the thyroid capsule and its visual thickening

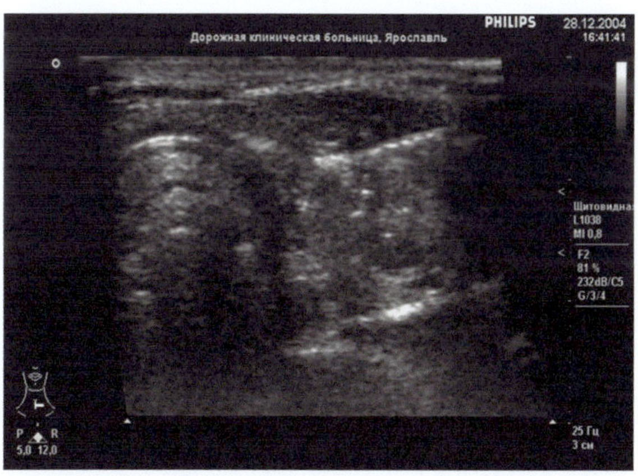

Fig. 15.31 PLA. The phenomenon of the motions of steam microbubbles in the needle lumen

reveals a linear hypoechoic structure with hyperechoic margins corresponding to the residual canal in nodule tissue. This structure is preserved after the withdrawal of the needle and the optical fiber. This image of a false needle can lead to mistakes (Fig. 15.34). Moving the needle or optical fiber in its lumen can easily highlight the true needle position: the true needle (optical fiber) moves in the corresponding direction on the screen while the false needle remains static.

The vaporization zone is normally accompanied by atypical posterior acoustic shadowing. Unlike classical paths behind high-density objects and large clumps of gas, it has moderately lowered echodensity and changes with depth (Fig. 15.35).

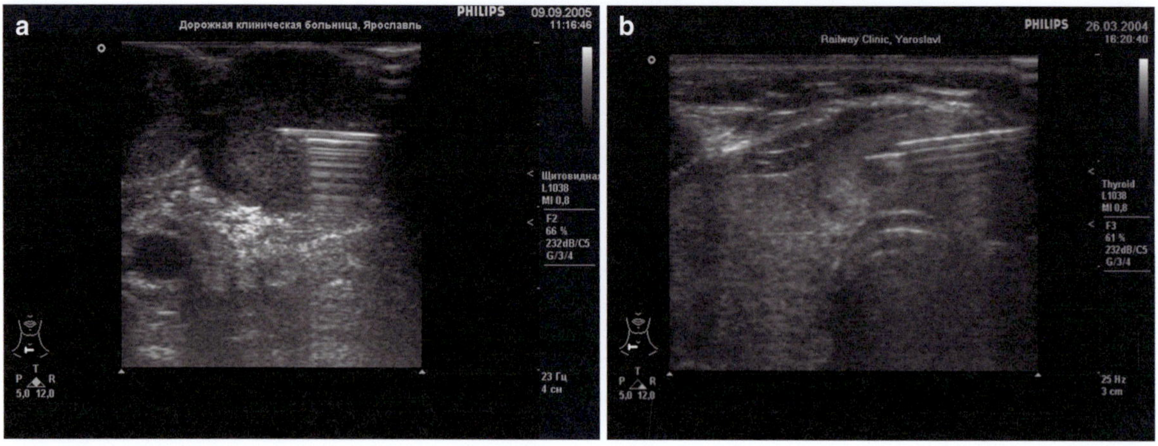

Fig. 15.32 (**a–b**) PLA. The artifact of multiple "false needles"

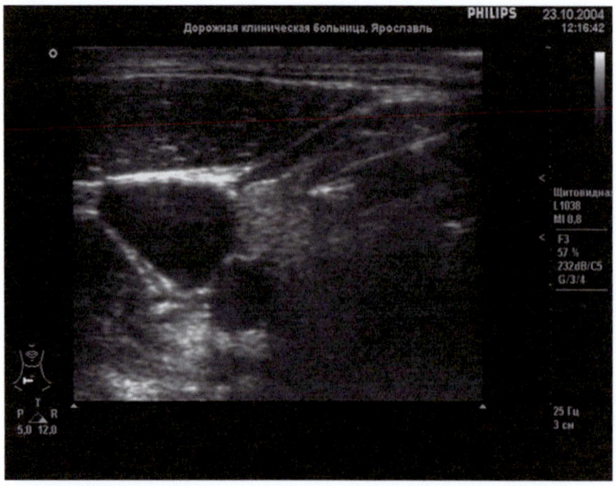

Fig. 15.33 PLA. The "fan" artifact at the needle end

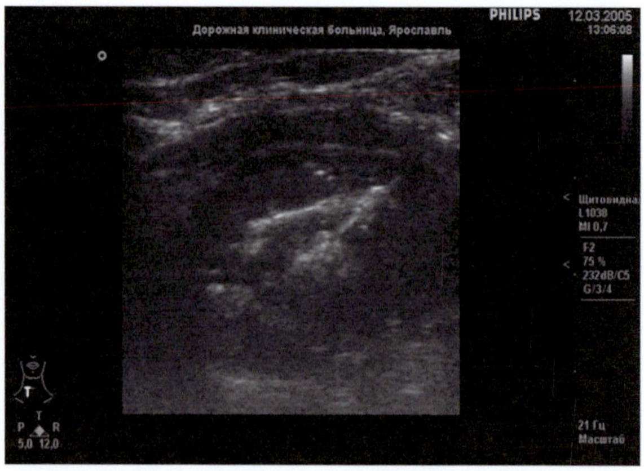

Fig. 15.34 PLA. The residual canal in nodule tissue

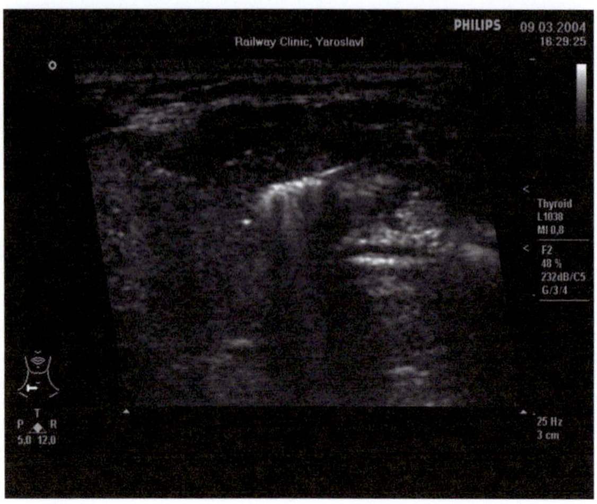

Fig. 15.35 PLA. The artifact of atypical posterior acoustic shadowing

This is due to the merging of reverberation effects from multiple microbubbles of boiling fluid. Color staining of the atypical acoustic shadowing is often observed in CDI and PDI modes. This is similar to the staining of the vaporization zone (Fig. 15.36).

Doppler staining along the needle is usually fragmentary and significantly less prominent than the staining of the vaporization zone, so it does not substantially affect the procedure.

The duration of the PLA session depends on nodule size, the health of the patient, the dynamics of the US image during the procedure, and can be 1–15 min. A control US scan of the nodule in B-mode, CDI, and PDI modes is performed 30–60 s after switching off the laser's power supply before withdrawing the optical fiber. When it depicts vascularized regions within the nodule, they must be processed by laser irradiation

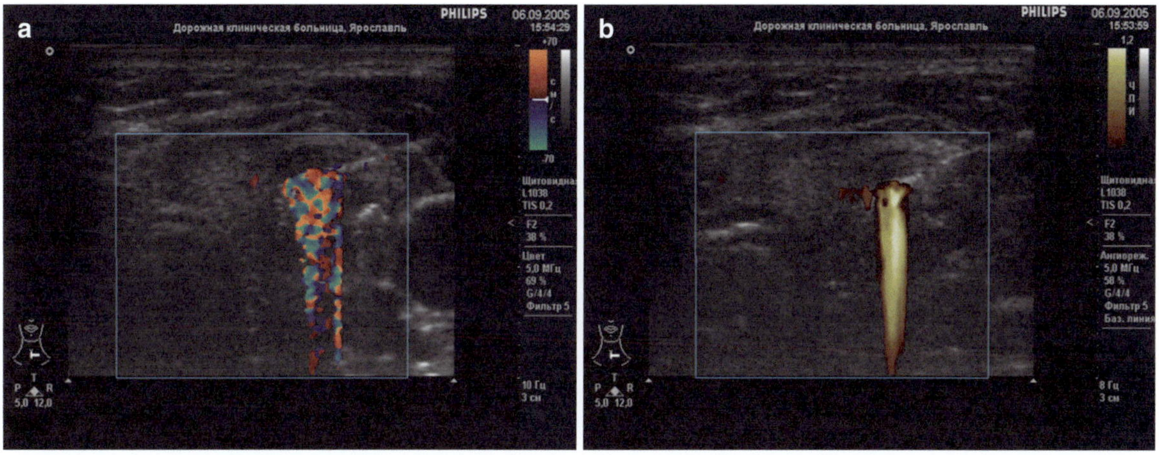

Fig. 15.36 (**a**, **b**) PLA. The artifact of Doppler staining of the atypical posterior acoustic shadowing

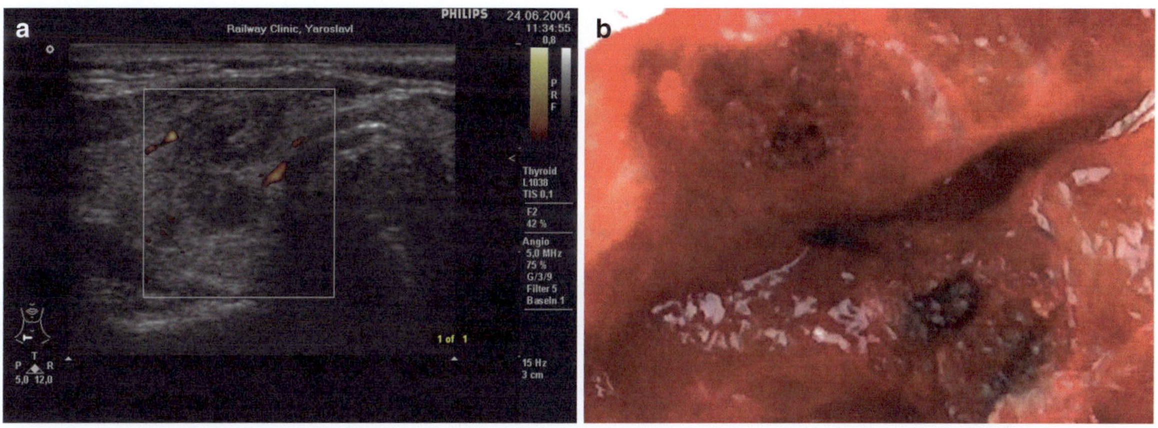

Fig. 15.37 (**a**, **b**) US and morphological zones of laser-induced damage

to eliminate the blood flow completely. If the nodule appears completely avascular, the optical fiber is withdrawn together with the needle as one unit.

Control US scans are expedient after 10–15 min, and 1, 3, 6, 12 months after PLA.

Beginning the second day after PLA, significant changes in the echostructure of the nodule can be seen. In some cases a hypoechoic zone with indistinct borders is detected in its place. Heterogeneity and a decrease in echodensity are morphologically associated with edema and aseptic inflammation. Infracentimetric nodules are normally enlarged and look like heterogeneous hypoechoic hypovascular lesions with indistinct irregular margins. Thus, the US picture may be similar to that of subacute thyroiditis due to common morphological changes that are characteristic of inflammatory processes (expressed infiltration). Irregularly shaped hypoechoic areas at the locations of ablation that are partially surrounded by hyperechoic rings are characteristic of large nodules.

US reveals a lesion with mixed echostructure 7–10 days after PLA. This is characterized by a small central hypoechoic region (the vaporization zone) surrounded by a hyperechoic ring (the carbonization zone) and exterior hypoechoic zone (the zone of coagulation necrosis) (Fig. 15.37).

US criteria for PLA efficacy are as follows (Table 15.4):

- Nodule size reduction (nodule fragmentation is possible)
- Change in echostructure
- Indistinct margins of the nodule
- Hypo- or avascularity in CDI and PDI modes

Table 15.4 Changes in the US features of nodules after PLA ($n=105$), M ± sd %

US features	Before PLA	After 1 month	After 6 months	After 12 months	Reliability of differences			
					p_{0-1}	p_{0-6}	p_{0-12}	p_{1-12}
Average maximal nodule size, (mm)	15.05 ± 2.1							
Character of size change:								
Unchanged		7.6 ± 2.6	9.5 ± 2.9	7.6 ± 2.6				
Decrease		74.3 ± 4.3	77.2 ± 4.1	73.4 ± 4.3				
Enlargement		16.2 ± 3.6	9.5 ± 2.9	3.8 ± 1.9				+
Scar		1.9 ± 1.3	3.8 ± 1.9	15.2 ± 3.2				+
Shape:								
Oval	66.7 ± 4.6	49.5 ± 4.9	55.2 ± 4.9	60.0 ± 4.8	+			
Spherical	29.5 ± 4.5	14.3 ± 3.4	16.2 ± 3.6	19.0 ± 3.8	+	+		
Irregular	3.8 ± 1.9	36.2 ± 4.7	28.6 ± 4.4	21.0 ± 4.0	+	+	+	+
Margins:								
Smooth	93.3 ± 2.4	10.5 ± 3.0	27.6 ± 4.4	40.95 ± 4.8	+	+	+	+
Rough	6.7 ± 2.4	89.5 ± 3.0	72.4 ± 4.4	59.05 ± 4.8	+	+	+	+
Contours:								
Well defined	98.1 ± 1.3	4.8 ± 2.1	34.3 ± 4.6	44.8 ± 4.9	+	+	+	+
Indistinct (or locally indistinct)	1.9 ± 1.3	95.2 ± 2.1	65.7 ± 4.6	55.2 ± 4.9	+	+	+	+
Echodensity:								
Hyper-	8.6 ± 2.7	4.8 ± 2.1	3.8%1.9	16.% ± 3.6				+
Iso-	68.6 ± 4.5	71.4 ± 4.4	75.2 ± 4.2	76.2 ± 4.2				
Hypo-	20.0 ± 3.9	18.0 ± 3.7	11.4 ± 3.1	6.7 ± 2.4				+
An-	2.8 ± 1.6	5.8 ± 2.3	9.6 ± 2.9	0.9 ± 0.9				
Echostructure:								
Homogeneous	41.9 ± 4.8	13.3 ± 3.3	8.6 ± 2.7	5.7 ± 2.3	+	+	+	
Heterogeneous	58.1 ± 4.8	86.7 ± 3.3	91.4 ± 2.7	94.3 ± 2.3	+	+	+	
Calcifications:								
Present	4.8 ± 2.1	10.5 ± 3.0	19.0 ± 3.8	31.4 ± 4.5			+	+
Absent	95.2 ± 2.1	89.5 ± 3.0	81.0 ± 3.8	68.6 ± 4.5			+	+
Fluid collections:								
Present	6.7 ± 2.4	3.8 ± 1.9	3.8 ± 1.9	4.8 ± 2.1				
Absent	93.3 ± 2.4	96.2 ± 1.9	96.2 ± 1.9	95.2 ± 2.1				
Vascularity:								
Hypervascular (including solid component)	37.1 ± 4.7	6.7 ± 2.4	7.6 ± 2.6	8.6 ± 2.7	+	+	+	
Hypovascular (including solid component)	44.8 ± 4.9	13.3 ± 3.3	15.2 ± 3.5	19.0 ± 3.8	+	+	+	
Avascular	18.% ± 3.8	80.0 ± 3.9	77.2 ± 4.1	72.4 ± 4.4	+	+	+	

+, differences significant at $p < 0.05$

Laser ablation is most effective in solid nodules (Fig. 15.38). Pacella et al. (2000) report that PLA efficacy decreases if big fluid or colloid collections are present.

PLA allows 38.6% of thyroid nodules to be cured completely, and achieves a positive result (a reduction in nodule volume by 50% or more) in 43.6% of cases (Fig. 15.39).

The efficacy of PLA is higher in small nodules (Fig. 15.40). Infracentimetric nodules decrease in volume by more than 50 % in 75–80% of cases and disappear in 30–40% of patients. In cases with nodules larger than 1–2 cm, the volume is halved in 50–60% of patients.

Complete disappearance of nodules larger than 2 cm is not observed. Fibrotic areas are formed in their place. These ultrasonically correspond to hypoechoic zones with hyperechoic centers and indistinct margins. The effect of PLA in solid nodules is inversely proportional to nodule size. PLA is efficacious (i.e., causes a reduction of 50% or more) within one year for solid nodules smaller than 10 mm in size in 79% of patients, 1–2 cm in size in 69% of patients, and 20 mm in size or larger in 55% of patients. The effect of the procedure is considered positive if nodule size decreases and the respective symptoms disappear. Therefore, it is not always expedient to achieve complete extinction of the nodule. In several cases it is enough to decrease its volume and to replace it with connective tissue. This prevents the nodule from progressing further and achieving functional autonomy.

The best PLA results are achieved in patients who have nodules with low or moderate intranodular vascular patterns. Smaller efficacies are seen for similar nodules with mixed and peripheral vascular patterns. The decrease in nodule size after PLA in such cases is typical enough and easily predicted. It allows the number of

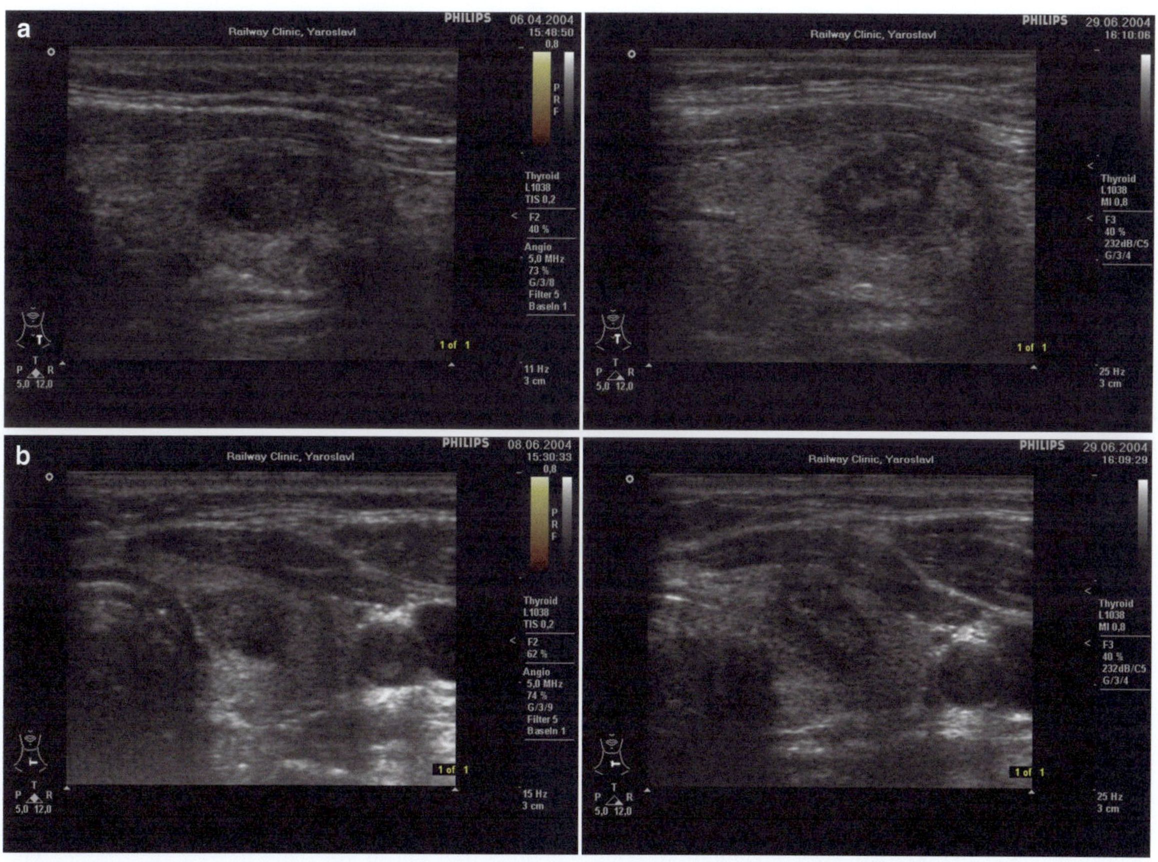

Fig. 15.38 (**a, b**) Change in the echostructure of the nodule three months after PLA. Nodule fragmentation

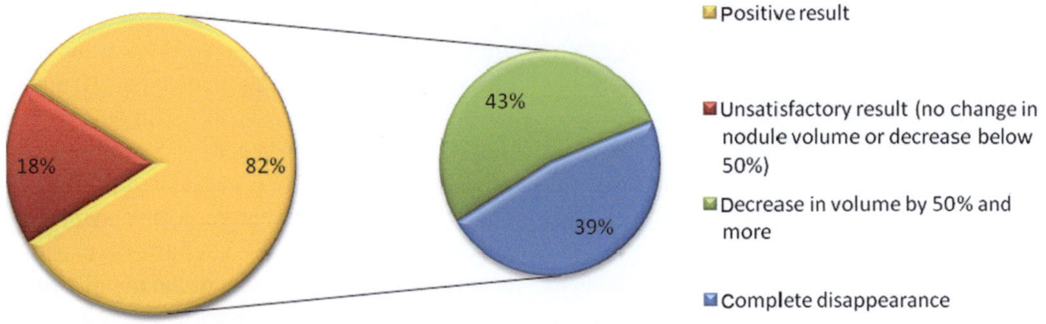

Fig. 15.39 Efficacy of PLA in benign thyroid nodules

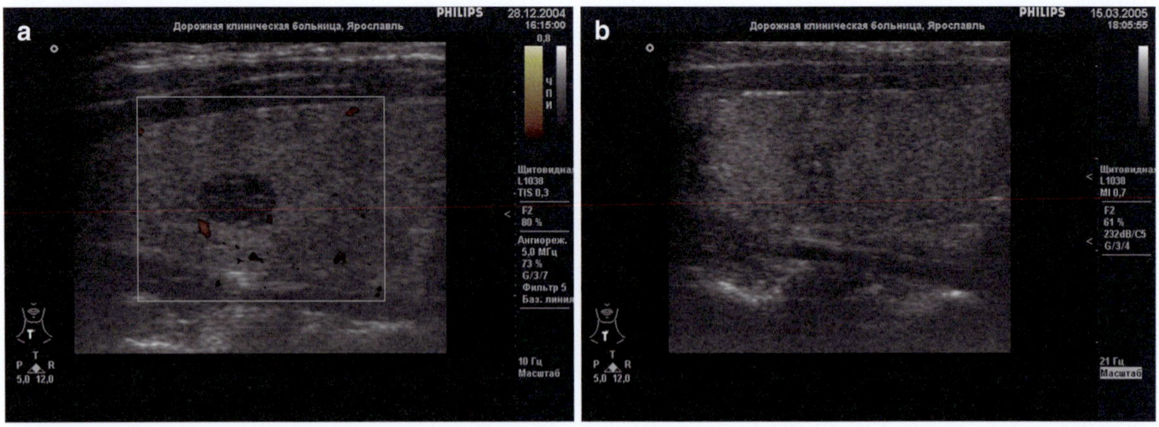

Fig. 15.40 (**a**, **b**) The change in nodule size three months after PLA

PLA sessions to be planned taking other predetermining factors into consideration (nodule size and so forth).

Hypervascular nodules normally demand more intense regimens and more PLA sessions. Two stages in their treatment are observed. The purpose of the first stage is the elimination of blood flow within the nodule. In most cases, especially in large nodules, one PLA session appears to be insufficient to reduce the intensity of the blood supply to a level comparable to the vascularization of surrounding tissue. Repeated sessions allow the blood flow to be reduced in fields with preserved hypervascularization. Considering the high reparative potential of well-vascularized tissue, it is expedient to decrease the interval between PLA sessions to 1–2 weeks. The main vessels that provide the primary blood supply of the nodule may sometimes be determined and exposed to laser coagulation. This helps to change the nodule from being hypervascular to hypovascular more effectively. A decrease in nodule size is usually not achieved during the first stage, and PLA efficacy is assessed only on color-flow Doppler data. Nodule size decreases only after the substantial reduction in its vascularity (Fig. 15.41). The second stage of PLA aims to shrink the nodule. This is similar to the management of hypovascular nodules described above. The procedure is expected to have the least effect on nodules with extreme hypovascularity (due to the prevalence of fibrous changes) or extreme hypervascularity (due to the difficulties involved in reducing the blood flow, and the fact that hemorrhages often occur within the nodule).

PLA allows the effective management of recurrent goiter. Positive dynamics are noted in 70% of patients with infracentimetric nodules, in 80% of patients with nodules 1–2 cm in size, and in 34% of patients with nodules larger than 2 cm in size. Seliverstov (2003)

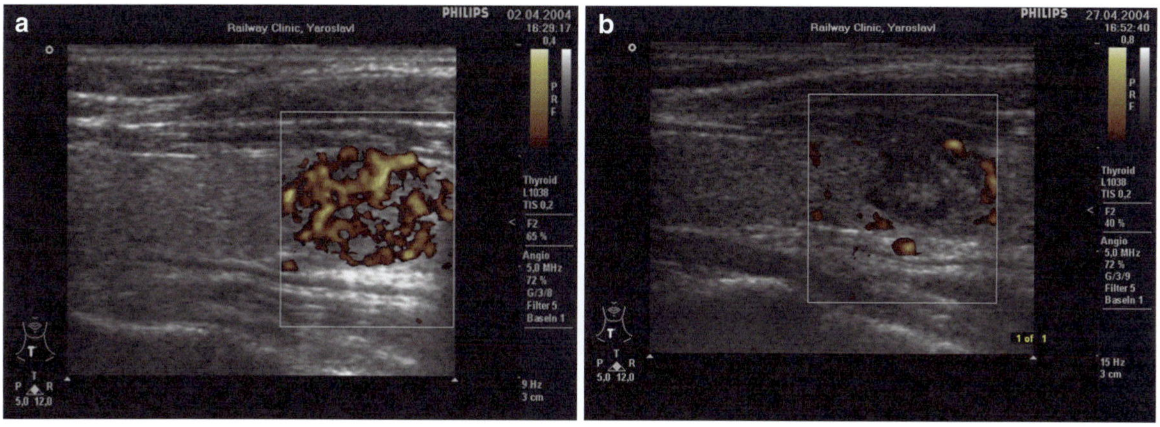

Fig. 15.41 (**a**, **b**) Nodule vascularity change one month after PLA

reports that a positive effect is observed within four years of PLA in 94.6% of patients with recurrent euthyroid nodular goiter (in 5.4% the nodules disappear, and in 89.2% the nodules show an average 4.7-fold decrease). A positive effect of PLA is seen in all patients with recurrent Graves' disease.

Any suspicion of thyroid malignancy is an absolute contraindication for PLA. However, there are individual publications regarding the utilization of PLA for unresectable locally extended cases of thyroid carcinoma (Pacella et al. 2000; Privalov et al. 2004). Those authors report that PLA reduces tumor size, constrains its growth, and decreases compression syndrome. At the same time, the relation between the US image and the actual volume of tumor necrosis is unpredictable. Because the tumor merges into the surrounding organs and tissues, it is only possible to achieve a partial decrease in volume instead of complete tumor ablation.

Easy management, variability of regimens, and local damage are characteristics of thyroid PLA. Nevertheless, many authors consider that PLA should only be performed in a specialized center, due to possible side-effects and complications. Complications may appear during nodule puncture, PLA performance, the early postoperative period, and the after-treatment stage.

Some complications are diagnosed clinically. Most of these can be detected with US (Figs. 15.42 and 15.43):

1. Nonspecific side-effects and complications are associated with inaccuracy of thyroid puncture (these are common side-effects and complications of FNAB): bleeding from large veins and arteries of the neck, from subcutaneous veins, and thyroid vessels; thrombosis of the jugular vein; injury to the carotid arteries with atherosclerotic plaque rupture, embolism or thrombosis; hemorrhage into nodule or cyst; hematoma; puncture of the nervous trunks and plexus; puncture of the trachea or esophagus.
2. Specific PLA complications include: dysphonia; optical fiber tip breakage with subsequent formation of granuloma; combustion of skin and neck organs (Table 15.5).

Most patients tolerate PLA well. Choosing the appropriate parameters for laser irradiation for each individual patient will help to minimize their discomfort. Iatrogenic damage during PLA is rare, and is strongly linked with the human factor: the accuracy and experience of the personnel. PLA demands that the indications are defined carefully and that the procedure is performed carefully.

15.4 Radiofrequency Ablation

Radiofrequency ablation (RFA) of thyroid nodules is one of the "youngest" modalities that demonstrated promising results. The first publications on RFA, which occurred in the late 1980s, referred to treatment of liver metastases, but RFA was quickly and successfully

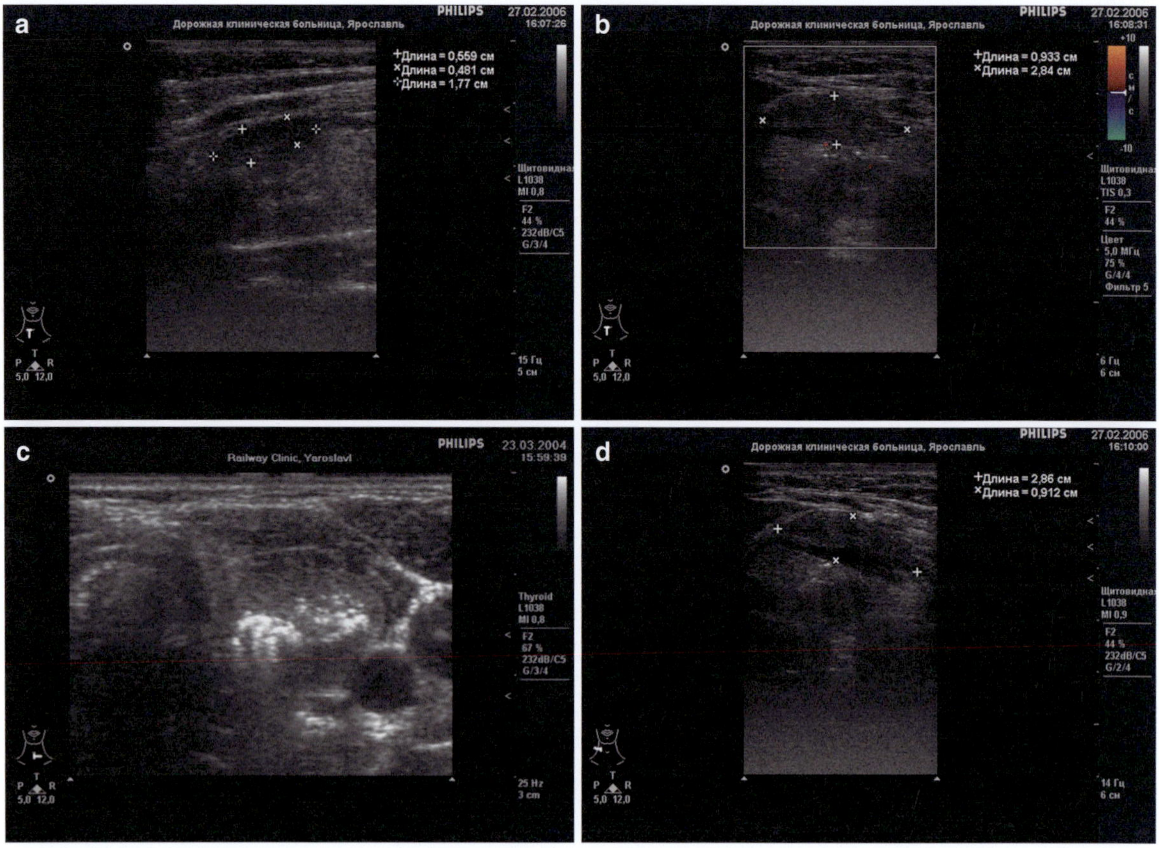

Fig. 15.42 (**a–d**) Complication of PLA. Subcapsular hematoma

applied to lesions in other organs too. RFA of thyroid nodules was introduced in 2004. The method is based on local hyperthermia of the thyroid nodule. The application of temperatures above 50°C leads to irreversible tissue changes with subsequent replacement of the necrotic area with connective tissue. Differences in RFA techniques, as reported by several authors, relate to power supply, exposure, and the geometry of the necrotic zone. It should be noted that this "young" method of treating thyroid nodules is carried out by experienced specialists using complex and expensive high-technology equipment.

The main group of patients that receive RFA is elderly people with bad concomitant diseases, usually of the cardiovascular system. The indications for thyroid surgery on the one hand and the objective difficulties involved in performing it on the other call for the implementation of minimally invasive procedures. According to Deandrea et al. (2008), RFA is indicated mainly for the treatment of patients with large autonomous thyroid nodules that cause thyrotoxicosis.

US-guided RFA is staged as follows:

1. Introduction of the needle into the thyroid nodule
2. Insertion of conductors with temperature sensors into the nodule under mild general anesthesia
3. Creation of a high-frequency electromagnetic field between the conductors
4. Heating and coagulation of the lesion
5. US follow-up after the procedure

The thyroid nodule can be heated during RFA up to temperature of 105°C within 2 min, which causes intracellular fluid to boil and results in the irreversible damage to the nodule cells. Applying a temperature of 50°C leads to cell destruction within 4–6 min, >60°C to instant coagulation, and ≥100°C to boiling and tissue carbonization. It is considered that the optimum temperature for RFA is 50–100°C.

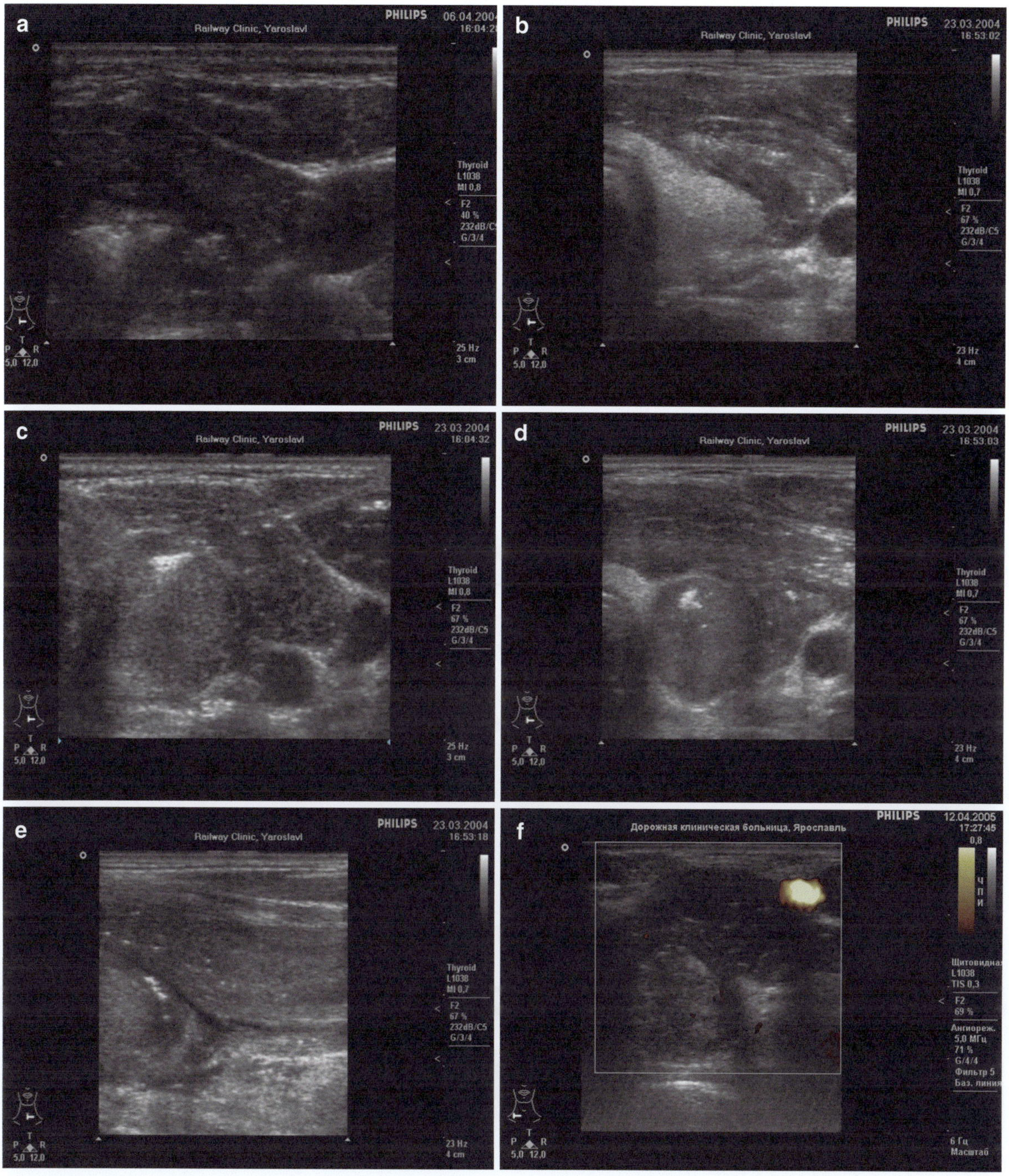

Fig. 15.43 (**a–e**) Complication of PLA. Interfascial hematoma

Table 15.5 Side-effects and complications of PLA

Side-effects and complications	References	Rate
Discomfort	Dossing et al. (2002) Our data (n=400)	Registered 55.25%
Cervical pain	Pacella et al. (2000) Dossing et al. (2002) Spiezia et al. (2003) Seliverstov and Fajzrahmanov (2004) Døssing et al. (2007) Papini et al. (2004) Our data (n=400)	Registered 6 of 16 4 of 12 In almost all cases 5 of 15 Registered 57%
Subfebrility	Pacella et al. (2000) Our data (n=400)	Registered 6.5%
Dysphonia	Pacella et al. (2004) Spiezia et al. (2003) Our data (n=400)	2 of 76 1 of 12 4.25%
Subcapsular hematoma	Cakir et.al. (2008)	Registered

Example of the US report at PLA:

First name, middle initial, last name:
Age:
Date:
A 19G needle was introduced into the 11x18x23 mm (volume 2.3cm3) heterogeneous hypovascular (in CDI and PDI) nodule in the middle compartment of the left lobe of the thyroid gland under US guidance with free hand technique in aseptic conditions.
US guided percutaneous laser ablation with a medical diode laser "LAMI" was performed.
Laser power 3.5W, impulse duration 200ms and interval 10ms, pulse number 2430.
Visualization during the procedure was satisfactory.
The patient tolerated the procedure satisfactory, somatic status without changes. Compression with aseptic bandage was applied to the puncture site for 10 minutes. The next visit is recommended in 4 weeks.
The surgeon (endocrinologist):
The US specialist:

Example of US report in 6 months after PLA:

First name, middle initial, last name:
Age:
Date:
6 months after PLA of the 11x18x23 mm (volume 2.3cm3) heterogeneous hypovascular (in CDI and PDI) nodule in the middle compartment of the left lobe of the thyroid gland. The nodule has decreased to 6*8*11 mm (volume 0.26 cm3), the form is irregular roundish, echostructure is heterogeneous hypoechoic with increased echodensity in the central compartment, with indistinct margins, avascular.
The next visit is recommended in 3 months.
The surgeon (endocrinologist):
The US specialist:

The morphological structure of tissue damage resulting from RFA differs from those obtained with PLA and PEI. RFA results in the formation of an area of total necrosis with practically unchanged tissue architectonics. The zone of total necrosis is surrounded by a thin zone of partial necrosis that corresponds to a transition to the outer zone of intact thyroid tissue. These morphological features mean that the US image after RFA differs from that after PLA.

Open, endoscopic, or percutaneous access can be used for RFA in thyroid nodules. Guidance is preferably performed by US with color-flow Doppler.

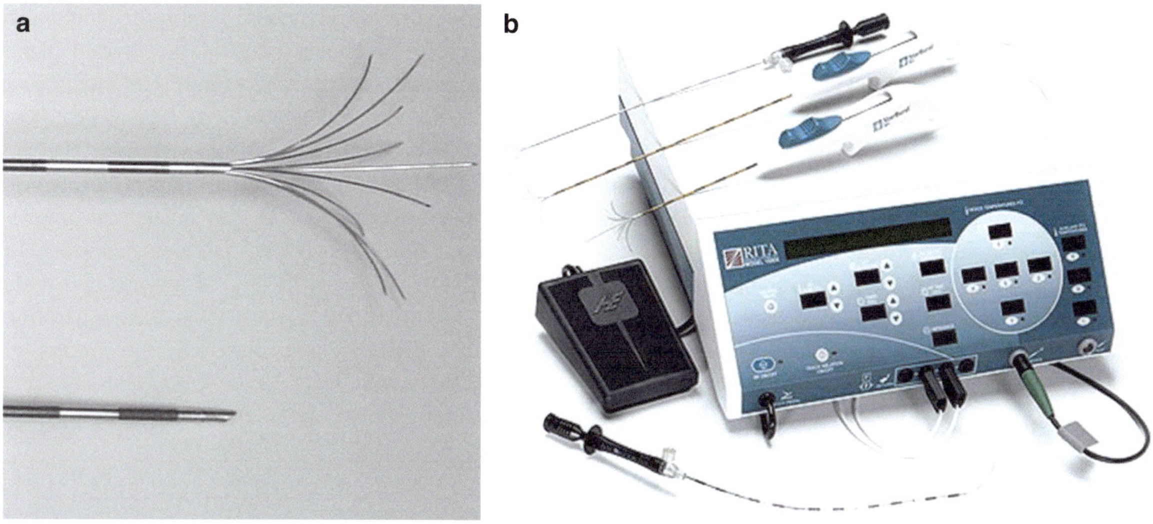

Fig. 15.44 "Umbrella-shaped" RFA device. (**a**) Radiofrequency generator (**b**)

Grayscale US reveals hyperechoic arc-shaped signals that originate proximal to the electrodes due to the appearance of steam during RFA. It is thought that this picture indicates correct RFA performance. Intensively stained hindrances of various sizes and shapes caused by gas bubbles are registered dorsal to the electrodes in CDI and PDI modes. On the whole, the US picture is close to that observed during PLA guidance.

The disadvantages of single-electrode RFA are irregular tissue heating due to the irregular resistance and blood supply of tissue, overheating of tissue adjacent to the electrode, and a maximum diameter of the locus of ablation of ≤16 mm. The situation is improved by using "umbrella-shaped" electrodes that can "warm up" nodules 50–60 mm or larger in size (Fig. 15.44).

When the procedure is finished, the conductors are pulled back into the needle and the needle is removed. Doppler mapping at this moment reveals a completely avascular spherical region where the RFA was applied, which contrasts with the mixed vascularity of the surrounding tissue. During RFA, constantly monitoring the temperature within the nodule makes the procedure safer and permits fast ablation of bigger nodules.

Subsequent monitoring of the reduction in the thyroid nodule is carried out with US. Changes in nodule size (volume), echodensity, echostructure, and vascularity, as well as the status of the surrounding thyroid tissue and neck organs are all assessed. It is reported that RFA decreases functional activity in 95% of all autonomous nodules 20–25 mm in size (Bubnov et al. 2008). This figure surpasses the results obtained with PEI and PLA. Sleptsov (2008) reports that a complete loss of functional activity in nodules up to 6 cm in size is possible using single-pass RFA.

RFA still has a number of disadvantages. The first is the high cost of the equipment and expendable material required. The second is the limited experience of this modality in thyroid surgery. The third is that RFA causes a large, high-temperature zone in the neck that can potentially result in serious complications. Therefore, according to the opinions of RFA pioneers, the method can only be safely performed in medical centers that have substantial MIP experience.

15.5 Conclusion

The diagnosis of thyroid disease is complicated by the difficulties, which are encountered during performance and interpretation of the results of modern examination techniques.

The diversity and variability of the diagnostic algorithms of thyroid disease as well as issues involving availability and cost of the corresponding diagnostic procedures contribute to the complexity in the field. The role of each individual diagnostic method, including sonography is actively debated in the current scientific literature. In spite of recent advances in the diagnostic arsenal, a rational algorithm of work-up, universally applicable to a wide variety of thyroid pathology has not been developed.

Comparative analysis of different methods demonstrates that even the most advanced diagnostic procedures and a combination thereof do not always allow to solve the problem of an early differential diagnosis of nodular goiter, adenomas, or thyroid cancer. Insufficient efficacy of the existing methods increases surgical intervention and expands the indications for surgery.

US, which utilizes all modern complex technologies, permits precise characterization of the thyroid gland and surrounding structures. Dynamic US monitoring allows to assess the efficacy of non-surgical treatment and the adequacy of surgical interventions. Thyroid ultrasound has already acquired an important position and exhibits further rapid advances in years to come.

This book introduces our current view on the role of sonography in diagnosis of thyroid disease to a wide audience. We are ready for discussion and cooperation with both individual specialists and the groups of experts in this field.

References

Abalmasov VG, Ionova EA (2007) To the question on preoperative ultrasound diagnosis of the nodular pathology of the thyroid gland. Vestnik roentgenologii i radiologii 6:9–17 (Article in Russian)

Abalmasov VG, Evmenova TD, Moshneguts SV (2002) Magnetic resonance tomography of nodular lesions of the thyroid gland: comparison to the data of histological examination. Visualizaciya v clinicke 21:18–21 (Article in Russian)

Abbasova EV, Parhomenko RA, Shcherbenko OI (2005) Echography in differential diagnosis of benign and malignant lymphadenopathies in children. Materials of the scientific forum "Radiology-2005", Moscow, pp 3–4 (Article in Russian)

Abdulhalimova MM, Mitkov VV, Bondarenko VO (1999) Utilization of CDI in complex ultrasound diagnosis of thyroid nodules. Ultrazvukovaya diagnostica 1:74–78 (Article in Russian)

Abdulhalimova MM, Mitkov VV, Bondarenko VO, Zubarev AR (1999) Diagnosis of thyroid nodules with the use of modern examination modalities. Ultrazvukovaya diagnostica 3:69–81 (Article in Russian)

Agamov AG, Alexandrov YK, Sencha AN (2003) Diagnosis, treatment, and postoperative follow-up of patients with the diagnosis of thyroid cancer. Informatsionniy bulletin, Yaroslavl 2:18–23 (Article in Russian)

Agapitov YN (1996) Ultrasound monitoring of thyroid pathology in endemic region (the Upper Volga region). PhD thesis. Obninsk (Book in Russian)

Ahmedova FB, Filatov AA (2003) Radiology of thyroid cancer. Medicinskaya radiologiya i radiacionnaya bezopasnost 3(48):41–46 (Article in Russian)

Ahuja A, Evans R (eds) (2000) The thyroid and parathyroid. Practical head and neck ultrasound. Greenwich Medical Media Ltd, London, pp 37–58

Ahuja A, Chick W, King W, Metreweli C (1996) Clinical significance of the comet tail artifact in thyroid ultrasound. J Clin Ultrasound 24(3):129–133

Alberti B, Campatelli A, Antonelly A et al (1994) Review of a case series of cervical cysts and evaluation of the efficacy of sclerotherapy with tetracycline hydrochloride in thyroid cystic lesions. Clin Ther 145(7):27–33

Alexandrov YK (1996) Puncture methods in diagnosis and treatment of the diseases of the thyroid gland. Yaroslavl (Book in Russian)

Alexandrov YK (1997) The system of early active revealing, surgical treatment, and rehabilitation of the patients with nodular goiter in the endemic area. PhD thesis. Moscow (Book in Russian)

Alexandrov YK, Mogutov MS (2003) Ultrasound assessment of the efficacy of laser destruction of thyroid nodules. Abstracts of the 4-d Congress of the Russian Association of experts in ultrasound diagnostics in medicine. Moscow, p 298 (Article in Russian)

Alexandrov YK, Agapitov YN, Kudryavtsev BA, Uryvchikov AV (2002) Ultrasound diagnosis of nodular goiter: preoperative and intraoperative stages. Materials of the 2nd Congress "Actual problems of thyroid diseases". Moscow, pp 123–124 (Article in Russian)

Alexandrov YK, Mogutov MS, Patrunov YN, Sencha AN (2004) Ultrasound guidance of laser destruction in nodular goiter: the criteria of the selection of the patients, the assessment of efficacy, and postoperative follow-up. Visualizaciya v clinicke 24–25:18–22 (Article in Russian)

Alexandrov YK, Mogutov MS, Sencha AN, Patrunov YN (2004) Ultrasound guided laser destruction of thyroid nodules: indications and selection of patients. Echographiya 4:346–351 (Article in Russian)

Alexandrov YK, Patrunov YN, Mogutov MS, Sencha AN (2004) The value of Doppler mapping for laser destruction of thyroid nodules. Materials of the scientific forum "Achievements and prospects of modern radiology" – "Radiology-2004", Moscow, pp 7–8 (Article in Russian)

Alexandrov YK, Mogutov MS, Patrunov YN, Sencha AN (2005a) Minimally invasive surgery of the thyroid gland. Moscow, Medicine (Book in Russian)

Alexandrov YK, Mogutov MS, Patrunov YN, Sencha AN (2005) Ultrasound effects during interstitial laser photocoagulation of benign thyroid nodules. Ultrazvukovaya i funkcionalnaya diagnostica 6:8–12 (Article in Russian)

Alexandrov YK, Mogutov MS, Sencha AN, Patrunov YN (2005) Ultrasound criteria of the efficacy of laser destruction of thyroid nodules and postoperative follow-up. Ultrazvukovaya i funkcionalnaya diagnostica 4:11–17 (Article in Russian)

Alexandrov YK, Sencha AN, Patrunov YN, Buydina TA, Leynova EV (2005) Ultrasound guided intraglandular injections of glucocorticoids in the treatment of subacute thyroiditis. Abstracts of the 12th International conference "Modern status of non-invasive diagnostics in medicine" – "Angiodop-2004", Sochi, 23–24 (Article in Russian)

Alexandrov YK, Mogutov MS, Sencha AN, Patrunov YN (2006) Complications and side-effects of minimally invasive procedures in thyroid nodules. Ultrazvukovaya i funkcionalnaya diagnostica 2:29–39 (Article in Russian)

Allahverdieva GF, Sinyukova GT, Sholokhov VN, Romanov IS (2005) Possibilities of complex ultrasound examination in diagnosis of metastatic lymph nodes of the neck. Ultrazvukovaya i funkcionalnaya diagnostica 1:18–22 (Article in Russian)

Altivilla G, Pascale M, Nenci I (1990) Fine needle aspiration cytology of thyroid gland diseases. Acta Cytol 34:251–256

Altunina VS (1996) Ultrasound diagnosis of thyroid cancer recurrences. PhD thesis. Obninsk (Book in Russian)

Anguissola R, Bozzini A, Campani R et al (1991) Role of color-coded duplex sonography in the study of thyroid pathology. Radiol Med 81(6):831

Antonelli A, Campatelli A, Di Vito A et al (1994) Comparison between ethanol sclerotherapy and emptying with injection of saline in treatment of thyroid cysts. Clin Investig 72(12): 971–974

Argalia G, De Bernardis S, Mariani D et al (2002) Ultrasonographic contrast agent: evaluation of time-intensity curves in the characterization of solitary thyroid nodules. Radiol Med (Torino) 103(4):407–413

Artyomov AM, Ignatkov VY (2001) Possibilities of ultrasound diagnostics in autoimmune thyroid. Actualniye problemy sovremennoy endocrinologii. Moscow, p 263 (Article in Russian)

Atabekova LA, Vasilchenko SA, Burkov SG (1999) Complex ultrasound and cytological assessment of proliferative processes in the thyroid gland. Sonoace International 4:60–65 (Article in Russian)

Atkov OY (2002) The basic tendencies of the development of ultrasound methods of diagnosis. Visualizaciya v clinicke 20:4–9 (Article in Russian)

Ayache S, Mardyla N, Tramier B, Strunski V (2006) Clinical signs and correlation with radiological extent in a series of 117 retrosternal goitre. Rev Laryngol Otol Rhinol (Bord) 127(4): 229–237

Bagley JS, Ewen SW, Swith FW. Krukowski ZH (1996) Magnetic resonance imaging of thyroid swellings. Br J Surg 83(6):828–829

Balter SA, Paches AI, Anohin BM et al (1989) Ultrasound tomography in diagnosis of thyroid diseases. Voprosy oncologii 35(8):920 (Article in Russian)

Barsukov AN (2003) Sclerosing therapy of solid nodules of the thyroid gland. Vrachebnoye delo 7:90–93 (Article in Russian)

Barsukov AN, Konoplyov OA, Chebotaryov NV, Tolpygo VA (2000) Clinical classification of cystic lesions of the thyroid gland. Materials of the IX (XI) Russian workshop on surgical endocrinology "Modern aspects of surgical endocrinology", Chelyabinsk, pp 50–52 (Article in Russian)

Barsukov AN, Konoplyov OA, Chebotaryov NV, Tolpygo VA (2000) Methods of treatment of benign thyroid lesions. Materials of the IX (XI) Russian workshop on surgical endocrinology "Modern aspects of surgical endocrinology", Chelyabinsk, pp 52–55 (Article in Russian)

Bashilov VP, Markova EN, Reshetnikov EA et al (2005) Ultrasound technologies in diagnosis and planning of operations in patients with thyroid nodules. Khirurgiya 3:4–9 (Article in Russian)

Baskin HJ, Duick DS, Levine RA (eds) (2008) Thyroid ultrasound and ultrasound-guided FNA. Springer, NewYork

Bataeva RS, Mitkov VV, Mitkova MD (2006) Evaluation of the reproducibility of the results of ultrasound volumetry of the thyroid gland. Ultrazvukovaya i funkcionalnaya diagnostica 1:37–43 (Article in Russian)

Becker D, Bair HJ et al (1997) Thyroid autonomy with color-coded image-directed Doppler sonography: internal hypervascularization for the recognition of autonomous adenomas. J Clin Ultrasound 25(2):63–69

Belashkin II, Kulikova AD, Kochetkov AV, Kulikov MP (2003) Value of the second tissue harmonic in diagnosis of colloid nodules of the thyroid gland. Abstracts of the 4-th Congress of the Russian Association of experts in ultrasound diagnosis in medicine. Moscow, p 209 (Article in Russian)

Belfiore A, La Rosa GL (2001) Fine-needle aspiration biopsy of the thyroid. Endocrinol Metab Clin North Am 30: 361–400

Bellantone R, Lombardi CP, Rafaelli M et al (2004) Management of cystic or predominantly cystic thyroid nodules:the role of ultrasound-guided fine-needle aspiration biopsy. Thyroid 14(1):143–150

Beloborodov VA (1996) Functional ultrasound dopplerography in diagnosis of nodular diseases of the thyroid gland. PhD thesis. Irkutsk (Book in Russian)

Beloborodov VA (2000) Differential diagnosis and surgical tactics in thyroid nodules. PhD thesis. Irkutsk (Book in Russian)

Blinov NN (2005) Methods of computed tomography in medicine. Zdravoohraneniye i medicinskaya technika 3(17):10–11 (Article in Russian)

Bogin YN, Manevich NA, Shapiro NA (1990) Complex diagnostics of nodular forms of thyroid diseases. Clinicheskaya medicina 5:70 (Article in Russian)

Bramley MD, Harrison BJ (1996) Papillary microcarcinoma of the thyroid gland. Br J Surg 83:1874–1883

Bronstein ME (1997) Thyroid cancer. Problemy endocrinologii 6:33–37 (Article in Russian)

Bubnov AN, Kuzmichyov AS, Grinyova EN, Trunin EM (2002) Thyroid diseases. Part I. Nodular goiter. St.Petersburg (Book in Russian)

Cantalamessa L, Baldini M et al (1999) Thyroid nodules in Graves' disease and the risk of thyroid carcinoma. Arch Intern Med 159(15):1705–1708

Carmeci C, Jeffrey RB, McDougall IR et al (1998) Ultrasound-guided fine-needle aspiration biopsy of thyroid masses. Thyroid 8(4):283–289

Cherenko SM (1998) The differential diagnosis of nodular formations of the thyroid. Lik Sprava 6:136–140

Chissov EY, Trofimova EY (2003) Ultrasound examination of lymph nodules in oncology. Strom, Moscow (Book in Russian)

Chlu WY, Chia NH, Wan SK (1998) The investigation and management of thyroid nodules – a retrospective review of 183 cases. Ann Acad Med Singapore 27(2):196–199

Chumakov AA, Sukhanov GA, Alexandrov YK et al (1999) Possibilities of two-staged instrumental screening in revealing of thyroid diseases in endemic area. Vestnik khirurgii imeni I I Grekova 158(2):9–12 (Article in Russian)

Cognetti DM, Pribitkin EA, Keane WM (2008) Management of the neck in differentiated thyroid cancer. Surg Oncol Clin North Am 1:157–173

Court-Payen M, Nygaard B et al (2000) Color Doppler ultrasound in the initial assessment of palpable thyroid nodules. Ultrasound Med Biol 26(2):a180

Cui Y, Zhang Z, Li S, Li L, Zhang H, Li Z (2002) Diagnosis and surgical management for retrosternal thyroid mass. Chin Med Sci J 17(3):173–177

Dedov II et al (1994) Computed tomography in diagnosis of substernal goiter. Problemy endocrinologii 40(5):26–28 (Article in Russian)

Dedov II, Troshina EA, Alexandrova GF (1999) Diagnosis, treatment, and prophylaxis of nodular forms of thyroid diseases. Moscow (Book in Russian)

Dedov II, Troshina EA, Yushkov PY, Alexandrova GF, Buhman AI, Ignatkov VY (2001) Diagnosis of thyroid diseases. Moscow, Vidar (Book in Russian)

Dedov II, Melnichenko GA, Gerasimov GA et al (2003) Clinical recommendations of the Russian Association of endocrinologists for diagnosis and treatment of autoimmune thyroiditis in adults. Problemy endocrinologii 6:50–51

Demidchik EP, Tsyb AF, Lushnikov EF (1996) Thyroid cancer in children. Moscow, Medicine (Book in Russian)

Drozd VM, Lyshchik AP, Rayners K, Terehova ZV (2000) Clinical value of three-dimensional reconstruction of the image of the thyroid gland for early verification of the diagnosis. Novosti luchevoy diagnostiki 2:64–65 (Article in Russian)

Dusmuratov AM, Yuldasheva NS, Hapizov HN (1998) Puncture with echography guidance: prophylaxis of complications and increase in efficacy. Ultrazvukovaya diagnostika 4: 14–19 (Article in Russian)

Dustov A (2007) Molecular nuclear medicine in the management of thyroid cancer. Radiother Oncol 82(1):32

Erbil Y, Barbaros U, Ozbey N et al (2008) Graves' disease, with and without nodules, and the risk of thyroid carcinoma. J Laryngol Otol 122:291–295

Ershov GI (2004) Ways of improvement of thyroid cancer diagnostics. Khirurgiya 12:47–49 (Article in Russian)

Esen G (2006) Ultrasound of superficial lymph nodes. Eur J Radiol 58(3):345–359

Evtyuhina AN, Strokova LA (2003) Ultrasound diagnostics and magnetic resonance tomography in assessment of local invasion of thyroid cancer. Abstracts of the 4th Russian scientific forum "Radiology-2003". Moscow, pp 90–91 (Article in Russian)

Fadeev VV (2002) Thyroid nodules: international algorithms and domestic clinical practice. Vrach 7:12–16 (Article in Russian)

Filatov AA, Vetshev PS, Filimonov GP, Ahmedova FB (2002) About the complexity of differential diagnosis of autoimmune thyroiditis. Ultrazvukovaya i funkcionalnaya diagnostika 4:40–43 (Article in Russian)

Filatov AA, Vetshev PS, Filimonov GP, Ahmedova FB (2002) Role of computed tomography in differential diagnosis of substernal goiter. Radiologiya-practicka 3:32–34 (Article in Russian)

Fish SA, Langer JE, Mandel SJ (2008) Sonographic imaging of thyroid nodules and cervical lymph nodes. Endocrinol Metab Clin North Am 37(2):401–417

Fomina IY (2003) Role of high-frequency echography in diagnosis of de Quervain's thyroiditis. PhD thesis. Nijniy Novgorod (Book in Russian)

Fujimoto Y, Oka A, Omoto R, Hirose M (1967) Ultrasound scanning of the thyroid gland as a new diagnostic approach. Ultrasonics 5:177

Fukunari N, Mimura T, Ito K, Ito Ku (2000) Clinical evaluation of color-Doppler guided thyroid PEI therapy with US contrast agent. Abstracts of the 9th Congress of World Federation for Ultrasound in Medicine and Biology. J Ultrasound Med Biol 26(2):A181

Gabuniya RI, Kolesnikov EK (1995) Computed tomography in clinical diagnostics. Medicine, Moscow (Book in Russian)

Garbuzov PI (2002) Algorithms of diagnosis and treatment of highly differentiated thyroid cancer. Materials of 2nd Congress "Actual problems of the diseases of the thyroid gland". Moscow: 65–76 (Article in Russian)

Gerasimov GA, Troshin EA (1998) Differential diagnosis and the choice of method of treatment of nodular goiter. Problemy endocrinologii 5(44):35–41 (Article in Russian)

Gillenwater AM, Weber RS (1997) Thyroid carcinoma. Cancer Treat Res 90:149–169

Giovagnorio F, Caiazzo R, Avitto A (1997) Evaluation of vascular patterns of cervical lymph nodes with power Doppler sonography. J Clin Ultrasound 25:71–76

Gooding GAW (1993) Sonography of the thyroid and parathyroid. Radiol Clin North Am 31:967–989

Goriyanov VF, Balatsky MV et al (1999) Color Doppler visualization of blood flow in differential diagnosis of thyroid lesions in children. Vizualizaciya v clinicke 8:1–4 (Article in Russian)

Graif M, Itzchak Y, Strauss S, Dolev E et al (1987) Parathyroid sonography: diagnostic accuracy related to shape location and texture of the gland. Br J Radiol 60:439–443

Grineva EN, Malakhov TV, Goryushkina EV (2005) Role of fine needle aspiration biopsy in diagnosis of thyroid nodules. Problemy endocrinologii 1:10–15 (Article in Russian)

Gritzmann N (2007) Ultrasound and US-guided biopsy. European Radiology. ECR 2007. European Congress of Radiology. Austria. Book of Abstracts. 17(1):129

Hadting T, Herfarth C (1997) Diagnosis and therapy of thyroid carcinoma. Dtsch Med Wochenschr 122(36):1077–1080

Hajek PC, Salomonowitz E, Turk R, Tscholakoff D, Kumpan W, Czembirek H (1986) Lymph nodes of the neck: evaluation with US. Radiology 158:739–742

Hara H, Igarashi A, Yano Y et al (2001) Ultrasonographic features of parathyroid carcinoma. Endocr J 48(2):213–217

Harchenko VP, Korobkina ES (2003) Computed and magnetic resonance tomography in algorithm of diagnostics of the head and neck tumors. Abstracts of the 4th Russian scientific forum "Radiology-2003" Moscow, pp 380–384 (Article in Russian)

Harchenko VP, Kotlyarov PM (2003) Thyroid cancer – value of predictive diagnosis with ultrasound. Abstracts of the 4th Russian scientific forum "Radiology-2003". Moscow, pp 320–322 (Article in Russian)

Harchenko VP, Smetanina LI et al (1998) Comparison of the efficacy of ultrasound and radionuclide scan in diagnosis of thyroid diseases. Lechashchiy vrach 2:20–22 (Article in Russian)

Harchenko VP, Kotlyarov PM, Smetanin LI (1999) Ultrasound diagnosis of thyroid diseases. Strom, Moscow (Book in Russian)

Harchenko VP, Kotlyarov PM, Zubarev AR (2002) Diagnosis of thyroid cancer according to the data of ultrasound examination. Moscow (Book in Russian)

Harchenko VP, Kotlyarov PM, Kamalova KC (2004) Differential diagnosis of nodular forms of chronic autoimmune thyroiditis and thyroid cancer according to the data of ultrasound examination. Abstracts of the Russian scientific forum "Achievements and prospects of modern radiology". Moscow, pp 253–254 (Article in Russian)

Harchenko VP, Snigireva RY, Smetanina LI, Mikheyev NV (2005) Diagnostics of chronic autoimmune thyroiditis with ultrasound and radionuclide scan. Abstracts of the Russian scientific forum "Radiology-2005". Moscow, pp 517–518 (Article in Russian)

Harchenko VP, Miheeva NV, Smetanina LI, Shadauri EV (2006) Differential diagnosis of nodular colloid (adenomatous) goiter and chronic autoimmune thyroiditis with ultrasound. Abstracts of the 7th Russian Scientific forum "Radiology-2006". Moscow, pp 254–255 (Article in Russian)

Harchenko VP, Tsallagova ZS, Kotlyarov PM, Mikheyev NV (2007) Ultrasound examination in differential diagnosis of thyroid lesions of different origin. Vestnik roentgenologii i radilogii 1:25–30 (Article in Russian)

Harchenko VP, Kotlyarov PM, Sencha AN, Mogutov MS, Buylov VM (2008) Radiological methods in diagnostics of diffuse pathology of the thyroid gland (diffuse hyperplasia, Graves' disease). Ultrazvukovaya I funkcionalnaya diagnostika 1:21–34 (Article in Russian)

Hatada T, Okada K et al (1998) Evaluation of ultrasound-guided fine-needle aspiration biopsy for thyroid nodules. Am J Surg 175(2):133–136

Helmann KD, Schmelzer A (1997) Ultrasound diagnosis of the thyroid gland. HNO 45(12):1029–1039

Holmgren L (1997) Malignant neovascularization. Eur J Ultrasound 6(6):11

Hopkins CR, Reading CC (1995) Thyroid and parathyroid imaging. Semin Ultrasound CT MR 16(4):279–295

Horli A, Takashima S et al (1998) Primary thyroid lymphoma associated with metastatic thyroid tumor discrimination with US. Eur J Ultrasound 7(3):199–203

Ignjatovic M (2001) Intrathoracic goiter. Vojnosanit Pregl 58(1):47–63

Ilyin AA (1995) Ultrasound morphometry of the thyroid gland. PhD thesis. Obninsk (Book in Russian)

Ilyin AA, Terentyev RO, Rumyantsev PO, Vtyurin BM, Parshin VS (2000) Results of sclerotherapy of thyroid cysts. Visualizaciya v clinicke 12:8–11 (Article in Russian)

Ilyin AA, Marchenko EV, Rumyantsev PO, Severskaya NV, Medvedev VS (2003) Role of sclerotherapy in treatment of nodular goiter. Mejdunarodniy Journal radiacionnoy medicini 5(3):56–58 (Article in Russian)

Ilyin AA, Rumyantsev PO, Isaev PA, Medvedev VS, Vtyurin BM, Drozdovsky YA, Garbuzov PI (2003) Sporadic and family variants of medullary cancer of the thyroid gland. Problemy endocrinologii 5:45–48 (Article in Russian)

Ionova EA, Tambovtseva NM, Abalmasov VG (2006) Preoperative diagnosis of nodular pathology of the thyroid gland with radiology methods. Abstracts of the 7th scientific forum "Radiology-2006", Moscow, pp 95–96 (Article in Russian)

Kabala JE (2007) CT and MR imaging of thyroid and parathyroid pathology. European Radiology. ECR 2007. European Congress of Radiology. Vienna, Austria. Book of Abstracts. 17(1):129

Kalinin AP, Filonenko AA, Mitkov VV (1990) Value of echography in diagnostics of thyroid and parathyroid diseases. Medicinskaya radiologiya 4:56 (Article in Russian)

Kamalova KC (2005) Complex ultrasound examination in diagnostics of thyroid cancer witht chronic autoimmune thyroiditis. Abstracts of scientific forum "Radiology-2005". Moscow, pp 158–159 (Article in Russian)

Kaplan EL, Yashiro T, Salti G (1992) Primary hyperparathyroidism in the 1990s. Choice of surgical procedures for this disease. Ann Surg 215:300–317

Karmazanovsky GG, Nikitaev NS (2005) Computed tomography of the neck: differential diagnosis of extraorgan lesions. Vidar, Moscow (Book in Russian)

Kasatkin YN, Ametov AS, Mitkov VV (1989) Ultrasound diagnosis of thyroid lesions. Medicinskaya radiologiya 1:14 (Article in Russian)

Kasatkina EP, Shilin DE, Pykov MI (1999) Thyroid ultrasound in children and teenagers. Moscow, Vidar (Book in Russian)

Kazakevich VI (2007) Possibilities of ultrasound examination of the mediastinum in substernal diffusion of thyroid neoplasm. Sonoace International 16:58–65 (Article in Russian)

Khurana KK, Richards VI et al (1998) The role of ultrasonography-guided fine-needle aspiration biopsy in the management of nonpalpable and palpable thyroid nodules. Thyroid 8(6):511–515

Klemens B, Wieler H, Kaiser KP (1997) Color-coded Doppler sonography in the differential diagnosis of nodular thyroid gland changes. Nuklermedizin 36(7):245–249

Kolokasidis I (1999) Magnetic resonance tomography in thyroid lesions. PhD thesis. Moscow (Book in Russian)

Kolokasidis I, Ahadov TA, Snegiryov RY (1999) Magnetic resonance tomography in diagnosis of thyroid diseases. Medicinskaya visualizaciya 1:11–15 (Article in Russian)

Kolosyuk VA (2000) Primary multiple tumors in patients with thyroid cancer. PhD thesis. St.Petersburg (Book in Russian)

Kononenko SN Early diagnosis and the differentiated treatment of thyroid cancer. Khirurgia (2000) 3:38–41 (Article in Russian)

Konovalov VA, Zubeev PS (2004) Possibilities of spectral dopplerography in differential diagnosis of thyroid lesions. Abstracts of the 8th Workshop with the international participation "Modern methods of instrumental diagnostics". Moscow: Strom, pp 264–265 (Article in Russian)

Kotlyarov PM (2000) Ultrasound features of malignancy. Abstracts of the 1st Scientific Forum "Radiology-2000". Moscow, pp 336–338 (Article in Russian)

Kotlyarov PM, Yanushpolskaya TO, Alexandrov YK, Agapitov YN, Sencha AN (2001) Ultrasound examination in diagnosis of thyroid cancer and its recurrences. Echographiya 4(2):349–354 (Article in Russian)

Kotova IV, Kalinin AP (2003) Modern methods of diagnosis of primary hyperparathyroidism. Problemy endocrinologii 6:46–50 (Article in Russian)

Kouvaraki MA, Shapiro SE, Fornage BD et al (2003) Role of preoperative ultrasonography in the surgical management of patients with thyroid cancer. Surgery 134(6):946–954

Kurzantseva OM, Murashkovskiy AL, Evmenova et al (2006) Experience of ultrasound examination with color Doppler mapping in diagnosis and differential diagnosis of thyroid lesions. Sonoace International 14:90–94 (Article in Russian)

Kuzmichyov AS (2002) Nodular goiter (diagnosis, treatment tactics). PhD thesis. St.Petersburg (Book in Russian)

Kuznetcov NA, Brontveyn AT, Abulov SE, Lapchenko MI, Nazarenko VA, Simeons IG (2002) Early diagnosis and the tactics of treatment of thyroid lesions. Russkiy medicinskiy Journal 3:13–16 (Article in Russian)

Lagalla R, Caruso J, Midiri M et al (1994) Vascular pattern of thyroid nodules: classification based on color Doppler imaging. Visualizaciya v clinicke 4:21–25 (Article in Russian)

Larson SM, Robbins R (2002) Positron emission tomography in thyroid cancer management. Semin Roentg 37(2):169–174

Laszlo H, Steen K (1998) Ultrasonography in the evaluation of cold thyroid nodules. Eur J Endocr 138:30–31

Lebedeva TP, Pashchevsky SA, Kotovich VM, Kuzmichev AS (2001) Fine needle biopsy in preoperative diagnosis of thyroid diseases. Materials of the 4th Russian Congress of Endocrinologists. St.Petersburg, p 332 (Article in Russian)

Lelyuk VG, Lelyuk SE (2007) Some methodological aspects of complex ultrasound examination of the thyroid gland. Moscow (Book in Russian)

Lelyuk VG, Lelyuk SE (2007b) Ultrasound angiology. Real time, Moscow (Book in Russian)

Lin JD, Huang BY et al (1997) Thyroid ultrasonography with fine-needle aspiration cytology for the diagnosis of thyroid cancer. J Clin Ultrasound 25(3):111–118

Lindenbraten LD, Zubarev AV, China VV, Shehter AI (1997) Dasic clinical syndromes and tactics of radiological examination. Vidar, Moscow (Book in Russian)

Lindop JE, Treece GM, Gee AH, Prager RW (2006) 3D elastography using freehand ultrasound. J Ultrasound Med Biol 32(4):529–545

Lippi F, Ferrari C, Manetti L et al (1996) Treatment of solitary autonomous thyroid nodules by percutaneous ethanol injection:results of an Italy multicenter study. The Multicenter Study Group. J Clin Endocrinol Metab 81(9):3261–3264

LiVolsi VA, Asa SL (2002) Endocrine Pathology. Elsevier Science, Philadelphia

Lushnikov EF, Vtyurin BM, Tsyb AF (2003) Thyroid microcarcinoma. Medicine, Moscow (Book in Russian)

Mack MG, Rieger J, Baghi M, Bisdas S, Vogl TJ (2008) Cervical lymph nodes. European J Radiol 66(3):493–500

Mackle T, Meaney J, Timon C (2006) Tracheoesophageal compression associated with substernal goitre. Correlation of symptoms with cross-sectional imaging findings. J Laryngol Otol 26:1–4

Manzone TA, Dam HQ, Intenzo CM et al (2008) Postoperative management of thyroid carcinoma. Surg Oncol Clin North Am 17(1):197–218

Marchenko EV (2003) Role of ultrasound guided sclerotherapy in treatment of nodular goiter. PhD thesis. Obninsk (Book in Russian)

Markova NV (2001) Value of ultrasound angiography in diagnosis of typical thyroid diseases. PhD thesis. Moscow (Book in Russian)

Markova EN (2004) Three-dimensional virtual tomography and ultrasound angiography in diagnosis of thyroid lesions. PhD thesis. Moscow (Book in Russian)

Markova NV, Zubarev AV et al (2001) Ultrasound examination of thyroid lesions. Khirurgiya 1:67–71 (Article in Russian)

Markova EN, Bashilov VP, Gazhonova VE, Minchenkov DV, Zubarev AV (2005) Complex ultrasound diagnosis of impalpable thyroid lesions. Abstracts of the Russian scientific forum "Radiology – 2005". Moscow, pp 253–254 (Article in Russian)

Martino E, Bogassi F (2000) Percutaneous ethanol injection for thyroid diseases. Thyroid Int 5:3–9

Masin EM, Alexandrov YK (2004) Ultrasound changes at laser destruction of benign thyroid nodules. Abstracts of the Russian scientific forum "Achievements and prospects of modern radiology" – "Radiology-2004". Moscow, pp 129–131 (Article in Russian)

Mazzaferri EL, Amdur RJ (eds) (2005) Essentials of thyroid cancer management. Springer, Berlin

Mazzaferri EL, Harmer C, Mallick UK, Kendall-Taylor P (eds) (2006) Practical management of thyroid cancer – a multidisciplinary approach. Springer, berlin

Mazzeo S, Toni MG, Pignatelli V et al (1991) The echo-guided percutaneous injection of ethanol: a therapeutic alternative in the "autonomous thyroid nodule". Our experience. Radiol Med (Torino) 82(6):776–781

Mazzeo S, Caramella D, Letncioni R et al (1997) Usefulness of echocolor Doppler in differentiating parathyroid lesions from other cervical masses. Eur Radiol 7(1):90–95

McDougall IR (2006) Management of thyroid cancer and related nodular disease. Springer, Berlin

Melnichenko GA (2002) Problems of classification and clinical diagnosis of nodular goiter. Materials of the 2nd Russian Congress "Actual problems of thyroid diseases", Moscow, pp 43–49 (Article in Russian)

Messina G, Viceconti N, Trinti B (1996) Echography and color Doppler in the diagnosis of thyroid carcinoma. Ann Ital Med Int 11(4):263–267

Mikheyeva NV (2003) Ultrasound examination and scintigraphy in diagnosis of thyroid lesions of various origin. PhD thesis. Moscow (Book in Russian)

Mikheyeva NV, Smetanina LI, Shadauri EV (2006) Differential diagnosis of acute (subacute) thyroiditis and thyroid cancer by ultrasound. Abstracts of the 7th Russian scientific forum "Radiology-2006". Moscow, pp 168–169 (Article in Russian)

Mitkov VV (ed) (1997) Clinical manual of ultrasound diagnostics, vol 2. Vidar, Moscow, pp 371–395 (Book in Russian)

Mitkov VV (ed) (2005) Practical manual of ultrasound diagnostics. General ultrasound diagnostics. Vidar, Moscow (Book in Russian)

Mitkov VV, Ignashin NS (1997) Echography of the parathyroids. In: Mitkov VV (ed) Clinical manual of ultrasound diagnosis, vol 4. Vidar, Moscow, pp 119–121 (Book in Russian)

Mitkov VV, Bataeva RS, Mitkova MD (2003) Three-dimensional echography in assessment of the volume of the thyroid gland. Ultrazvukovaya i funkcionalnaya diagnostica 4:35–41 (Article in Russian)

Mogutov MS (2007) Efficacy of interstitial laser photocoagulation in the treatment of nodular goiter. Annaly khirurgii 3:23–27 (Article in Russian)

Mogutov MS (2009) Ultrasound-assisted operations for thyroid diseases. PhD thesis. Moscow (Book in Russian)

Mogutov MS, Alexandrov YK, Goldobin VA, Sencha AN (2004) Complex ultrasound diagnosis of metastatic lymph nodes of the neck in thyroid cancer. Abstracts of the 11th International conference "Modern status of non-invasive diagnosis in medicine" – Angiodop – 2004, Sochi, pp 244–246 (Article in Russian)

Mogutov MS, Alexandrov YK, Goldobin VA, Sencha AN, Patrunov YN (2006) Sonographic visualization at interstitial laser photocoagulation of benign thyroid nodules. Ultrasound in medicine and biology. Abstracts of the 11th Congress of WFUMB. Seoul. Korea. 32(5):184

Mogutov MS, Alexandrov YK, Patrunov YN, Sencha AN, Mitkov VV (2006) Ultrasound effects at interstitial laser photocoagulation in nodular goiter. Ultrasound in medicine and biology. Abstracts of the 11th Congress of WFUMB. Seoul. Korea, 32(5):185

Mogutov MS, Alexandrov YK, Sheverdova EA (2007) The system of surgical aid for patients with thyroid lesions. Annaly khirurgii 6:14–17 (Article in Russian)

Moon WJ, Jung SL, Lee JH et al (2008) Benign and malignant thyroid nodules: US differentiation-multicenter retrospective study. Radiology 247(3):762–770

Morozov DA (1997) Optimization of differential diagnosis of thyroid lesions in children. PhD thesis. Moscow (Book in Russian)

Nakahara H, Noguchi S, Murakami N et al (1997) Gadolinium-enhanced MR imaging of thyroid and parathyroid masses. Radiology 3:202–203

Narhova NP (2004) Methodology and efficacy of ultrasound screening in early diagnosis of cancer and nontumor diseases of the thyroid gland. PhD thesis. Obninsk (Book in Russian)

Nazarenko GI, Krasnova TV, Zykova NA, Hitrova AN, Konovalov AY, Kuchin GA (2004) Technological aspects of diagnosis of parathyroid tumors by means of radiological methods. Ultrazvukovaya i funkcionalnaya diagnostika 4:15–22 (Article in Russian)

Neff RL, Farrar WB, Kloos RT, Burman KD (2008) Anaplastic thyroid cancer. Endocr Metab Clin North Am 37(2): 525–538

Nicolaeva ST, Gachilova R et al (2000) Is there any place of the contrast ultrasound of the thyroid gland in differential diagnosis of the small sized solid lesions. Ultrasound in medicine and biology. Abstracts of the 9th Congress of WFUMB. Florence. Italy, 26(2):a181

Noma S, Kanaoka M et al (1988) Thyroid masses: MR imaging and pathologic correlation. Radiology 168(3):759–764

Oertli D, Udelsman R (2007) Surgery of the thyroid and parathyroid glands. Springer, Berlin

Ogawa Y, Kato Y, Ikeda K et al (2001) The value of ultrasound-guided fine-needle aspiration cytology for thyroid nodules: an assessment of its diagnostic potential and pitfalls. Surg Today 31(2):97–101

Olshansky VO, Sergeev SA et al (1996) Primary multiple tumors in patients with thyroid neoplasms. Khirurgiya endocrinnih zhelez. St.Petersburg, pp 80–82 (Article in Russian)

Orlov SA, Zelenin AA, Trusov VV (2004) Preoperative radionuclide scan of thyroid cancer. Abstracts of the Russian scientific forum "Achievements and prospects of modern radiology". Moscow, pp 158–159 (Article in Russian)

Pacella CM, Papini E, Bizzarri G, Fabbrini R, Anelli V, Rinaldi R, Valle D, Nardi F (1995) Assessment of the effect of percutaneous ethanol injection in autonomously functioning thyroid nodules by colour-coded duplex sonography. Eur Radiol 5:395–400

Pacella CM, Gugliemi R et al (1998) Papillary carcinoma in small hypoechoic thyroid nodules: predictive value of echocolor Doppler evaluation. Preliminary results. J Exp Clin Cancer Res 1:127–128

Paches AI, Propp RM (1995) Thyroid cancer. Moscow (Book in Russian)

Parshin VS (1994) Ultrasound diagnosis of thyroid diseases (the data of clinical and screening examinations). PhD thesis. Obninsk (Book in Russian)

Parshin VS, Terentyev RO et al (1998) The possibilities of echography in preoperative diagnosis of thyroid cancer expansion out of the thyroid capsule. Visualizaciya v clinicke 12:16–20 (Article in Russian)

Parshin VS, Tarasova GP et al (1999) Ultrasound screening in diagnosis of thyroid diseases. Methodical aspects and efficacy. Visualizaciya v clinicke 14–15:1–8 (Article in Russian)

Parshin VS, Yamasita S, Tsyb AF (2000) Goiter. Ultrasound diagnostics. The clinical atlas. Nagasaki-Obninsk (Book in Russian)

Parshin VS, Tsyb AF, Tarasova GP (2001) Ultrasound diagnosis of diffuse euthyroid goiter. Actualniye problemy sovremennoy endocrinologii. Obninsk, p 358 (Article in Russian)

Parshin VS, Tsyb AF, Yamasita S (2002) Ultrasound diagnosis. Clinical atlas: Chernobyl data. Obninsk (Book in Russian)

Pashchevsky SA (2004) Possibilities of ultrasonography in complex radiological diagnostics and treatment of thyroid diseases. PhD thesis. St.Petersburg (Book in Russian)

Pashchevsky SA, Bubnov AN, Trunin EN et al (2001) Ultrasound semiotics of thyroid lesions. Materials of the 4th Russian Congress of Endocrinologists. St.Petersburg, p 359 (Article in Russian)

Pinsky SV, Dvornichenko VV, Beloborodov VA (1999) Thyroid tumors. Irkutsk (Book in Russian)

Pinsky SV, Kalinin AP, Beloborodov VA (2005) Diagnosis of thyroid diseases. Medicine, Moscow (Book in Russian)

Pishchik VG (2008) Mediastinal neoplasms: the principles of differential diagnosis and surgical treatment. PhD thesis. S-Petersburg (Book in Russian)

Pleshkov VG, Barsukov AN, Konoplyov OA et al (1999) Possibilities of sclerosing therapy for benign thyroid nodules. Abstracts of VIII (X) Russian workshop on surgical endocrinology "Modern aspects of surgical endocrinology". Kazan, pp 245–248 (Article in Russian)

Pleshkova NM (1997) Dynamic and static scintigraphy with ^{99m}Tc-Pertechnetate in thyroid lesions. Actualniye voprosy endocrinologii. Perm, p 88 (Article in Russian)

Podvyaznikov SO (1998) Thyroid cancer (clinic, diagnosis, treatment). Russkiy medicinsky Journal 10(6):658–668 (Article in Russian)

Portnoy LM (2001) The role of algorithms in modern radiologys. Abstracts of the 8th Russian Congress of roentgenologists and radiologists "Algorithms in radiological diagnostics and programs of nuclear and complex treatment of patients" – "Radiology-2001". Moscow, pp 312–317 (Article in Russian)

Pripachkina AP (1997) The possibilities of ultrasound in diagnosis of thyroid tumors. PhD thesis. Moscow (Book in Russian)

Privalov VA, Seliverstov OV, Revel-Muroz ZhA et al (2001) Percutaneous laser induced thermotherapy of nodular goiter. Khirurgiya 4:10–13 (Article in Russian)

Privalov VA, Seliverstov OV, Kochneva EV et al (2004) Laser technologies in the treatment of locally extended thyroid cancer. Abstracts the 12(14) Russian workshop on surgical endocrinology with international participation "Modern aspects of surgical endocrinology". Yaroslavl, pp 207–210 (Article in Russian)

Pykov MI, Vatolin KV (1998) Clinical of ultrasound diagnostics in pediatrics. Vidar, Moscow (Book in Russian)

Pykov MI, Vatolin KV (eds) (2001) Clinical manual of ultrasound diagnostics in pediatrics. Ultrasound examination of the thyroid gland. Vidar, Moscow , pp 556–591 (Book in Russian)

Pykov MI, Shilin DE et al (1997) Thyroid gland in healthy children:quantitative parameters of echodensity and blood flow. Visualizaciya v clinicke 10:15–20 (Article in Russian)

Rago T, Vitti P et al (1998) Role of conventional ultrasonography and color flow Doppler sonography in predicting malignancy in cold thyroid nodules. Eur J Endocrinol 138(1): 41–46

Randel SB, Gooding GAW, Clark OH et al (1987) Parathyroid variants: US evaluation. Radiol 165:191–194

Ravetto C, Colombo L, Dottorini ME (2000) Usefulness of nine-needle aspiration in the diagnosis of thyroid carcinoma: a retrospective study in 37, 895 patients. Cancer 90(6): 357–363

Reading CC, Charboneau WJ, James EM et al (1982) High resolution parathyroid sonography. AJR 139:539–546

Revel-Muroz ZhA (1999) Dynamics of reparative and adaptive processes in the thyroid gland after influence of high-intensive laser radiation of near infrared range. PhD thesis. Chelyabinsk (Book in Russian)

Romanchishen AF, Gostimsky AV (1996) Diagnosis and principles of surgical treatment of thyroid carcinomas in children and teenagers. Abstracts of the 5-th Russian workshop on surgical endocrinology. Ulyanovsk, pp 113–118 (Article in Russian)

Romanko SI (1997) Echosemiotics of solitary solid thyroid lesions. PhD thesis. Obninsk (Book in Russian)

Romanko SI, Zhelonkina NV, Solovyeva LP (2003) Role of ultrasound guided fine needle aspiration biopsy in differential diagnosis of nodular pathology of the thyroid gland. Abstracts of the 4th Congress of the Russian Association of experts in ultrasound diagnosis in medicine. Moscow, pp 310–311 (Article in Russian)

Rubello D, Pelizzo MR, Al-Nahhas A et al (2006) The role of sentinel lymph node biopsy in patients with differentiated thyroid carcinoma. Eur J Surg Oncol 32(9):917–921

Rusakov VF (1994) To the question on diagnostic value of various methods of examination of thyroid diseases. PhD thesis. St.Petersburg (Book in Russian)

Rutherford GC, Franc B, O'Connor A (2008) Nuclear medicine in the assessment of differentiated thyroid cancer. Clin Radiol 63(4):453–463

Salvatori M, Raffaelli M, Castaldi P et al (2007) Evaluation of the surgical completeness after total thyroidectomy for differentiated thyroid carcinoma. Eur J Surg Oncol 33: 648–654

Sandrikov VA, Fisenko EP, Struchkova TY (2008) Complex ultrasound examination of the thyroid gland. Strom, Moscow (Book in Russian)

Sciume C, Geraci G, Pisello F, LiVolsi F, Facella T, Modica G (2005) Substernal goitre. Personal experience. Ann Ital Chir 76(6):517–521

Sekach NS, Hlyavin VI, Rzheutsky VA (1997) Perspective directions in ultrasound diagnosis of thyroid diseases. Medicinskiye novosti 9:26–27 (Article in Russian)

Seliverstov OV, Fayzrahmanov AB (2004) Use of high-intensive laser radiation in the treatment of thyroid diseases. Abstracts of the 12(14) Russian workshop on surgical endocrinology with the international participation "Modern aspects of surgical endocrinology". Yaroslavl, pp 235–238 (Article in Russian)

Seliverstov OV, Privalov VL, Demidov AK (1999) Sclerotherapy of postoperative recurrent goiter. Abstracts of VIII (X) Russian workshop on surgical endocrinology "Modern aspects of surgical endocrinology". Kazan, pp 282–284 (Article in Russian)

Semenov VD, Ivanova NV, Diomidova VN (2001) Choice of radiology method in the program of examination of patients with thyroid diseases. Abstracts of the 8th Russian Congress of roentgenologists and radiologists "Algorithms in radiological diagnostics and programs of nuclear and complex treatment of patients" – "Radiology-2001". Moscow, p 159 (Article in Russian)

Semenov VD, Sverchkova LA, Pavlova YN (2006) Ultrasound diagnosis of thyroid lesions. Abstracts of the 7th Russian Scientific forum "Radiology-2006". Moscow, pp 217–218 (Article in Russian)

Semikov VI (2004) Therapeutic and diagnostic strategy in thyroid nodules. PhD thesis. Moscow (Book in Russian)

Sencha AN (2001) Diagnosis of thyroid cancer by ultrasound. PhD thesis. Moscow (Book in Russian)

Sencha AN (2006) Three-dimensional reconstruction of the ultrasound image in diagnosis of thyroid cancer. Ultrazvukovaya i funkcionalnaya diagnostica 3:117 (Article in Russian)

Sencha AN (2008) Radiological methods in diagnosis and treatment of thyroid diseases. PhD thesis. Moscow (Book in Russian)

Sencha AN (2008) Radiological methods in diagnosis of thyroid cancer. Ultrazvukovaya i funkcionalnaya diagnostica 2:30–36 (Article in Russian)

Sencha AN (2008) Ultrasound visualization of malignant tumors of the thyroid gland. Ultrazvukovaya i funkcionalnaya diagnostica 2:20–29 (Article in Russian)

Sencha AN, Belyaev DV, Neapolitanskiy VY (2005) Ultrasound diagnosis of parathyroid hyperplasia in patients with dialysis stage of chronic kidney failure. Abstracts of the Russian scientific forum "Radiology-2005". Moscow, pp 409–411 (Article in Russian)

Sencha AN, Alexandrov YK, Mogutov MS, Patrunov YN, Belyaev DV (2006) Ultrasound aspects of diapevtic procedures on the thyroid gland. Ultrazvukovaya i funkcionalnaya diagnostica 6:122–123 (Article in Russian)

Sencha AN, Alexandrov YK, Mogutov MS, Builov VM, Patrunov YN (2007a) Ultrasound-guided interstitial laser photocoagulation in patients with nodular goiter: indications, efficacy and follow-up principles. Eur Radiol 17(1):234

Sencha AN, Mogutov MS, Patrunov YN, Bahtin AL, Chuprin AG, Ignatovich MY (2007) Radiological visualization of neck lymph nodes in thyroid cancer. Abstracts of the Russian Congress of radiologists "Radiology-2007". Moscow, pp 333–334 (Article in Russian)

Sencha AN, Patrunov YN, Karpov AY, Sotskova NI (2007) Electroimpedance imaging as a method of diagnosis of thyroid diseases. Collection of proceedings. Neva radiological forum "New horizons". St.Petersburg, pp 502–503 (Article in Russian)

Severskaya NV (2002) Assessment of the value of radiological and non-radiological methods in diagnosis of thyroid cancer. PhD thesis. Obninsk (Book in Russian)

Shilin DE (2000) Clinical aspects of ultrasound diagnosis of thyroid diseases. Sonoace International 8:3–10 (Article in Russian)

Shilin DE, Pykov MI, Okminyan GF (2002) Ultrasound parameters of the thyroid gland in children. To the question on specifications the WHO. Ultrazvukivaya i funkcionalnaya diagnostica 2:59–64 (Article in Russian)

Shulutko AM, Semikov VI, Kulikov IO (2001) Application of sclerotherapy for the treatment of nodular goiter. Abstracts of the 4th Russian Congress of endocrinologists. St.Petersburg, p 418 (Article in Russian)

Shulutko AM, Semikov VI, Mironov MV et al (2004) Possibilities of ultrasound and FNAB in verification of morphological structure of thyroid lesions. Abstracts of the 12(14) Russian workshop on surgical endocrinology with international participation "Modern aspects of surgical endocrinology". Yaroslavl, pp 283–286 (Article in Russian)

Sigematsu I, Yamasita S, Ito M, Nagataki S (1996) Diagnosis of thyroid diseases. Tokyo

Sihuralidze EN (2001) Assessment of the efficacy of surgical method of local chemical destruction of benign thyroid nodules. PhD thesis. Yaroslavl (Book in Russian)

Smetanina LI (1998) Thyroid ultrasound. Lechashchiy vrach 2:18–20

Solbiati L, Rizzatto G, Ballarati E et al (1993) Practical implications of color doppler sonography of parathyroid gland: study of 203 tumors. Radiology 198:210

Spiezia S, Colao A et al (1996) Usefulness of color echo Doppler wish power Doppler in the diagnosis of hypoechoic thyroid nodules: work in progress. Radiol Med (Torino) 9(5): 616–621

Spiezia S, Farina R et al (2000) Analysis of time intensity enhancement curves after echocontrast agents injection in thyroid nodules evaluation: preliminary report. Ultrasound in medicine and biology. Abstracts of the 9th Congress of WFUMB. Florence. Italy, 26(2):a181

Standring S (2004) Gray's anatomy, 40th edn. Elsevier Science, Philadelphia

Struchkova TY (2003) Parameters of blood flow in the inferior and upper thyroid arteries. Standard values. Abstracts of the 4th Congress of the Russian Association of experts in ultrasound diagnostics in medicine. Moscow, pp 221–222 (Article in Russian)

Struchkova TY, Vetshev PS (2003) Blood flow parameters in differential diagnosis of nodular goiter and thyroid adenoma. Abstracts of the 4th Congress of the Russian Association of experts in ultrasound diagnostics in medicine. Moscow, p 222 (Article in Russian)

Svinarev MY (2000) Ultrasound examination of the thyroid gland in the assessment of severity of iodine deficient status (to the question on specifications of thyroid volume in children). Ultrazvukovaya diagnostica 2:69 (Article in Russian)

Sviridenko NY (1999) Iodine deficiency associated diseases (epidemiology, diagnosis, prophylaxis, and treatment). PhD thesis. Moscow (Book in Russian)

Tanaka K, Fukunari N, Igarashi T et al (2006) Evaluation of thyroid malignant tumor using real-time tissue elastography. Ultrasound in medicine and biology. Abstracts of the 11th Congress of WFUMB. Seoul. Korea, 32(5):93

Trofimova E (1999) Intraoperative ultrasonography in thyroid cancer. Abstracts of the 8th Congress on interventional ultrasound. Copenhagen, p 65

Trofimova EY (2008) Ultrasound examination of lymph nodes. Sonoace Ultrasound 18:59–64 (Article in Russian)

Trofimova EY, Novozhilova EN (1997) Role of ultrasound in diagnosis of residual tumors after inadequate operations for thyroid cancer. Abstracts of the Conference "Actual questions of radiology". Chelyabinsk, pp 16–18 (Article in Russian)

Trofimova EY, Shamatava NE (2000) Technique of intraoperational ultrasound in patients with thyroid nodules. Ultrazvukovaya i funkcionalnaya diagnostica 3:25–31 (Article in Russian)

Trofimova EY, Franc GA et al (1999) Puncture of the tumors of superficial organs and soft tissues under the ultrasound guidance. Rossiyskiy oncologicheskiy Journal 4:39–43 (Article in Russian)

Trofimova EY, Volchenko NN et al (2000) Ultrasound diagnosis of thyroid cancer. Visualizaciya v clinicke 17:37–45 (Article in Russian)

Trofimova EY, Parshin VS, Shamatava NE (2001) Algorithm of ultrasound examination in patients with thyroid tumors. Abstracts of the 8th Russian Congress of roentgenologists and radiologists "Algorithms in radiological diagnostics and programs of nuclear and complex treatment of patients" – "Radiology-2001". Moscow, pp 175–176 (Article in Russian)

Trofimova EY, Parshin VS, Shamatava NE (2001) Fine needle aspiration puncture under ultrasound guidance. Abstracts of the 8th Russian Congress of roentgenologists and radiologists "Algorithms in radiological diagnostics and programs of nuclear and complex treatment of patients" – "Radiology-2001". Moscow, pp 176–177 (Article in Russian)

Trofimova EY, Struchkova TY, Parshin VS (2002) Technique and report of ultrasound examination of the thyroid gland. Visualizaciya v clinicke 20:57–59

Troshina EA (2002) Diagnosis, treatment and monitoring of nodular forms of thyroid diseases. PhD thesis. Moscow (Book in Russian)

Tsyb AF, Parshin BC, Nestayko GV et al (1997) Ultrasound diagnosis of thyroid diseases. Medicine, Moscow (Book in Russian)

Tsyb AF, Oleynik NA, Davidov GP, Matveenko EG (2000) Assessment of possibilities of scintigraphy with technetril (MIBI) in differential diagnosis of thyroid tumors. Abstracts of the (1st Russian forum with international participation – "Radiology-2000". Moscow, pp 647–648 (Article in Russian)

Urso M, Angelillis L, Ambrosio GB (1996) Vascularization of single thyroid nodule as an indication of malignant neoplasm:a study using echo-color Doppler. Ann Ital Med Int 11(3):175–179

Uryvchikov AV (2004) Application of minimally invasive methods in treatment of postoperative recurrent nodular goiter. PhD thesis. Yaroslavl (Book in Russian)

Vagapova GR, Mihaylov IM, Hamzina FT (2006) Dopplerography in diagnosis of autoimmune thyroid disease. Ultrazvukovaya i funkcionalnaya diagnostica 3:77–84 (Article in Russian)

Valdina EA (2001) Thyroid diseases. Piter, St.Petersburg (Book in Russian)

Valdina EA, Puchkov YG (1988) Puncture biopsy in diagnosis of thyroid diseases. Vestnik khirurgii 10:154 (Article in Russian)

Vanushko VE, Kuznetsov MS, Kim IV, Artemova AM, Soldatov TV (2004) Optimization of preoperative diagnosis of thyroid cancer. Abstracts of VIII workshop with the international participation "Modern methods of instrumental diagnosis" . Strom, Moscow, pp 257–261 (Article in Russian)

Vetshev PS, Kuznetsov MS et al (1997) Intraoperative ultrasound in surgical treatment of euthyroid nodules of the thyroid gland. Problemy endocrinologii 4 (43):7–8 (Article in Russian)

Vetshev PS, Chilingaridi KE, Cherepenin MY (2002) Minimally invasive technologies in the treatment of benign lesions of the thyroid gland. Khirurgiya 5:7–12 (Article in Russian)

Vetshev PS, Chilingaridi KE, Gabaidze DI, Saliba MB (2005) Thyroid adenomas. Khirurgiya 7:4–8 (Article in Russian)

Vlasov PV (2006) Radiological diagnosis of the diseases of the organs of the thorax. Vidar, Moscow (Book in Russian)

Vnotchenko SL et al (1993) Fine needle puncture biopsy and the methods of visualization of the thyroid gland in diagnosis of nodular forms of goiter. Problemy endocrinologii 6(39): 30–33 (Article in Russian)

Voskoboynikov VV, Vanushko VE, Artyomov AM et al (2001) Diagnosis, tactics, and surgical treatment of patients with multinodular euthyroid goiter. Problemy endocrinologii 2(47):5–12 (Article in Russian)

Vuytsik NB (2008) Differential diagnosis of inflammatory diseases, solid tumors, and cystic lesions of head and neck with complex ultrasound examination. PhD thesis. Moscow (Book in Russian)

Wu CH, Shih JC, Chang YL, Lee SY, Hsieh FJ (1998) Two-dimensional and three-dimensional power Doppler sonographic classification of vascular patterns in cervical lymphadenopathies. J Ultrasound Med 17(7):459–464

Yamada H, Katob A, Isbinaga H (2000) Ultrasonographic screening for thyroid cancer in the screening. Nippon Jibiinkoka Gakka:Kaibo 103:13–18

Yano Y, Shibuya H, Kitagawa W et al (2007) Recent outcome of Graves' disease patients with papillary thyroid cancer. Eur J Endocrinol 157:325–329

Yanovskaya ME, Alexandrov YK, Agapitov YN, Sencha AN (2001) Influence of urban factors to the development of thyroid pathology. Actualniye problem sovremennoy endocrinologii. St.Petersburg, p 424 (Article in Russian)

Zabolotskaya NV (1994) Basic aspects of ultrasound diagnosis of thyroid diseases. Ultrazvukovaya diagnostika v akusherstve, gynecologii i pediatrii 3:127–136 (Article in Russian)

Zabolotskaya NV (1999) Utilization of ultrasound for assessment of the status of superficial lymph nodes. Sonoace International 5:46–50 (Article in Russian)

Zimin VV (2004) Radiology in diagnosis and monitoring of thyroid diseases during the treatment. PhD thesis. Nijniy Novgorod (Book in Russian)

Zubarev AV (1997) Three dimensional and contrast echography. Medicinskaya visualizaciya 4:3–8 (Article in Russian)

Zubarev AV, Bashilov VP et al (2000) Value of ultrasound angiography and three-dimensional reconstruction of vessels in diagnostics of thyroid lesions. Medicinskaya visualizaciya 3:57–62 (Article in Russian)

Zubovsky GA (1992) Ultrasound diagnostics and acupuncture. Moscow, Medicine (Book in Russian)

Zubovsky GA, Sarkisyan KY, Volohov AB (1986) Ultrasound and stsintigraphy in diagnosis of thyroid diseases. Medicinskaya radiologiya 10:45–51 (Article in Russian)

Index